MEDICAL GENETICS

Lynn B. Jorde, PhD
Professor and Associate Chairman
Department of Human Genetics
University of Utah Health Sciences Center
Salt Lake City, Utah

John C. Carey, MD
Professor and Director, Division of Medical Genetics
Department of Pediatrics
University of Utah Health Sciences Center
Salt Lake City, Utah

Raymond L. White, PhD
Chairman, Department of Oncological Sciences
Director, Huntsman Cancer Institute
University of Utah Health Sciences Center
Salt Lake City, Utah

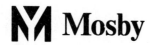 Mosby

St. Louis Baltimore Berlin Boston Carlsbad Chicago London Madrid
Naples New York Philadelphia Sydney Tokyo Toronto

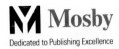

A Times Mirror
Company

Editor: Emma D. Underdown

Project Manager: Mark Spann

Production Coordinator: Diane B. Oehler, Publishers Services, Inc.

Production Editor: Melissa Martin

Designer: David Zielinski

Manufacturing Supervisor: Betty Richmond

Artist: Carol Cassidy

Printed in the United States of America
Composition by Black Dot Graphics
Printing/binding by Von Hoffman Press

Mosby–Year Book, Inc.
11830 Westline Industrial Drive
St. Louis, Missouri 63146

Library of Congress Cataloging in Publication Data

Jorde, Lynn B.
    Medical genetics / Lynn B. Jorde, John C. Carey, Raymond L. White.
        p.   cm.
    Includes bibliographical references and index.
    ISBN 0-8016-6414-4
    1. Medical genetics. I. Carey, John C., 1946-   . II. White,
Raymond L., 1943-   . III. Title.
    [DNLM: 1. Hereditary Diseases—genetics.   QZ 50 J82m 1994]
RB155.J67   1994
616' .042—dc20
DNLM/DLC
for Library of Congress   94-13013
                                                                      CIP

97 98 99   /   9 8 7 6 5 4 3

MEDICAL GENETICS

To our families—

Eileen and Alton Jorde

Leslie, Patrick, and Andrew Carey

Joan, Juliette, and Jeremy White

Preface

This textbook evolved from courses we teach for medical students, nursing students, and graduate and undergraduate students in human genetics. These students are the primary audience for this book, but it should also be useful for students in genetic counseling and biology and for house staff, physicians, and other health care professionals who wish to become more familiar with medical genetics.

Medical genetics is a rapidly progressing field. No textbook can remain factually current for long, so we have attempted to emphasize the central principles of genetics and their clinical application. In particular, this textbook integrates recent developments in molecular genetics with clinical practice.

Basic principles of molecular biology are introduced early in the book so that they can be discussed and applied in subsequent chapters. The chapters on autosomal and X-linked disorders include discussions of recent developments such as genomic imprinting, anticipation, and expanded repeat mutations. The chapter on cytogenetics highlights recent molecular advances in this area. Gene mapping and cloning, a central focus of modern medical genetics, is treated at length. Chapters are included on the rapidly developing fields of immunogenetics and cancer genetics. Departing somewhat from tradition, this book gives special emphasis to the genetics of common adult diseases such as diabetes, cancer, and heart disease. Although such diseases are more refractory to genetic analysis than many of the pediatric diseases usually emphasized in medical genetics textbooks, their impact on public health is enormous. Fortunately, they too are beginning to yield to newer methods of genetic analysis. The book concludes with chapters on genetic diagnosis (again emphasizing current molecular approaches) and clinical genetics and genetic counseling.

We have incorporated several pedagogical aids in this book. Brief, bold-faced summaries are placed on nearly every page to help the reader understand and summarize important concepts. Study questions provided at the end of each chapter will further aid the reader in review and comprehension. Key references are listed at the end of each chapter, and a detailed glossary is included at the end of the book. We have augmented our clinical photographs by referring to the excellent color illustrations in the Slice of Life series, available on CD-ROM in most medical libraries. References to the Slice of Life photographs are placed parenthetically in the text. For example "(SOL 3)" refers to Slice of Life illustration 3 in the Appendix. The illustration is displayed by scanning bar code 3 in the appendix.

Many of our colleagues have generously donated their time and expertise in reading and commenting on portions of this book. We extend our sincere gratitude to Michael Bamshad, MD; Arthur Brothman, PhD; Peter Byers, MD; William Carroll, MD; Ruth Foltz, MS; Sandra Hasstedt, PhD; James Kushner, MD; Jean-Marc Lalouel, MD, DSc; Mark Leppert, PhD; William McMahon, MD; James Metherall, PhD; Thérèse Tuohy, PhD; Scott Watkins, BS; John Weis, PhD; and Rebekha Zenger, BS. In addition, a number of colleagues provided photographs; they are acknowledged individually in the figure captions. We wish to thank Peeches Cedarholm, RN, for her help in obtaining and organizing the photographs. The karyotypes in Chapter 6 were provided by Arthur Brothman, PhD and Bonnie Issa, BS. The illustrations were ably generated by Carol Cassidy. Our editors at Mosby-Year Book, Robert Farrell and Emma Underdown, offered ample encouragement and displayed a surprising amount of patience. Finally, we wish to acknowledge the thousands of students with whom we have interacted during the past two decades. Teaching involves communication in both directions, and we have undoubtedly learned as much from our students as they have learned from us.

Lynn B. Jorde
John C. Carey
Raymond L. White
June 1994

■ NOTES ON THE 1997 EDITION

This revision of our first edition is being published less than two years after the original first edition was published. Although this is a relatively brief interval, medical genetics has seen a number of significant new developments during this time. Consequently, we have taken the opportunity to incorporate this new information in this revision. A complete revision is planned for the second edition of this book, to appear in two years.

REVIEWERS:

Susan Berry, MD
Associate Professor, Department of Pediatrics
Division of Genetics and Metabolism and the Institute of Human Genetics
University of Minnesota Hospital
Minneapolis, Minnesota

Joe C. Christian, MD, PhD
Chairman, Department of Medical and Molecular Genetics
Indiana University School of Medicine
Indianapolis, Indiana

Linda A. Corey, PhD
Associate Professor, Department of Human Genetics
Medical College of Virginia
Richmond, Virginia

Eric P. Hoffman, PhD
Assistant Professor, Department of Molecular Genetics and Biochemistry
University of Pittsburgh School of Medicine
Pittsburgh, Pennsylvania

Warren G. Sanger, PhD
Director, Cytogenetics Laboratories
Professor, Departments of Pediatrics and Pathology/Microbiology
University of Nebraska Medical Center
Omaha, Nebraska

Lisa S. Steinberg, MS
Section of Medical Genetics
St. Christopher's Hospital for Children
Philadelphia, Pennsylvania

Contents

1 Introduction

Genetics is playing an increasingly important role in the practice of clinical medicine. Medical genetics, once largely confined to relatively rare diseases seen only by a few specialists, is now becoming a central component of our understanding of most major diseases. These include not only the pediatric diseases but also common adult diseases such as heart disease, diabetes, many cancers, and many psychiatric disorders. Because all components of the human body are influenced by genes, genetic disease is relevant to all medical specialties. Today's practicing physician must understand the science of medical genetics.

■ WHAT IS MEDICAL GENETICS?

Medical genetics involves any application of genetics to medical practice. It thus includes studies of the inheritance of diseases in families, the mapping of disease genes to specific locations on chromosomes, analyses of the molecular mechanisms through which genes cause disease, and the diagnosis and treatment of genetic disease. As a result of rapid progress in molecular genetics, gene therapy, the insertion of normal genes into patients to correct genetic diseases, has recently been initiated. Medical genetics also includes genetic counseling, the communication of information regarding risks, prognoses, and treatment to patients and their families.

■ WHY IS A KNOWLEDGE OF MEDICAL GENETICS IMPORTANT FOR TODAY'S PRACTICING PHYSICIAN?

There are several answers to this question. Genetic diseases compose a large proportion of the total disease burden, both in the pediatric and adult populations (Table 1-1). This proportion will continue to grow as our understanding of the genetic basis of diseases grows. In addition, modern medicine is placing an increasing emphasis on

the importance of prevention. Because genetics provides a basis for understanding the fundamental biologic makeup of the organism, it naturally leads to a better understanding of the disease process. In many cases this knowledge can lead to the actual prevention of the disorder. It also leads to more effective disease treatment. Prevention and effective treatment are among the highest goals of medicine. In the chapters to follow, we will see many examples of the ways in which genetics contributes to these goals, but first we will review the foundations upon which current practice is built.

■ A BRIEF HISTORY

The inheritance of physical traits has been a subject of curiosity and interest for thousands of years. The ancient Hebrews and Greeks, as well as later Medieval scholars, described many genetic phenomena and proposed theories to account for them. Many of these theories were incorrect. Gregor Mendel (Fig. 1-1), an Austrian monk who is usually considered to be the "father" of genetics, advanced the field significantly by performing a series of cleverly designed experiments upon living organisms (garden peas). He then used this experimental information to formulate a series of fundamental principles of heredity.

Mendel published the results of his experiments in 1865 in a relatively obscure journal. It is one of the ironies of biologic science that his discoveries, which still form the foundation of genetics, received virtually no recognition for 35 years. During this time, Charles Darwin formulated his theories of evolution, and his cousin, Francis Galton, performed an extensive series of family studies (concentrating especially on twins) in an effort to understand the influence of heredity on various human traits. Neither scientist was aware of Mendel's work.

Table 1-1 ■ A partial list of some important genetic diseases

Disease	Approximate prevalence
Chromosome abnormalities	
Down syndrome	1/700 to 1/1000
Klinefelter syndrome	1/1000 males
Trisomy 13	1/10,000
Trisomy 18	1/6000
Turner syndrome	1/2500 to 1/10,000 females
Single-gene disorders	
Adenomatous polyposis coli	1/6000
Adult polycystic kidney disease	1/1000
α_1-Antitrypsin deficiency	1/2500 to 1/10,000 whites
Cystic fibrosis	1/2000 to 1/4000 whites
Duchenne muscular dystrophy	1/3500 males
Familial hypercholesterolemia	1/500
Fragile X syndrome	1/1500 males; 1/2500 females
Hemochromatosis (hereditary; symptomatic)	1/5000
Hemophilia A	1/10,000 males
Hereditary nonpolyposis colorectal cancer	up to 1/200
Huntington disease	1/20,000 whites
Marfan syndrome	1/10,000 to 1/20,000
Myotonic dystrophy	1/7000 to 1/20,000 whites
Neurofibromatosis type 1	1/3000 to 1/5000
Osteogenesis imperfecta	1/5000 to 1/10,000
Phenylketonuria	1/10,000 to 1/15000 whites
Retinoblastoma	1/20,000
Sickle cell disease	1/400 to 1/600 African-Americans; up to 1/50 in central Africa
Tay-Sachs disease	1/3000 Ashkenazi Jews
Thalassemia	1/50 to 1/100 (South Asian and circum-Mediterranean population)
Multifactorial disorders	
Congenital malformations	
Cleft lip with/without cleft palate	1/500 to 1/1000
Club foot (talipes)	1/1000
Congenital heart defects	1/200 to 1/500
Neural tube defects (spina bifida, anencephaly)	1/200 to 1/1000
Pyloric stenosis	1/300
Adult diseases	
Alcoholism	1/10 to 1/20
Alzheimer disease	1/10 (Americans over age 65)
Bipolar affective disorder	1/100 to 1/200
Cancer (all types)	1/3
Diabetes (types I and II)	1/10
Heart disease/stroke	1/3 to 1/5
Schizophrenia	1/100
Mitochondrial diseases	
Kearns-Sayre disease	Rare
Leber hereditary optic neuropathy (LHON)	Rare
Mitochondrial encephalopathy, lactic acidosis, and strokelike episodes (MELAS)	Rare
Myoclonic epilepsy and ragged-red fiber disease (MERRF)	Rare

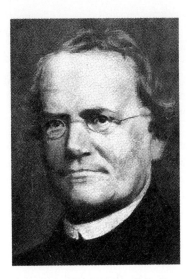

Figure 1-1 ■ **Gregor Johann Mendel.** (From Raven PH and Johnson GB: Biology, ed 3, St Louis, 1992, Mosby.)

Genetics as we know it today is largely the result of research done during this century. Mendel's principles were independently rediscovered in 1900 by three different scientists working in three different countries. This was also the year in which Landsteiner discovered the ABO blood group. In 1902 Archibald Garrod described alkaptonuria as the first "inborn error of metabolism." In 1909 Johannsen coined the term **gene** to denote the basic unit of heredity.

The next several decades were a period of considerable experimental and theoretical work. Several organisms, including *Drosophila* (fruit flies) and *Neurospora* (bread mold), served as useful experimental systems in which to study the actions and interactions of genes. For example, H.J. Muller demonstrated the genetic consequences of ionizing radiation in the fruit fly. During this period much of the theoretical basis of population genetics was developed by three central figures, Ronald Fisher, J.B.S. Haldane, and Sewall Wright. In addition, the modes of inheritance of several important genetic diseases, including phenylketonuria, sickle cell disease, Huntington disease, and cystic fibrosis, were established. In 1944 Oswald Avery showed that genes are composed of **DNA (deoxyribonucleic acid)**.

Probably the most significant achievement of the 1950s was the specification of the physical structure of DNA by James Watson and Francis Crick in 1953. Their seminal paper, which was only one page in length, formed the basis for what is now known as **molecular genetics** (the study of the structure and function of genes at the molecular

level). Another significant accomplishment in this decade was the correct specification of the number of human chromosomes. Since the early 1920s it had been thought that humans have 48 chromosomes in each cell. Only in 1956 was the correct number, 46, finally determined. The ability to count and identify chromosomes led to a flurry of new findings in cytogenetics, including the discovery in 1959 that Down syndrome is caused by an extra copy of chromosome 21.

Technologic developments since 1960 have brought about significant achievements at an ever-increasing rate. The most spectacular have occurred in the field of molecular genetics. During the past decade more than 3000 genes have been mapped to specific chromosome locations. The Human Genome Project, a large collaborative venture begun in 1991, hopes to provide a complete map of all human genes by the year 2005 (the term "**genome**" refers to all of the genes in an organism). Important developments in computer technology will aid in deciphering the barrage of data being generated by this and related projects. In addition to mapping genes, molecular geneticists have pinpointed the molecular defects underlying a number of important genetic diseases. This research has contributed greatly to our understanding of the ways in which gene defects can cause diseases, opening the path to more effective treatment and potential cures. The next decade promises to be a time of great excitement and fulfillment.

■ TYPES OF GENETIC DISEASES

Each human is estimated to have approximately 50,000 to 100,000 different genes. Alterations in these genes, or in combinations of them, can produce genetic disorders. These disorders are classified into several major groups: (1) **Chromosome disorders**, in which entire chromosomes, or large segments of them, are missing, duplicated, or otherwise altered. These disorders include diseases such as Down syndrome and Turner syndrome. (2) Disorders in which single genes are altered (often termed "Mendelian" conditions, or **single-gene disorders**). Well-known examples include cystic fibrosis, sickle cell disease, and hemophilia. (3) **Multifactorial disorders**, which are due to a combination of multiple genetic as well as environmental causes. Many birth defects, such as cleft lip and/or cleft palate, as well as many adult disorders, including heart disease and diabetes, belong to this category. (4) **Mitochondrial disorders**, a relatively small number of diseases due to alterations in the small cytoplasmic mitochondrial chromosome. Table 1-1 provides some examples of each of these types of diseases.

Of these major types of diseases, the single-gene disorders have probably received the greatest amount of attention. These disorders are classified according to the way in which they are inherited in families (autosomal dominant, autosomal recessive, and X-linked). These modes of inheritance will be discussed extensively in Chapters 4 and 5. As Table 1-2 shows, the number of defined single-gene traits has grown considerably during recent years, with a total of more than 6600 conditions presently defined. With continued advances, this number is certain to increase.

Whereas some genetic disorders, particularly the single-gene conditions, are strongly determined by genes, many others are the result of multiple genetic and nongenetic factors. We can therefore think of genetic diseases lying along a continuum (Fig. 1-2), with disorders such as cystic fibrosis and Duchenne muscular dystrophy situated at one end (strongly determined by genes), and conditions such as measles situated at the other (strongly determined by environment). Many of the most prevalent disorders, such as many birth defects and common diseases, including diabetes, hypertension, heart disease, and cancer, lie somewhere in the middle of the continuum. These diseases are the product of varying degrees of both genetic and environmental influences.

■ CLINICAL IMPACT OF GENETIC DISEASE

Genetic diseases are sometimes perceived as being so rare that the average physician will seldom encounter them. This is far from the truth, which is becoming increasingly evident as our knowledge and technology progress. Less than a century ago, diseases of largely nongenetic causation (diseases caused by malnutrition, unsanitary conditions, and contagions) accounted for the great majority of deaths in children. During this century, however, public health has vastly improved. As a result, genetic diseases have come to account for an ever-increasing proportion of pediatric deaths in developed countries. For example, the percentage of deaths due to genetic causes in various hospitals in the United Kingdom has increased from 16.5% in 1914 to 50% in 1976 (Table 1-3).

In addition to contributing to a large proportion of childhood deaths, genetic diseases also account for a large share of admissions into pediatric hospitals. A survey of Seattle hospitals showed that 27% of all pediatric inpatients presented with a genetic disorder, and a survey of admissions into a major pediatric hospital in Mexico showed that 37.8% had a disease that was either genetic or partly genetic.

Another way to assess the importance of genetic diseases is to ask, "What proportion of individuals

Table 1-2 ■ Number of entries representing loci identified mainly by mendelizing phenotypes*

MIM edition	Autosomal dominant	Autosomal recessive	X-linked	Total	Grand total
1966(ed 1)	269(+568)†	237(+294)	68(+51)	574(+913)	1487
1968(ed 2)	344(+449)	280(+349)	68(+55)	692(+853)	1545
1971(ed 3)	415(+528)	365(+418)	86(+64)	866(+1010)	1876
1975(ed 4)	583(+635)	466(+481)	93(+78)	1142(+1194)	2336
1978(ed 5)	736(+753)	521(+596)	107(+98)	1364(+1447)	2811
1983(ed 6)	934(+893)	588(+710)	115(+128)	1637(+1731)	3368
1986(ed 7)	1172(+1029)	610(+810)	124(+162)	1906(+2001)	3907
1988(ed 8)	1442(+1117)	626(+851)	139(+171)	2207(+2139)	4346
1990(ed 9)	1864(+1183)	631(+923)	161(+175)	2656(+2281)	4937
1992(ed 10)	2470(+1241)	647(+984)	190(+178)	3307(+2403)	5710
1994(ed 11)	4458	1730	412	6678‡	6678
1996 (online edition)	7430§		461	7975	7975

*From McKusick VA: Mendelian inheritance in man: catalogs of autosomal dominant, autosomal recessive, and X-linked phenotypes, ed 11, Baltimore, 1994, Johns Hopkins University Press.
†Values in parentheses refer to loci not fully identified or validated and include 121 number-signed entries. Increasingly loci identified by molecular and cellular genetic methods are included despite the lack of mendelian variation in phenotype.
‡The total for the 1994 edition includes 19 Y-linked loci and 59 mitochondrial loci not shown in the table.
§This number includes both autosomal dominant and autosomal recessive traits, which are not separated in the online edition. The grand total for 1996 includes 24 Y-linked and 60 mitochondrial loci.

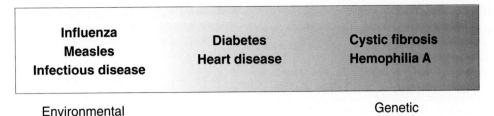

Influenza Measles Infectious disease	Diabetes Heart disease	Cystic fibrosis Hemophilia A

Environmental   Genetic

Figure 1-2 ■ Continuum of genetic diseases. Some diseases (e.g., cystic fibrosis) are strongly determined by genes, whereas others (e.g., infectious disease) are strongly determined by environment.

Table 1-3 ■ Percentages of childhood deaths in United Kingdom hospitals attributable to nongenetic (e.g., infections) and genetic causes*

	London 1914	London 1954	Newcastle 1966	Edinburgh 1976
Nongenetic	83.5	62.5	58.0	50.0
Genetic				
Single-gene	2.0	12.0	8.5	8.9
Chromosomal	—	—	2.5	2.9
Multifactorial	14.5	25.5	31.0	38.2

*From Emery AEH and Rimoin DL, editors: Principles and practice of medical genetics, ed 2, Edinburgh, 1990, Churchill Livingstone.

in the population will be diagnosed with a genetic disorder?" This is not as simple a question as it may seem. A variety of factors can influence the answer. For example, some diseases are found more frequently in certain ethnic groups. Cystic fibrosis is especially common among whites, whereas sickle cell disease is especially common among Africans. Also, some diseases are more common in older individuals. Colon cancer, breast cancer, and Alzheimer disease, for example, are each caused in part by genes and are not usually seen until later in life. The prevalence estimates for these diseases would be higher in a more aged population. Variations in diagnostic and recording practices can also cause prevalence estimates to vary. Accordingly the prevalence data shown in Table 1-4 are given as rather broad ranges. Keeping these sources of variation in mind, it is notable that 3% to 7% of the population will be diagnosed with a recognizable genetic disease. This tabulation does not include most cases of the more common adult diseases, such as heart disease, diabetes, and cancer. However-

er, it is known that these diseases also have genetic components. If we include these diseases in our assessment, the clinical impact of genetic disease is considerable indeed.

Table 1-4 ■ Approximate prevalence of genetic disease in the general population

Type of genetic disease	Lifetime prevalence per 1000
Autosomal dominant	3-9.5
Autosomal recessive	2-2.5
X-linked	0.5-2
Chromosome disorders*	6-9
Congenital malformation†	20-50
TOTAL	31.5-73

*The upper limit of this range is obtained when newer chromosome banding techniques (see Chapter 6) are used.
†Congenital means "present at birth." Most congenital malformations are thought to be multifactorial and thus likely have both genetic and environmental components.

■ **ADDITIONAL READING**

Baird PA, Anderson TW, Newcombe HB, and Lowry RB: Genetic disorders in children and young adults: a population study, Am J Hum Genet 42:677–693, 1988.

Dunn LC: A short history of genetics, New York, 1965, McGraw-Hill.

Emery AEH and Rimoin DL, editors: Principles and practice of medical genetics, ed 2, Edinburgh, 1990, Churchill Livingstone.

McKusick VA: Medical genetics: a 40-year perspective on the evolution of a medical specialty from a basic science, JAMA 270:2351–2356, 1993.

McKusick VA: Mendelian inheritance in man: catalogs of autosomal dominant, autosomal recessive, and X-linked phenotypes, ed 11, Baltimore, 1994, Johns Hopkins University Press.

Seashore MS, Wappner RS: Genetics in primary care and clinical medicine, Stamford, CT, 1996, Appleton & Lange.

Scriver CR, Beaudet AL, Sly WS, and Valle D, editors: The metabolic basis of inherited disease, ed 7, New York, 1995, McGraw-Hill.

Watson JD and Crick FHC: Molecular structure of nucleic acids: a structure for deoxyribose nucleic acid, Nature 171:737, 1953.

World Health Organization: Prevention of avoidable mutational disease: memorandum from a WHO meeting, Bull WHO 64:205–216, 1986.

2 Basic Cell Biology: Structure and Function of Genes and Chromosomes

All genetic diseases involve defects at the level of the cell. For this reason one must understand basic cell biology to understand genetic disease. Errors may occur in the replication of genetic material or in the translation of genes into proteins. These errors commonly produce single-gene disorders. In addition, errors occurring during cell division can lead to disorders involving entire chromosomes. To provide the basis for understanding these errors and their consequences, this chapter focuses on the processes through which genes are replicated and translated into proteins, as well as the process of cell division.

In the nineteenth century, microscopic studies of cells led scientists to suspect that the nucleus of the cell (Fig. 2-1) contained the important mechanisms of inheritance. They found that **chromatin**, the substance that gives the nucleus a granular appearance, is observable in the nuclei of non-dividing cells. Just before a cell undergoes division, the chromatin condenses to form discrete, dark-staining bodies, called **chromosomes** (from the Greek for "colored bodies"). With the rediscovery of Mendel's breeding experiments at the beginning of this century, it soon became apparent that chromosomes contained **genes**. Genes are transmitted from parent to offspring and are considered to be the basic unit of inheritance. It is through the transmission of genes that physical traits, such as eye color, are inherited in families. Diseases can also be transmitted through genetic inheritance.

Physically genes are composed of **deoxyribonucleic acid (DNA)**. DNA provides the genetic "blueprint" for all proteins in the body. Thus genes ultimately influence all aspects of body structure and function. The human is estimated to have 50,000 to 100,000 **structural genes** (genes that code for proteins). An error (or **mutation**) in one of these genes often leads to a recognizable genetic disease. To date approximately 5700 single-gene traits have been identified; most of these represent disease conditions (see Table 1-1).

Genes, the basic unit of inheritance, are contained in chromosomes and consist of DNA.

Each human **somatic cell** (cells other than the **gametes**, or sperm and egg cells) contains 23 pairs of different chromosomes, for a total of 46. One member of each pair is derived from one's father, while the other member is derived from one's mother. One of the chromosome pairs consists of the **sex chromosomes**. In normal males the sex chromosomes are a Y chromosome inherited from the father and an X chromosome inherited from the mother. Two X chromosomes are found in normal females, one inherited from each parent. The other 22 pairs of chromosomes are termed **autosomes**. The members of each pair of autosomes are said to be **homologs**, or **homologous**, because their DNA is very similar. The X and Y chromosomes are not homologs of one another.

Somatic cells, having two of each chromosome, are termed **diploid** cells. Gametes have the **haploid** number of chromosomes, 23. The diploid number of chromosomes is maintained in successive generations of somatic cells by the process of **mitosis**, whereas the haploid number is obtained through a process known as **meiosis**. Both of these processes will be discussed in detail in the latter part of this chapter.

Somatic cells are diploid, having 23 pairs of chromosomes (22 autosomes and one pair of sex chromosomes). Gametes are haploid and have a total of 23 chromosomes.

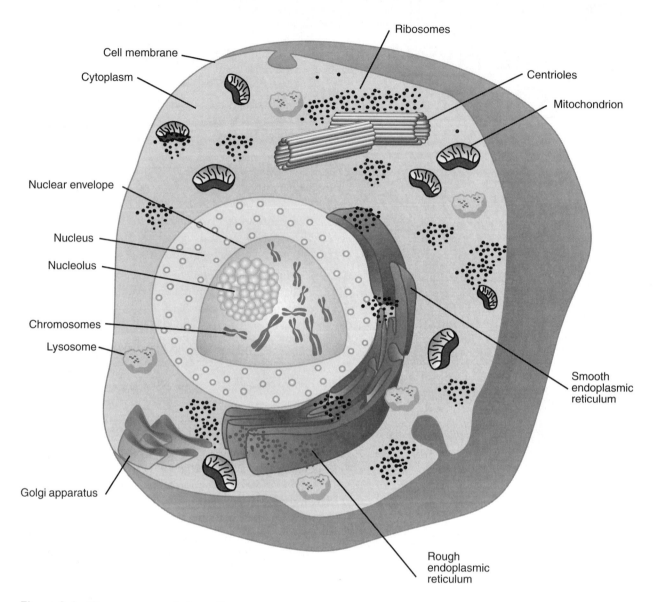

Ribosomes

Centrioles

Mitochondrion

Cell membrane

Cytoplasm

Nuclear envelope

Nucleus

Nucleolus

Chromosomes

Lysosome

Golgi apparatus

Smooth
endoplasmic
reticulum

Rough
endoplasmic
reticulum

Figure 2-1 ■ The anatomy of the cell. See color plate 1.

■ DNA, RNA, AND PROTEINS: HEREDITY AT THE MOLECULAR LEVEL
DNA
Composition and Structure of DNA

The DNA molecule has three basic components: the pentose sugar, deoxyribose; a phosphate group; and four types of nitrogenous **bases** (so named because they can combine with hydrogen ions in acidic solutions). Two of the bases, **cytosine** and **thymine**, are single carbon–nitrogen rings called **pyrimidines**. The other two bases, **adenine** and **guanine**, are double carbon–nitrogen rings called

purines (Fig. 2-2). The four bases are commonly represented by their first letters: C, T, A, and G.

One of Watson and Crick's contributions was to demonstrate how these three components are physically assembled to form DNA. They proposed the now-famous **double helix** model, in which DNA can be envisioned as a twisted ladder with chemical bonds as its rungs (Fig. 2-3). The two sides of the ladder are composed of the sugar and phosphate components, held together by strong phosphodiester bonds. Projecting from each side of the ladder, at regular intervals, are the

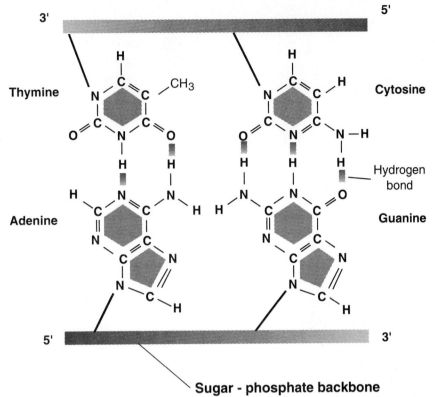

Figure 2-2 ■ Chemical structure of the four bases, showing hydrogen bonds between base pairs. Three hydrogen bonds are formed between cytosine-guanine pairs, and two bonds are formed between adenine-thymine pairs.

nitrogenous bases. The base projecting from one side is bound to the base projecting from the other by a relatively weak hydrogen bond. The paired nitrogenous bases therefore form the rungs of the ladder.

Figure 2-3 (page 10) illustrates the chemical bonds between bases and shows that ends of the ladder terminate in either 3′ or 5′. These labels are derived from the order in which the five carbon atoms composing deoxyribose are numbered. Each DNA subunit, consisting of one deoxyribose, one phosphate group, and one base, is called a **nucleotide**.

As we shall see, different sequences of nucleotide bases (e.g., ACCAAGTGC) specify different proteins. Specification of the body's many proteins must require a great deal of genetic information. Indeed, each human cell contains approximately 3 billion nucleotides, more than enough information to specify the composition of all of our proteins.

The most important constituent of DNA is the four nucleotide bases, adenine, thymine, cytosine, and guanine. DNA has a double helix structure.

Replication of DNA

As cells divide to make copies of themselves, identical copies of DNA must be made and incorporated into the new cells. This is essential if DNA is to serve as the basic genetic material. DNA **replication** consists basically of the breaking of the weak hydrogen bonds between the bases, leaving a single DNA strand with each base unpaired. The consistent pairing of adenine with thymine and guanine with cytosine, known as **complementary base pairing**, is the key to accurate replication. The principle of complementary base pairing dictates that the unpaired base will attract a free nucleotide only if the nucleotide has the proper complementary base. Thus a portion of a single strand with the base sequence ATTGCT will bond with a series of free nucleotides with the bases TAACGA. The single strand is said to be a **template** upon which a complementary strand is built. When replication is complete, a new double-stranded molecule identical to the original is formed (Fig. 2-4, page 10).

Several different enzymes are involved in DNA replication. One enzyme unwinds the double helix, one holds the strands apart, and others perform

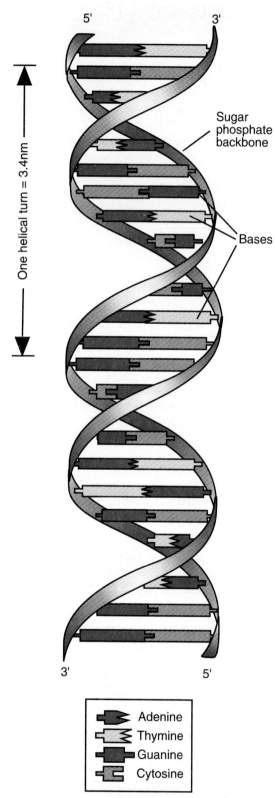

Figure 2-3 ■ The DNA double helix, with sugar-phosphate backbone and nitrogenous bases.

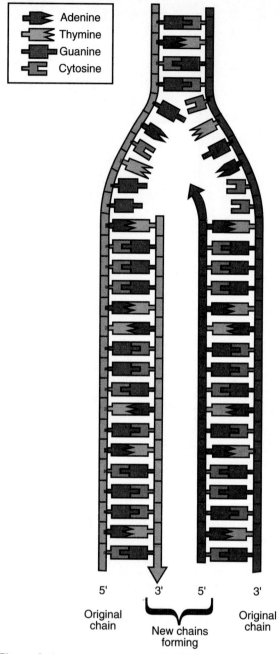

Figure 2-4 ■ DNA replication. The hydrogen bonds between the two original strands are broken, allowing the bases in each strand to undergo complementary base pairing with free bases. This process, which proceeds 5′ to 3′ on each strand, forms two new double strands of DNA.

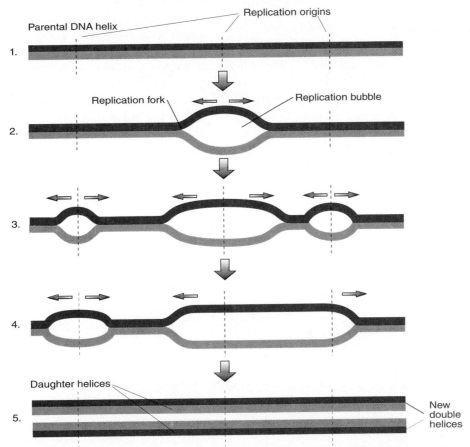

Figure 2-5 ■ Replication bubbles form at multiple points along the DNA strand, allowing replication to proceed more rapidly.

other distinct functions. **DNA polymerase** is one of the key replication enzymes. It travels along the single DNA strand, adding free nucleotides to the 3′ end of the new strand. Nucleotides can be added only to this end of the strand, so replication always proceeds from the 5′ to the 3′ end. When referring to the orientation of sequences along a gene, the 5′ direction is termed "upstream," whereas the 3′ direction is termed "downstream."

In addition to adding new nucleotides, DNA polymerase performs part of a **proofreading** procedure, in which a newly added nucleotide is checked to make certain that it is in fact complementary to the template base. If not, the nucleotide is excised and replaced with a correct complementary nucleotide base. This process substantially enhances the accuracy of DNA replication. When a DNA replication error is not successfully repaired, a mutation has occurred. As will be seen in Chapter 3, many such mutations cause genetic diseases.

DNA replication is critically dependent upon the principle of complementary base pairing. This allows a single strand of the double-stranded DNA molecule to form a template for the synthesis of a new, complementary strand.

The rate of DNA replication in humans, about 40 to 50 nucleotides per second, is comparatively slow. In bacteria the rate is much higher, reaching 500 to 1000 nucleotides per second. Given that some human chromosomes have as many as 250 million nucleotides, replication would be an extraordinarily time-consuming process if it proceeded linearly from one end of the chromosome to the other (for a chromosome of this size, a single round of replication would require nearly 2 months). Instead replication begins at many different points along the chromosome, termed **replication origins**. The resulting multiple separations of the DNA strands are called **replication bubbles** (Fig. 2-5). By occurring simultaneously at many different sites along the chromosome, the replication process can proceed much more quickly.

Replication bubbles allow DNA replication to take place at multiple locations on the chromosome, greatly speeding the replication process.

From Genes to Proteins

While DNA is formed and replicated in the cell nucleus, protein synthesis takes place in the cytoplasm. The information contained in DNA must thus be transported somehow to the cytoplasm and then used to dictate the composition of proteins. This involves two processes, **transcription** and **translation**. Briefly the DNA code is **transcribed** into messenger RNA, which then leaves the nucleus to be **translated** into proteins. These processes, summarized in Figure 2-6, will be discussed at length herein. Transcription and translation are both mediated by **ribonucleic acid (RNA)**, a type of nucleic acid that is chemically similar to DNA. Like DNA, RNA is composed of sugars, phosphate groups, and nitrogenous bases. It differs from DNA in that the sugar is ribose instead of deoxyribose and in that uracil rather than thymine is one of the four bases. Uracil is structurally similar to thymine, so, like thymine, it can pair with adenine. Another difference between RNA and DNA is that whereas DNA usually occurs as a double strand, RNA usually occurs as a single strand.

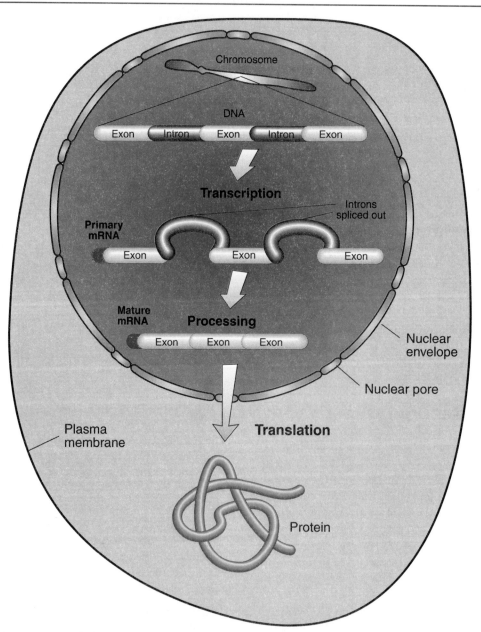

Figure 2-6 ■ A summary of the steps leading from DNA to proteins. Replication and transcription occur in the cell nucleus, after which the mRNA is transported to the cytoplasm, where translation of the mRNA into amino acid sequences composing a protein occurs.

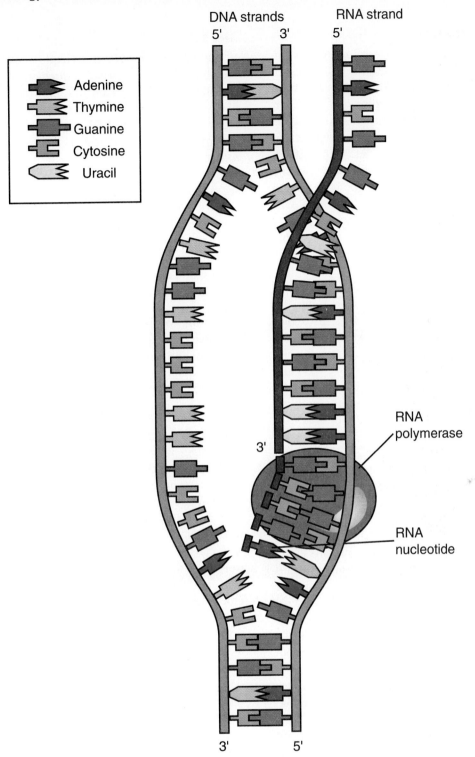

DNA strands   RNA strand

Adenine
Thymine
Guanine
Cytosine
Uracil

RNA polymerase

RNA nucleotide

Figure 2-7 ■ Transcription of DNA to mRNA. RNA polymerase II proceeds along the DNA strand in the 3′ to 5′ direction, assembling a strand of mRNA nucleotides that is complementary to the DNA template strand.

DNA sequences encode proteins through the processes of transcription and translation. These both involve ribonucleic acid, a single-stranded molecule similar to **DNA** except that it has a ribose sugar and has a uracil base rather than thymine.

Transcription

Transcription is the process by which an RNA sequence is formed from a DNA template (Fig. 2-7). The type of RNA produced by the transcription process is termed **messenger RNA (mRNA)**. To initiate transcription, one of the **RNA polymer-**

ase enzymes (RNA polymerase II) binds to a **promoter** site on the DNA (a promoter is a nucleotide sequence that specifies the beginning of a gene). The RNA polymerase then pulls a portion of the DNA strands apart from one another, exposing unattached DNA bases. One of the two DNA strands then provides the template for the sequence of mRNA nucleotides. Although either DNA strand could in principle serve as the template for mRNA synthesis, only one is chosen to do so in a given region of the chromosome. This choice is determined by the promoter sequence, which orients the RNA polymerase in a specific direction along the DNA sequence. Because mRNA can be synthesized only in the 5′ to 3′ direction, the promoter, by specifying directionality, determines which DNA strand serves as the template. RNA polymerase moves in the 3′ to 5′ direction along the DNA template strand, assembling the complementary mRNA strand from 5′ to 3′ (Fig. 2-7). Because of complementary base pairing, the mRNA sequence is identical to that of the DNA strand that does not serve as the template (except, of course, for the substitution of uracil for thymine).

Soon after RNA synthesis begins, the 5′ end of the growing RNA molecule is "capped" by the addition of a chemically modified guanine nucleotide. This **5′ cap** appears to help to prevent the RNA molecule from being degraded during synthesis, and it later helps to indicate the starting position for translation of the mRNA molecule into protein. Transcription continues until a DNA sequence called a **termination sequence** is reached. Near this point a series of 100 to 200 adenine bases are added to the 3′ end of the RNA molecule. This structure, known as the **poly-A tail**, may be involved in stabilizing the mRNA molecule so that it is not degraded when it reaches the cytoplasm. RNA polymerase usually continues to transcribe DNA for several thousand additional bases, but the mRNA bases following the poly-A tail are eventually lost. Finally the DNA strands and RNA polymerase separate from the RNA strand, leaving a transcribed single mRNA strand. This mRNA molecule is termed the **primary transcript**.

> **In the process of transcription RNA polymerase II binds to a promoter site near the 5′ end of a gene on the non-template strand and, through complementary base pairing, helps to produce an mRNA strand from the template DNA strand.**

Gene Splicing

The primary mRNA transcript is exactly complementary to the base sequence of the DNA template. In **eukaryotes*** an important step takes place before this RNA transcript leaves the nucleus. Sections of the RNA are removed by nuclear enzymes, and the remaining sections are spliced together to form the functional mRNA that will migrate to the cytoplasm. The excised sequences are called **introns**, and the sequences that are left to code for proteins are called **exons** (Fig. 2-8). Only when gene splicing is completed does the **mature transcript** move out of the nucleus into the cytoplasm. Errors in gene splicing, like replication errors, are a form of mutation that can lead to genetic disease.

> **Introns are spliced out of the primary mRNA transcript before the mature transcript leaves the nucleus. Exons contain the mRNA that specifies proteins.**

The Genetic Code

Proteins are composed of one or more **polypeptides**, which are in turn composed of sequences of **amino acids**. The body contains 20 different types of amino acids, and the amino acid sequences that make up polypeptides must in some way be designated by the DNA after transcription into mRNA.

Because there are 20 different amino acids and only four different RNA bases, a single base could not specify each amino acid. Similarly, specific amino acids could not be defined by couplets of bases (e.g., adenine followed by guanine, uracil followed by adenine) because only 16 (4 × 4) different couplets are possible. If triplet sets of bases are translated into amino acids, however, 64 (4 × 4 × 4) combinations can be achieved, more than enough to specify each different amino acid. Conclusive proof that amino acids are specified by these triplets of bases, or **codons**, was obtained by manufacturing synthetic nucleotide sequences and allowing them to direct the formation of polypeptides in the laboratory. The correspondence between specific codons and amino acids, known as the **genetic code**, is shown in Table 2-1.

---

*Eukaryotes are organisms that have a defined cell nucleus, as opposed to **prokaryotes**, which lack a defined nucleus.

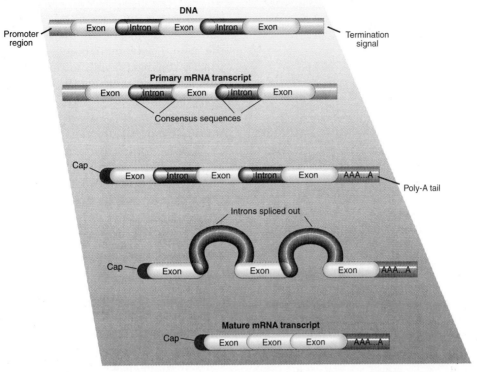

Figure 2-8 ■ Gene splicing. Introns are precisely removed from the primary mRNA transcript to produce a mature mRNA transcript. Consensus sequences mark the sites at which splicing occurs.

Table 2-1 ■ **The genetic code*** †

1st position (5′ end) ↓	2nd position				3rd position (3′ end) ↓
	U	**C**	**A**	**G**	
U	Phe	Ser	Tyr	Cys	U
U	Phe	Ser	Tyr	Cys	C
U	Leu	Ser	STOP	STOP	A
U	Leu	Ser	STOP	Trp	G
C	Leu	Pro	His	Arg	U
C	Leu	Pro	His	Arg	C
C	Leu	Pro	Gln	Arg	A
C	Leu	Pro	Gln	Arg	G
A	Ile	Thr	Asn	Ser	U
A	Ile	Thr	Asn	Ser	C
A	Ile	Thr	Lys	Arg	A
A	Met	Thr	Lys	Arg	G
G	Val	Ala	Asp	Gly	U
G	Val	Ala	Asp	Gly	C
G	Val	Ala	Glu	Gly	A
G	Val	Ala	Glu	Gly	G

*Examples: UUG is translated into leucine; UAA is a stop codon; GGG is translated into glycine. Under some circumstances the UGA codon can specify an amino acid called *selenocysteine*. This is often termed the "21st" amino acid.
†Phe, phenylalanine; Ser, serine; Tyr, tyrosine; Cys, cysteine; Leu, leucine; Trp, tryptophan; Pro, proline; His, histidine; Arg, arginine; Gln, glycine; Ile, isoleucine; Thr, threonine; Asn, asparagine; Lys, lysine; Met, methionine; Val, valine; Ala, alanine; Asp, aspartic acid; Gly, glutamic acid; Glu. glutamine.

Of the 64 possible codons, three signal the end of a gene and are known as **stop codons**. These are UAA, UGA, and UAG. The remaining 61 all specify amino acids. This means that most amino acids can be specified by more than one codon, as Table 2-1 shows. The genetic code is thus said to be "degenerate." Whereas a given amino acid may be specified by more than one codon, each codon can designate only one amino acid.

Individual amino acids, which compose proteins, are encoded by units of three mRNA bases, termed codons. There are 64 possible codons and only 20 amino acids, so the genetic code is degenerate.

A significant feature of the genetic code is that it is universal: virtually all living organisms use the same codons to specify amino acids. One known exception to this rule is in **mitochondria**, cytoplasmic organelles that are the sites of cellular respiration (see Fig. 2-1). The mitochondria have their own extranuclear DNA molecules. Several codons of mitochondrial DNA encode different amino acids than do the same nuclear DNA codons.

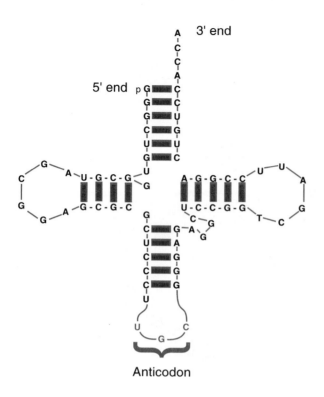

Figure 2-9 ■ The structure of tRNA. In two
dimensions the tRNA has a cloverleaf shape. Note
the 3′ site of attachment for an amino acid. The
anticodon pairs with a complementary mRNA
codon.

Translation

Translation is the process in which mRNA provides a template for the synthesis of a polypeptide. mRNA cannot, however, bind directly to amino acids. Instead, it interacts with **transfer RNA (tRNA),** a cloverleaf-shaped RNA strand of about 80 nucleotides. As Figure 2-9 illustrates, the tRNA molecule has a site at its 3′ end for the attachment of an amino acid by a covalent bond. At the opposite end of the cloverleaf is a sequence of three nucleotides, called the **anticodon**. This sequence undergoes complementary base pairing with an appropriate codon in the mRNA. The mRNA thus specifies the sequence of amino acids by acting through the tRNA.

The cytoplasmic site of protein synthesis is the **ribosome**, which consists of roughly equal parts of enzymatic proteins and **ribosomal RNA (rRNA).** The function of rRNA is to help bind mRNA and tRNA to the ribosome. During translation, depicted in Figure 2-10, the ribosome first binds to an initiation site on the mRNA sequence. This site consists of a specific codon, AUG, which specifies the amino acid methionine (this amino acid is usually removed from the polypeptide before the completion of polypeptide synthesis). The ribosome then binds the tRNA to its surface so that base pairing can occur between tRNA and mRNA. The ribosome moves along the mRNA sequence, codon by codon, in the usual 5′ to 3′ direction. As each codon is processed, an amino acid is translated by the interaction of mRNA and tRNA.

In this process the ribosome provides an enzyme that catalyzes the formation of covalent bonds between the adjacent amino acids, resulting in a growing polypeptide. When the ribosome arrives at a stop codon on the mRNA sequence, translation and polypeptide formation cease. The amino (NH_2) terminus of the polypeptide corresponds to the 5′ end of the mRNA strand, and the carboxyl (COOH) terminus corresponds to the 3′ end. With synthesis completed the mRNA, ribosome, and polypeptide separate from one another. The polypeptide is then released into the cytoplasm.

> In the process of translation, the mRNA sequence serves as a template to specify sequences of amino acids. These sequences, which form polypeptides, are assembled by ribosomes. tRNA and rRNA interact with mRNA in the translation process.

Before a newly synthesized polypeptide can begin its existence as a functional protein, it often undergoes further processing, termed **posttranslational modification**. These modifications can take a variety of forms, including cleavage into smaller polypeptide units or combination with other polypeptides to form a larger protein. Other possible modifications include the addition of carbohydrate side chains to the polypeptide. These modifications are needed, for example, to produce proper folding of the mature protein or to stabilize its structure. An example of a clinically important protein that undergoes considerable posttranslational modification is given by type 1 collagen (Clinical Commentary 2-1, page 18).

> Posttranslational modification consists of various chemical changes that occur in proteins shortly after they are translated.

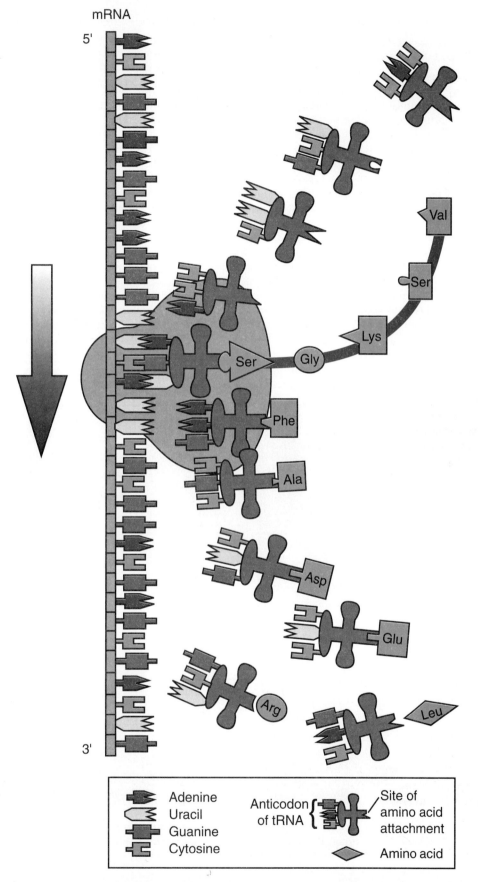

mRNA

5'

3'

Adenine
Uracil
Guanine
Cytosine

Anticodon of tRNA {

Site of amino acid attachment

Amino acid

Figure 2-10 ■ Translation of mRNA to amino acids. The ribosome moves along the mRNA strand in the 5′ to 3′ direction, assembling a growing polypeptide chain. In this example the mRNA sequence GUG-AGC-AAG-GGU-UCA has assembled five amino acids, Val, Ser, Lys, Gly, and Ser, into a polypeptide.

Clinical Commentary 2-1. Osteogenesis Imperfecta, an Inherited Collagen Disorder

As its name implies, osteogenesis imperfecta is a disease caused by defects in the formation of bone. This disorder, sometimes known as brittle bone disease, affects approximately 1 in 10,000 individuals in all ethnic groups.

Nearly all cases of osteogenesis imperfecta are caused by defects in type I collagen, a major component of bone that provides much of its structural stability (Table 2-2). The function of collagen in bone is analogous to that of the steel bars incorporated in reinforced concrete. This is perhaps an especially apt analogy because the tensile strength of collagen fibrils is roughly equivalent to that of steel wires.

When type I collagen is improperly formed, the bone loses much of its strength and thus fractures easily (Fig. 2-11). Patients with osteogenesis imperfecta may suffer hundreds of bone fractures, or they may suffer only a few. The disease is highly variable in its expression (reasons for this will be discussed in Chapter 4). In addition to bone fractures, patients may have short stature, hearing loss,

Table 2-2 ■ Characteristics of osteogenesis imperfecta

OI type	Disease features
I	Mild bone fragility, blue sclerae, hearing loss in 50% of patients, normal stature, few bone deformities
II	Severest form, with extreme bone fragility, long bone deformities, compressed femurs; lethal in the perinatal period (most die of respiratory failure)
III	Severe bone fragility, very short stature, variably blue sclerae, progressive bone deformities, dentinogenesis imperfecta common
IV	Short stature, normal sclerae, mild to moderate bone deformity, hearing loss in some patients, dentinogenesis imperfecta common; bone fragility variable

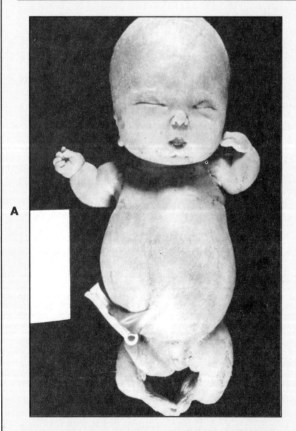
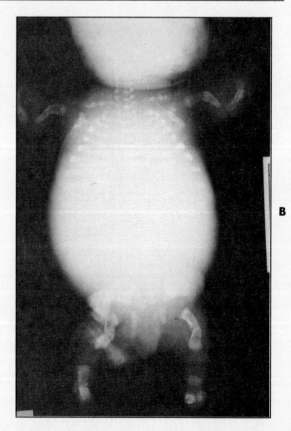

Figure 2-11 ■ (A) A stillborn infant with type II osteogenesis imperfecta (the perinatal lethal form). The infant had a type I procollagen mutation and presents with short, slightly twisted limbs. (B) Radiograph of the infant shown in A. Note rib fractures and bowed, thickened femurs. (*SOL* 1, 2, 3, 4)*

SOL refers to the Slice of Life bar codes included in Appendix.

abnormal tooth development (dentiogenesis imperfecta), thin and easily scarring skin, bluish sclerae, and various bone deformities. Osteogenesis imperfecta is commonly classified into four types, as shown in Table 2-2. There is currently no cure for this disease, and patient management consists largely of the repair of fractures and, in some cases, the use of external or internal bone support (e.g., surgically implanted rods). Physical rehabilitation also plays an important role in clinical management.

Type I collagen is a trimeric protein (having three subunits) with a triple helix structure (Fig. 2-12). It is formed from a precursor protein, type I procollagen. Two of the three subunits of type 1 procollagen [labeled proα1(I) chains] are encoded by a gene on chromosome 17 that is about 18,000 base pairs (18 kb) in length. The third subunit, the proα2(I) chain, is encoded by a gene on chromosome 7 that is 38 kb in size. Each of these genes contains more than 50 exons. After transcription and splicing, the mature mRNA formed from each gene is only 5 to 7 kb in length. The mature mRNAs proceed to the cytoplasm, where they are translated into polypeptide chains by the ribosomal machinery of the cell.

At this point the polypeptide chains undergo a series of posttranslational modifications. Many of the proline and lysine residues* are hydroxylated (i.e., hydroxyl groups are added) to form hydroxyproline and hydroxylysine, respectively. The three polypeptides, two proα1(I) and one proα2(I) chain, begin to associate with one another at their COOH-termini. This association is stabilized by sulfide bonds that form between the chains near the COOH-termini. The triple helix then forms, in zipperlike fashion, beginning at the COOH-terminus and proceeding toward the NH$_2$-terminus. Some of the hydroxylysines are glycosylated [i.e., sugars are added, a modification that commonly occurs in the rough endoplasmic reticulum (see Fig. 2-1), where the chains reside for a time]. The hydroxyl groups in the hydroxyprolines help to connect the three chains by forming hydrogen bonds, which then stabilize the triple helix. Critical to the proper folding of the helix is the presence of a glycine in every third position of each polypeptide. This is because every third residue must fit into the center of the helix, and only glycine is small enough to do so.

Once the protein has folded into a triple helix, it moves from the endoplasmic reticulum to the Golgi apparatus (see Fig. 2-1) and is then secreted from the cell. Yet another modification then takes place: the procollagen is cleaved by proteases near both the NH$_2$- and COOH-termini of the triple helix, removing some amino acids at each end. These amino acids performed essential functions earlier in the life of the protein (e.g., helping to form the triple helix structure, helping to thread the protein through the endoplasmic

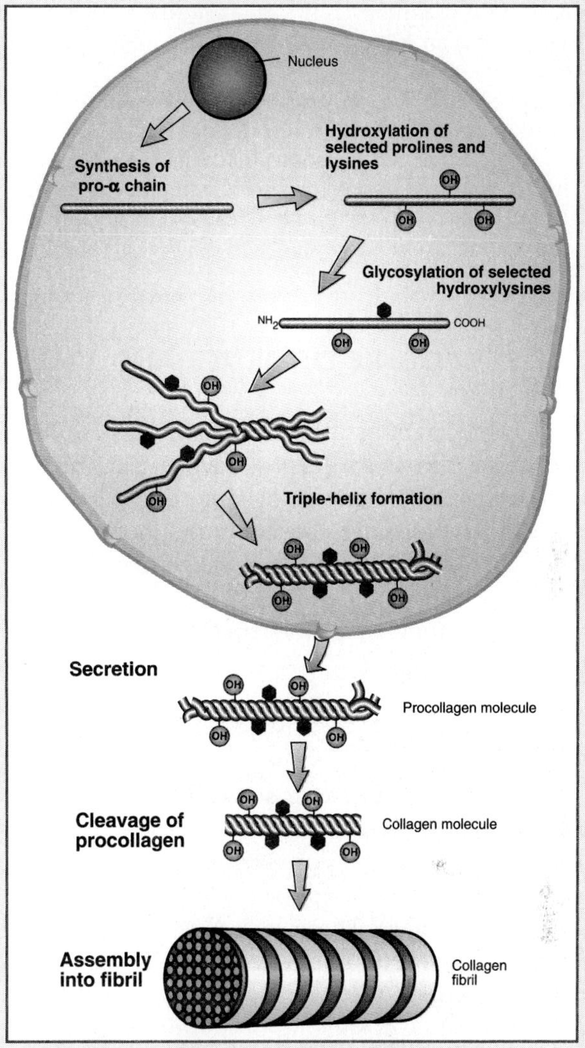

Figure 2-12 ■ **The process of collagen fibril formation. After the pro-α polypeptide chain is formed, a series of posttranslational modifications takes place, including hydroxylation and glycosylation. Three polypeptide chains assemble into a triple helix, which is secreted outside the cell. Portions of each end of the procollagen molecule are cleaved, resulting in the mature collagen molecule. These molecules then assemble into collagen fibrils.**

reticulum) but are no longer needed. This cleavage results in the mature protein, type I collagen. The collagen then assembles itself into fibrils, which react with adjacent molecules outside the cell, forming covalent cross-links that impart tensile strength to the fibrils.

The path from the DNA sequence to the mature collagen protein involves many steps. The com-

*A residue is an amino acid that has been incorporated into a polypeptide chain.

Continued.

> **Clinical Commentary 2-1. Osteogenesis Imperfecta, an Inherited Collagen Disorder—Cont.**
>
> plexity of this path provides many opportunities for mistakes (in replication, transcription, translation, or posttranslational modification) that can cause disease. One common mutation produces a replacement of glycine by another amino acid. Because only glycine is small enough to be accommodated in the center of the helix structure, substitution of a different amino acid will cause instability of the structure and thus poorly formed fibrils. This type of mutation is seen in most cases of type II osteogenesis imperfecta. Other mutations can cause excess posttranslational modification of the polypeptide chains, again producing abnormal fibrils. Other examples of disease-causing mutations are given in the reviews listed at the end of this chapter.

■ THE STRUCTURE OF GENES AND THE GENOME

Some aspects of gene structure, such as the existence of introns and exons, have already been touched upon. Alterations of different parts of genes can have distinct consequences in terms of genetic disease. It is therefore necessary to describe more fully the details of gene structure. A schematic diagram of gene structure is given in Figure 2-13.

Promoters and Enhancers: Regulators of Transcription

As mentioned, a promoter sequence defines the location on the DNA sequence where transcription into mRNA begins. RNA polymerase II, the enzyme responsible for transcription, binds tightly to promoter sequences. These sequences are usually located within several hundred base pairs (usually abbreviated **bp**) of the site at which transcription begins. A number of specific promoter sequences have been identified. Some of the most common ones (often referred to as "boxes") are GC, TATA, and CCAAT. In some human genes, such as the one that can cause Duchenne muscular dystrophy, several different promoters exist and are located in different parts of the gene. Thus transcription of the gene can start in different places, producing somewhat different proteins. This allows the same gene sequence to code for variations of a protein in different tissues (e.g., muscle tissue vs. brain tis-

sue). As will be discussed in Chapter 3, mutations in promoter sequences usually lead to decreased levels of transcription of the associated gene.

Enhancers are a second type of regulatory sequence. Whereas promoters are always located close to the transcription initiation site, enhancer sequences may be thousands of base pairs upstream or downstream from the initiation site. Enhancers increase transcriptional activity by interacting with promoters. Often specific enhancers are active only in the cells of certain tissues. Thus they are partly responsible for tissue-specific expression of genes. Because cells usually have certain specialized functions (i.e., they produce only certain gene products), fewer than 10% of the genes in most cells are transcriptionally active at any given time.

> **Promoters and enhancers are DNA sequences that help to regulate the transcription of genes. Mutations in these regulatory sequences usually lead to decreased levels of transcription.**

If enhancers can be located thousands of base pairs away from a promoter, how can they interact with it? One mechanism that allows this interaction is **DNA looping**. Proteins binding to the enhancer and promoter sites can also bind to one another, generating a loop in the DNA. Formation of more complex loops can permit the simultaneous interaction of several regulatory elements. Enhancer–promoter interaction may also be accomplished

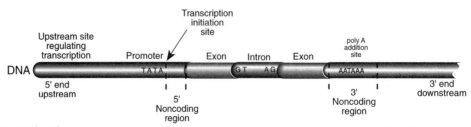

Figure 2-13 ■ Details of gene structure, showing promoter and upstream regulation (enhancer) sequences and a poly-A addition site.

when a regulatory protein first binds to an enhancer sequence and then slides down the DNA to locate and bind the promoter. Although evidence supports the existence of these and other mechanisms, the relative importance of each mechanism in facilitating enhancer–promoter interactions is not yet established.

Other types of regulatory elements exist as well. These include, for example, **chromatin openers**, which can decondense sections of chromatin. Decondensation can make a gene accessible to RNA polymerase. A number of other regulators of transcription have also been described; they are discussed further in some of the additional readings listed at the end of this chapter.

Introns and Exons

The intron–exon structure of genes, discovered in 1977, is one attribute that distinguishes eukaryotes from prokaryotes. Introns form the major portion of most eukaryotic genes. As noted, introns are spliced out of the mRNA before it is transported out of the nucleus. This splicing must be under precise control, or there would be an intolerable amount of variation in the amino acid sequences produced from mRNA. Splicing is controlled by DNA sequences known as **consensus sequences** (so named because the sequences are common in all eukaryotic organisms) that are located adjacent to each exon.

Because most eukaryotic genes are composed primarily of introns, it is natural to ask whether introns might have some function. At present this is largely material for speculation. One interesting hypothesis is that introns, by lengthening genes, encourage the shuffling of genes when homologous chromosomes exchange material during meiosis. It has also been suggested that introns have evolved to modify the amount of time required for DNA replication and transcription.

The intron–exon structure is a key feature of most eukaryotic genes. Presently the function of introns, if any, is unknown.

A surprising feature of at least a few introns is that they contain transcribed genes that are apparently unrelated to the gene in which the introns are contained. For example, introns of the human neurofibromatosis type 1 (NF1) gene contain three genes that are transcribed in the direction opposite that of the NF1 gene itself. These genes appear to have no functional relationship to the NF1 gene. Similar gene inserts have been found within the factor VIII gene on the human X chromosome.

Types of DNA

Although most of the emphasis in genetics is given to DNA that codes for proteins, it is important to note that less than 10% of the 3 billion nucleotides in the human genome actually performs this role. Most of our genetic material has no known function. To better understand the nature of all types of DNA we will briefly review the several categories into which they are classified (Fig. 2-14).

The first, and most common, class of DNA is termed **single-copy** DNA. As the name implies, single-copy DNA sequences are seen only once (or possibly a few times) in the genome. Single-copy DNA composes about 75% of the genome and

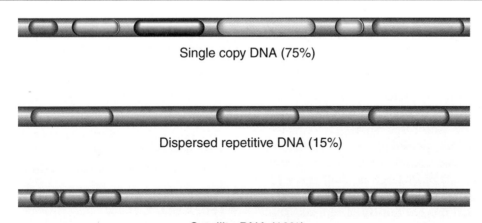

Single copy DNA (75%)

Dispersed repetitive DNA (15%)

Satellite DNA (10%)

Figure 2-14 ■ Single-copy DNA sequences are unique and dispersed throughout the genome. Satellite DNA sequences are repetitive elements that occur together in clusters, whereas dispersed repeats are similar to one another but do not cluster together.

includes the protein-coding genes. However, protein-coding DNA represents only a small proportion of all single-copy DNA. Most of it is found in introns or in DNA sequences that lie between genes.

The remaining 25% of the genome consists of **repetitive DNA**, sequences that are repeated over and over again in the genome, often thousands of times. There are two major classes of repetitive DNA, **dispersed repetitive DNA** and **satellite DNA**. Satellite repeats are clustered together in certain chromosome locations, where they occur in **tandem** (i.e., the beginning of one repeat occurs immediately adjacent to the end of another). Dispersed repeats, as the name implies, tend to be scattered singly throughout the genome (they do not occur in tandem).

The term satellite is derived from the fact that these sequences, because of their composition, can be easily separated by centrifugation in a cesium chloride density gradient. The DNA appears as a "satellite," separate from the other DNA in the gradient. This term is not to be confused with the "satellites" that can be observed microscopically on certain chromosomes (Chapter 6). Satellite DNA composes approximately 10% of the genome and can be further subdivided into several categories. **Alpha-satellite** DNA occurs as tandem repeats of a 171-bp sequence that can extend several million base pairs or more in length. This type of satellite DNA is found near the centromeres of chromosomes. **Minisatellites** are blocks of tandem repeats, the total length of which is much less. These repeats, which are 20 to 70 bp in length, usually have a total length of a few thousand base pairs. A final category, **microsatellites**, are smaller still: the repeat units are usually only 2, 3, or 4 bp in length, and the total length of the array is usually less than a few hundred base pairs. Minisatellites and microsatellites are of special interest in human genetics because they vary in length among individuals, making them highly useful for gene mapping (see Chapter 7).

Dispersed repetitive DNA makes up about 15% of the genome, and these repeats fall into two major categories, **SINEs** (short interspersed elements) and **LINEs** (long interspersed elements). Individual SINEs range in size from 90 to 500 bp, whereas individual LINEs can be as large as 7000 bases (7 **kilobases, or kb**). One of the most important types of SINEs is termed the *Alu* **family** of repeats. The term *Alu* derives from the fact that these repeat units, which are about 300 bp in size, contain a DNA sequence that can be cut by the *Alu* restriction enzyme (see Chapter 3 for further discussion). The

Alu repeats are a family of genes, meaning that all of them have highly similar DNA sequences. About 300,000 to 500,000 *Alu* repeats are scattered throughout the genome; these repeats thus constitute about 2% to 3% of all human DNA. A remarkable feature of *Alu* sequences is that they can generate copies of themselves, which can then insert into other parts of the genome. This insertion can sometimes interrupt a protein-coding gene, causing genetic disease (examples will be discussed in Chapter 4).

> **There are several major types of DNA, including single-copy DNA, satellite DNA, and dispersed repetitive DNA. The latter two categories are both classes of repeated DNA sequences. Less than 10% of our DNA actually encodes proteins.**

DNA Coiling

Textbook illustrations usually depict DNA as a double-helix molecule that continues in a long straight line. However, if the DNA in a cell were actually stretched out in this way, it would be about 2 m in length. To package all of this DNA into a tiny cell nucleus, it is coiled at several levels. First, the DNA is wound around a **histone** protein core to form a **nucleosome** (Fig. 2-15). About 140 to 150 DNA bases are wound around each histone core, and then 20 to 60 bases form a "spacer" element before the next nucleosome complex. The nucleosomes in turn form a helical **solenoid**; each turn of the solenoid includes about six nucleosomes. The solenoids themselves are organized into **chromatin loops**, which are attached to a protein scaffold. Each of these loops contains approximately 100 kb of DNA. The end result of this coiling and looping is that the DNA, when at its maximum stage of condensation, is only about 1/10,000th the length it would be if it were fully stretched out. Specific patterns of coiling may be related to the regulation of gene activity.

> **DNA is a tightly coiled structure. This coiling occurs at several levels, the nucleosome, the solenoid, and 100-kb chromatin loops.**

■ THE CELL CYCLE

During the course of development, each human progresses from a single-cell **zygote** (an egg cell fertilized by a sperm cell) to a marvelously complex organism containing approximately 100 tril-

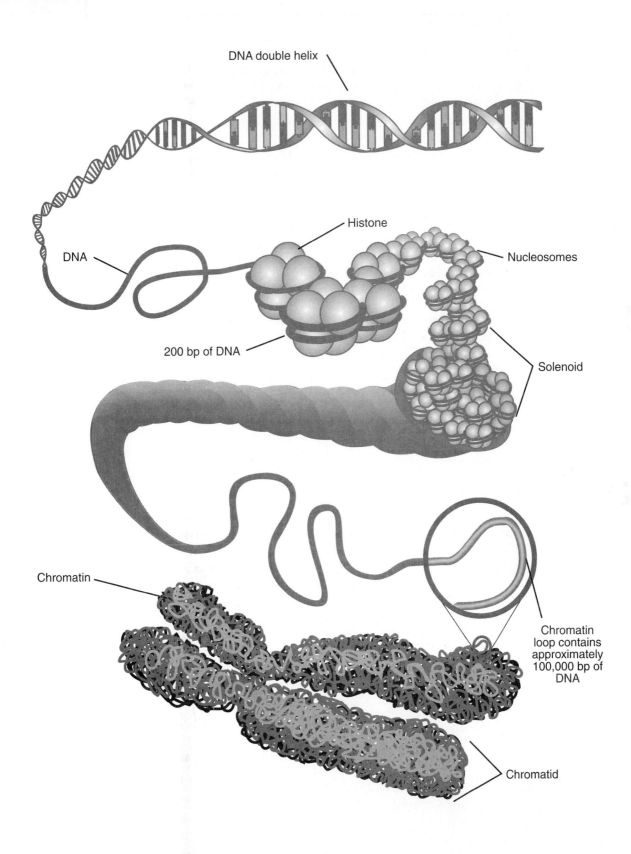

Figure 2-15 ■ Patterns of DNA coiling. DNA is wound around histones to form nucleosomes. These are organized into solenoids, which in turn compose chromatin loops. See color plate 2.

lion (10^{14}) individual cells. Because few cells last for an individual's entire lifetime, new ones must be generated continuously to replace those that die. Both of these processes, development and repair, require the manufacture of new cells. The cell division processes responsible for the creation of new diploid cells from existing ones are termed **mitosis** (nuclear division) and **cytokinesis** (cytoplasmic division). Before dividing, a cell must duplicate its contents, including its DNA; this occurs during **interphase**. The alternation of mitosis and interphase is referred to as the **cell cycle**.

As Figure 2-16 shows, a typical cell spends most of its life in interphase. This portion of the cell cycle is divided into three phases, **G1, S,** and **G2.** During G1 (gap 1) synthesis of RNA and proteins takes place. DNA replication occurs during the S (synthesis) phase. During G2 some DNA repair takes place, and the cell prepares for mitosis. By the time G2 has been reached, the cell contains two identical copies of each of the 46 chromosomes. These identical chromosomes are referred to as **sister chromatids**. Sister chromatids often exchange material during or after the S phase, a process known as **sister chromatid exchange**.

> **The cell cycle consists of the alternation of cell division (mitosis and cytokinesis) and interphase. DNA replication and protein synthesis take place during interphase.**

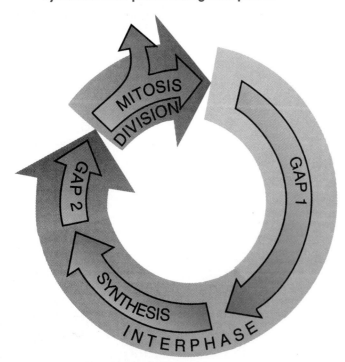

Figure 2-16 ■ Major phases of the mitotic cell cycle, showing the alternation of interphase and mitosis (division).

The length of the cell cycle varies considerably from one cell type to another. In rapidly dividing cells, such as those of epithelial tissue (e.g., found in the lining of the intestines and lungs), the cycle may be completed in fewer than 10 hours. Other cells, such as those of the liver, may divide only once each year or so. Some cell types, such as skeletal muscle cells and neurons, completely lose their ability to divide and replicate in adults. Although the lengths of all stages of the cell cycle vary somewhat, the great majority of this variation is due to differences in the length of the G1 phase. When cells stop dividing for a long period, they are often said to be in the G0 stage.

Mitosis

Although mitosis usually requires only 1 to 2 hours to complete, this portion of the cell cycle involves many critical and complex processes. Mitosis is divided into several phases (Fig. 2-17). During **prophase**, the first mitotic stage, the chromosomes become visible under a light microscope as they condense and coil (chromosomes are not clearly visible during interphase). The two sister chromatids of each chromosome lie together, attached at a point called the **centromere**. The nuclear membrane, which surrounds the nucleus, disappears during this stage. **Spindle fibers** begin to form. These radiate from two **centrioles** located on opposite sides of the cell. The spindle fibers become attached to the centromeres of each chromosome and eventually pull the two sister chromatids in opposite directions.

The chromosomes reach their most highly condensed state during **metaphase**, the next stage of mitosis. Because they are highly condensed, they are easiest to visualize microscopically during this phase. For this reason clinical diagnosis of chromosome disorders is usually based on metaphase chromosomes. During metaphase the spindle fibers begin to contract and pull the centromeres of the chromosomes, which are now arranged along the middle of the spindle (the **equatorial plane** of the cell).

During **anaphase**, the next mitotic stage, the centromeres of each chromosome split, allowing the sister chromatids to separate. The chromatids are then pulled by the spindle fibers, centromere first, toward opposite sides of the cell. At the end of anaphase the cell contains 92 separate chromosomes, half lying near one side of the cell and half lying near the other side. If all has proceeded correctly, the two sets of chromosomes are identical.

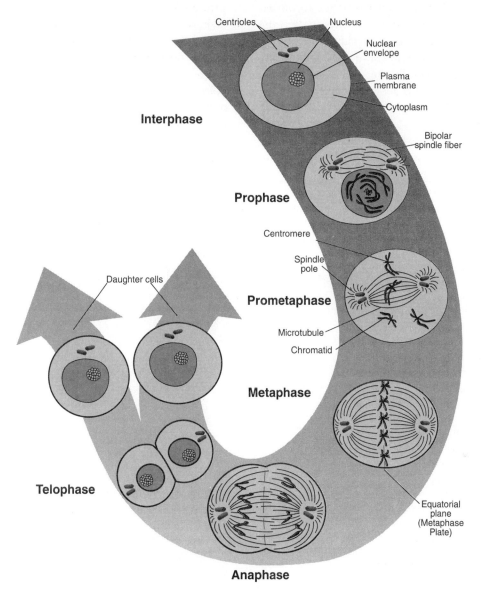

Figure 2-17 ■ The stages of mitosis, during which two identical diploid cells are formed from one original diploid cell.

Telophase, the final stage of mitosis, is characterized by the formation of new nuclear membranes around each of the two sets of 46 chromosomes. Also the spindle fibers disappear, and the chromosomes begin to decondense. Cytokinesis generally occurs after nuclear division and results in a roughly equal division of the cytoplasm into two parts. When telophase is completed, two diploid **daughter cells**, both identical to the original cell, have been formed.

Mitosis is the process through which two diploid identical daughter cells are formed from a single diploid cell.

Meiosis

When an egg cell and sperm cell unite to form a zygote, their chromosomes are combined into a single cell. Because humans are diploid organisms, there must be a mechanism to reduce the number of chromosomes in gametes to the haploid state. Otherwise the zygote would have 92, instead of the normal 46, chromosomes. The primary mechanism by which haploid gametes are formed from diploid precursor cells is termed **meiosis**.

Two cell divisions occur during meiosis. Each meiotic division has been divided into stages with the same names as those of mitosis, but the processes involved in some of the stages are different (Fig. 2-18). During meiosis I, often called the **reduction division** stage, two haploid cells are formed from a diploid cell. These diploid cells are the **oogonia** in females and the **spermatogonia** in males. Following meiosis I a second meiosis, the **equational division**, takes place, and each haploid cell is replicated.

The first stage of meiosis is **interphase I**. During this phase, as in mitotic interphase, important processes such as replication of chromosomal DNA take place. The second phase of meiosis I, **prophase I**, is complex and includes many of the key events that distinguish meiosis from mitosis. Prophase I begins as the chromatin strands coil and condense, causing them to become visible as chromosomes. During a process called **synapsis** the homologous chromosomes pair up, side by side, lying together in perfect alignment (in males, the X and Y chromosomes, being mostly nonhomol-

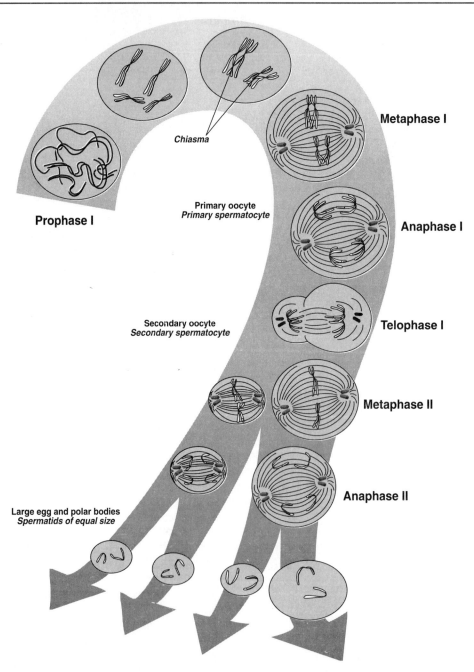

Figure 2-18 ■ The stages of meiosis, during which haploid gametes are formed from a diploid stem cell. For brevity, prophase II and telophase II are not shown. Note the relationship between meiosis and spermatogenesis and oogenesis.

ogous, line up end to end). This pairing of homologous chromosomes is an important part of the cell cycle that does not occur in mitosis. As prophase I continues, the chromatids of the two chromosomes intertwine. Each pair of intertwined homologous chromosomes is called a **bivalent** (indicating two chromosomes) or **tetrad** (indicating four chromatids in the unit).

A second key feature of prophase I is the formation of **chiasmata** (the singular is **chiasma**), cross-shaped structures that mark attachments between the homologous chromosomes (Fig. 2-19). Each chiasma indicates a point at which the homologous chromosomes exchange genetic material. This process, called **crossing over**, results eventually in chromosomes consisting of combinations of parts of the original chromosomes. This chromosomal "shuffling" is important because it greatly increases the possible combinations of genes in each gamete and thereby increases the number of possible combinations of human traits. Also as noted in Chapter 8, this phenomenon is critically important in assessing the order of genes along chromosomes. At the end of prophase I the bivalents begin to move toward the equatorial plate, a spindle apparatus begins to form in the cytoplasm, and the nuclear membrane dissipates.

Metaphase I is the next phase. Like mitotic metaphase, this stage is characterized by the completion of spindle formation and the alignment of the bivalents, which are still attached at the chiasmata in the equatorial plate. The two centromeres of each bivalent now lie on opposite sides of the equatorial plate.

During **anaphase I**, the next stage, the chiasmata disappear, and the homologous chromosomes are pulled by the spindle fibers toward opposite poles of the cell. The key feature of this phase is that,

unlike the corresponding phase of mitosis, the centromeres *do not duplicate and divide,* so that only half of the original number of chromosomes migrate toward each pole. The chromosomes migrating toward each pole thereby consist of one member of each pair of autosomes and one of the sex chromosomes.

The next stage, **telophase I**, begins when the chromosomes reach opposite sides of the cell. The chromosomes uncoil slightly, and a new nuclear membrane begins to form. The two daughter cells each contain the haploid number of chromosomes, each represented as a bivalent. In humans cytokinesis also occurs during this phase. The cytoplasm is divided approximately equally between the two daughter cells in the gametes formed in males. In those formed in females nearly all of the cytoplasm goes into one daughter cell, which will later form the egg. The other daughter cell becomes a **polar body**, a small nonfunctional cell that eventually degenerates.

> **Meiosis I (reduction division) includes a prophase I stage in which homologous chromosomes line up and exchange material (crossing over). During anaphase I the centromeres do not duplicate and divide, so that only one member of each pair of chromosomes migrates to each daughter cell.**

The equational division, meiosis II, then begins with **interphase II;** this is a brief phase. The important feature of interphase II is that, unlike interphase I and mitotic interphase, *no replication of DNA occurs.* **Prophase II**, the next stage, is similar to mitotic prophase, except that the cell nucleus contains only the haploid number of chromosomes. During prophase II the chromosomes thicken as they coil, the nuclear membrane disappears, and new spindle fibers are formed. Following this phase is **metaphase II**, during which the spindle fibers pull the chromosomes into alignment at the equatorial plate.

Anaphase II then follows. This stage resembles mitotic anaphase in that the centromeres split, each carrying a single chromatid toward a pole of the cell. The bivalents have now separated, but as Figure 2-19 shows, chiasma formation and crossing over mean that the two sister chromatids that have just separated may not be identical.

Telophase II, like telophase I, begins when the chromosomes reach opposite poles of the cell. There they begin to uncoil, new nuclear membranes are formed around each group of chromosomes, and cytokinesis occurs. In gametes formed

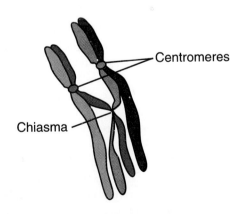

Figure 2-19 ■ The process of chiasma formation and crossing over results in the exchange of genetic material between homologous chromosomes.

Centromeres

Chiasma

in males, the cytoplasm is again divided equally between the two daughter cells. The end result of male meiosis is thus four functional daughter cells, each of which has an equal amount of cytoplasm. In female gametes unequal division of the cytoplasm again occurs, forming the egg cell and another polar body. The polar body formed during meiosis I sometimes undergoes a second meiosis, so three polar bodies may be present when the second stage of meiosis is completed.

> **Meiosis is a specialized cell division process in which a diploid cell gives rise to haploid gametes. This is accomplished by combining two rounds of division with only one round of DNA replication.**

Most chromosome disorders are caused by errors that occur in meiosis. Gametes can be created that contain missing or additional chromosomes or chromosomes with altered structures. In addition, mitotic errors that occur early in the life of the embryo can affect enough of the body's cells to produce clinically significant disease. Mitotic errors occurring at any point in one's lifetime can, under some circumstances, cause cancer. Cancer genetics will be discussed in Chapter 9, and chromosome disorders will be the subject of Chapter 6.

Relationship between Meiosis and Gametogenesis

The stages of meiosis can be related directly to stages in **gametogenesis**, the formation of gametes (see Fig. 2-17). In mature males the seminiferous tubules of the testes are populated by spermatogonia, which are diploid cells. After going through several mitotic divisions, the spermatogonia produce **primary spermatocytes**. Each primary spermatocyte, which is also diploid, undergoes meiosis I to produce a pair of **secondary spermatocytes**, each of which contains 23 double-stranded chromosomes. These undergo meiosis II, and each produces a pair of **spermatids** that contain 23 single-stranded chromosomes. The spermatids then lose most of their cytoplasm and develop tails for swimming as they become mature **sperm** cells. This process, known as **spermatogenesis**, continues throughout the life of the mature male.

> **In spermatogenesis, each diploid spermatogonium produces four haploid sperm cells.**

Oogenesis, the process in which female gametes are formed, differs in several important ways from spermatogenesis. Whereas the cycle of spermatogenesis is constantly recurring in males, much of female oogenesis is completed before birth. Diploid oogonia divide mitotically to produce **primary oocytes** by the third month of fetal development. More than 2 million primary oocytes are formed during gestation, and these are suspended in prophase I by the time the female is born. Meiosis continues only when a mature primary oocyte is ovulated. In meiosis I the primary oocyte produces one **secondary oocyte** (containing the cytoplasm) and one polar body. The secondary oocyte then emerges from the follicle and proceeds down the fallopian tube, with the polar body attached to it. Meiosis II begins only if the secondary oocyte is fertilized by a sperm cell. If so, one haploid **mature ovum**, containing the cytoplasm, and another haploid polar body are produced. The polar bodies eventually disintegrate. About 1 hour after fertilization, the nuclei of the sperm cell and ovum fuse, forming a diploid **zygote**. The zygote then begins its development into an embryo through a series of mitotic divisions.

> **In oogenesis one haploid ovum and three haploid polar bodies are produced meiotically from a diploid oogonium. Unlike spermatogenesis, which continues throughout the mature male's life, the first phase of oogenesis is completed before the female is born and is then halted until ovulation occurs.**

■ STUDY QUESTIONS

1. Consider the following double-stranded DNA sequence:
   5′-CAG AAG AAA ATT AAC ATG TAA-3′
   3′-GTC TTC TTT TAA TTG TAC ATT-5′
   What is the mRNA sequence produced by transcription of this DNA sequence? What is the amino acid sequence produced by translation of the mRNA sequence?

2. Arrange the following terms according to their hierarchical relationship to one another: genes, chromosomes, exons, codons, nucleotides, genome.

3. Less than 10% of our DNA codes for proteins. Furthermore, in a given cell type only 10% of the coding DNA actively encodes proteins. Explain these statements.

4. What are the major differences between mitosis and meiosis?

5. The human body contains approximately 10^{14} cells. Starting with a single-cell zygote, how many mitotic cell divisions, on average, would be required to produce this number of cells?

6. How many mature sperm cells will be produced by 100 primary spermatocytes? How many mature egg cells will be produced by 100 primary oocytes?

■ ADDITIONAL READING

Alberts B and Stillman B: *Molecular biology of the cell, ed 3,* New York, 1994, Garland Publishing.

Byers PH: Disorders of collagen biosynthesis and structure. In Scriver CR, Beaudet AL, Sly WS, and Valle D, editors: The Metabolic and Molecular Bases of Inherited Disease ed. 7, New York, 1995, McGraw-Hill.

Clayton DA: Structure, replication, and transcription of DNA. In Leder P, Clayton DA, Rubenstein E, editors: Introduction to Molecular Medicine, New York, 1994, Scientific American.

Gardiner K: Human genome organization. Curr Opin Genet Dev 5:315–322, 1995.

Kelman Z and O'Donnel M: DNA replication: enzymology and mechanisms, Curr Opin Genet Dev 4:185–195, 1994.

Latchman DS: Transcription-factor mutations and disease, N Eng J Med 334:28–33, 1996.

Müller R: Transcriptional regulation during the mammalian cell cycle. Trends Genet 11:173–178, 1995.

Murray A, Hunt T: The cell cycle: an introduction, Oxford, 1994, Oxford University Press.

Papavassiliou AG: Transcription factors, N Eng J Med 332: 45–47, 1995.

Tsipouras P: Osteogenesis imperfecta. In Beighton P, editor: McKusick's heritable disorders of connective tissue, ed 5, St Louis, 1993, Mosby.

Tyler-Smith C and Willard HF: Mammalian chromosome structure, Curr Opin Genet Dev 3:390–397, 1993.

Watson JD, Hopkins NH, Roberts JW, Steitz JA, and Weiner AM: Molecular biology of the gene, ed. 4, Menlo Park, Calif, 1987, Benjamin/Cummings.

3 Genetic Variation: Its Origin and Detection

Humans display a remarkable degree of genetic variation. This is seen in traits such as height, blood pressure, and skin color. Included in the spectrum of genetic variation are disease states, such as cystic fibrosis or type 1 neurofibromatosis (see Chapter 4). This aspect of genetic variation is the focus of medical genetics.

All genetic variation originates from the process known as **mutation**, which is defined as a change in DNA sequence. Mutations can affect either somatic or **germline** cells (cells that produce gametes). Mutations in **somatic** cells (all cells other than germline cells) can lead to cancer and are thus of significant concern. However, our attention in this chapter will be directed primarily to germline mutations because these can be transmitted from one generation to the next.

As a result of mutations, a gene may differ among individuals in terms of its DNA sequence. The differing sequences are referred to as **alleles**. A gene's location on a chromosome is termed a **locus** (from the Latin for "place"). Thus we might say that an individual has a certain allele at the β-globin locus on chromosome 11. If an individual has the same allele on both members of a chromosome pair, he or she is said to be a **homozygote**. If the alleles differ in DNA sequence, the individual is a **heterozygote**. The alleles that are present at a given locus are referred to as the individual's **genotype**. Some **loci** (plural of locus) vary considerably among individuals. If a locus has two or more alleles, the frequencies of which each exceed 1% in a population, the locus is said to be **polymorphic** ("many forms"). The polymorphic locus is often termed a **polymorphism**.

In this chapter we examine mutation as the source of genetic variation. We discuss the different types of mutations, as well as the causes and consequences of mutation. In addition, we discuss biochemical and molecular techniques that are

now used to detect genetic variation in human populations.

■ MUTATION: THE SOURCE OF GENETIC VARIATION

Types of Mutation

Some mutations consist of an alteration of the number or structure of chromosomes in a cell. These major chromosome abnormalities can be observed microscopically and are the subject of Chapter 6. Here we focus on mutations that affect only single genes and are not microscopically observable. Most of our discussion centers on mutations that take place in coding DNA or in regulatory sequences because mutations occurring in other parts of the genome usually have no clinical consequences.

One important type of **single-gene mutation** is the **base pair substitution**, in which one base pair is replaced by another.* This can result in a change in amino acid sequence, although, because of the redundancy of the genetic code, many of these mutations do not change the amino acid sequence and thus have no consequence. The latter are called **silent substitutions**. Nonsilent base pair substitutions consist of two basic types: **missense mutations** produce a change in a single amino acid, whereas **nonsense mutations** produce one of the three stop codons in the mRNA: UAA, UAG, or UGA (Fig. 3-1, *A, B*). These codons terminate translation of the mRNA and thus result in a premature termination of the polypeptide chain. Conversely when a stop codon is altered so that it encodes an amino acid, an abnormally elongated polypeptide is produced. Alterations of amino acid sequences can

---

*In molecular genetics, base pair substitutions are also termed **point mutations**. The latter term, however, was used in classical genetics to denote any mutation small enough to be unobservable under a microscope.

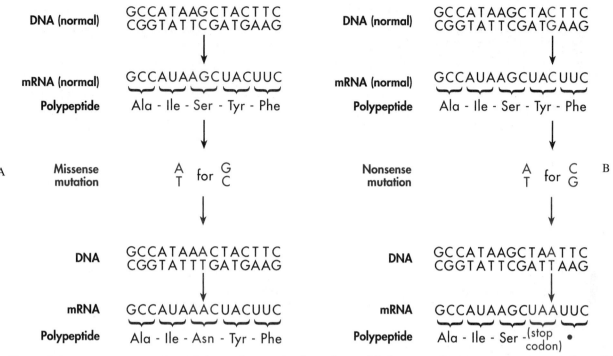

Figure 3-1 ■ Missense mutations (A) produce a single amino acid change, whereas nonsense mutations (B) produce a stop codon in the mRNA. Stop codons terminate translation of the polypeptide.

have profound consequences. Many of the serious genetic diseases to be discussed later are the result of base pair substitutions.

A second major type of mutation consists of **deletions** or **insertions** of one or more base pairs. These mutations, which can produce extra or missing amino acids in a protein, are often detrimental. An example of such a mutation is a 3-bp deletion that causes most cases of cystic fibrosis seen in whites (see Chapter 4 for further details). Deletions and insertions tend to be especially harmful when the number of missing or extra base pairs is not a multiple of three. Because codons consist of groups of 3 bp, such insertions or deletions can alter all of the downstream codons. For example, a single-base insertion (an A in the second codon) could convert a sequence read as 5'-ACT GAT TGC GTT-3' to 5'-ACT GAA TTG CGT-3'. This would convert an amino acid sequence from Thr-Asp-Cys-Val to Thr-Glu-Leu-Arg. These mutations, illustrated further in Figure 3-2, are known as **frameshift mutations**.

Other types of mutations can alter the regulation of transcription or translation. A **promoter mutation** can decrease the affinity of RNA polymerase for a promoter site, often resulting in reduced production of mRNA. The final result is decreased

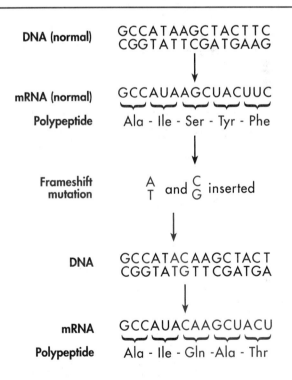

Figure 3-2 ■ Frameshift mutations result from the insertion or deletion of a number of bases (not a multiple of 3). This alters all of the codons downstream from the site of insertion or deletion.

production of a particular protein. **Enhancer mutations** can have similar effects.

Mutations may also interfere with the splicing of introns as mature mRNA is formed from the primary mRNA transcript. **Splice site mutations**, occurring at intron–exon boundaries, alter the splicing signal necessary for proper excision of an intron. These may occur at the GT sequence that always defines the **5′ donor site** or at the AG sequence that defines the **3′ acceptor site**. They may also occur in the sequences that lie near the donor and acceptor sites; i.e., the consensus se-

quences defined in Chapter 2. When such mutations take place, the excision will often take place within the next exon, at a splice site located in the exon. These splice sites, the DNA sequences of which differ slightly from those of normal splice sites, are ordinarily unused and "hidden" within the exon and thus termed **cryptic splice sites**. The use of a cryptic site for splicing results in partial deletion of the exon. In other cases an entire exon can be deleted. As Figure 3-3 shows, splice site mutations can also result in the abnormal inclusion of part or all of an intron in the mature mRNA. It is

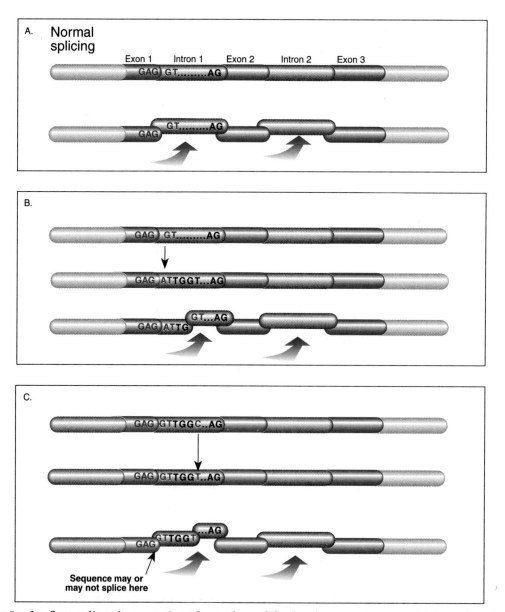

Figure 3-3 ■ In the first splice site mutation shown here (B), the donor sequence, GT, is replaced with AT. This results in an incorrect splice that leaves part of the intron in the mature mRNA transcript. In the second mutation (C), a second GT donor site is created in the first intron, resulting in a combination of abnormally and normally spliced mRNA products.

also possible for a mutation to occur at a cryptic splice site, causing it to appear as a normal splice site, thus competing with the normal splice site.

There are several types of DNA sequences that are capable of propagating copies of themselves; these copies are then inserted in other locations on chromosomes. The insertion of these **transposons** (or **mobile elements**) can cause frameshift mutations. Until recently, it was not clear whether this phenomenon, which has been well documented in experimental animals such as fruit flies, occurred in humans. The insertion of mobile elements has now been shown to cause isolated cases of type 1 neurofibromatosis and hemophilia A (a clotting disorder) in humans.

The final type of mutation to be considered here has been discovered recently and affects tandem repeated DNA sequences (see Chapter 2) that occur within or near certain disease genes. A normal individual will have a relatively small number of these tandem repeats (e.g., 20 to 40). For reasons that are not yet understood, the number of repeats can increase dramatically during meiosis or possibly during early fetal development, so that a newborn may have hundreds or even thousands of repeats. When this occurs in certain regions of the genome, it causes genetic disease. Like other mutations, these **expanded repeats** can be transmitted to the patient's offspring. At least seven genetic diseases are now known to be caused by expanded repeats. These will be discussed further in Chapter 4.

> **Mutations are the ultimate source of genetic variation. Some mutations result in genetic disease, whereas others have no physical effects. The principal types of mutations include missense, nonsense, frameshift, promoter, and splice site mutations. There is also evidence for mutations caused by the random insertion of mobile elements, and several genetic diseases are known to be caused by expanded repeats.**

Clinical Consequences of Mutation: The Hemoglobin Disorders

Genetic disorders of human hemoglobin are the most common group of single-gene disorders: an estimated 5% of the world's population carries one or more mutations of the genes involved in hemoglobin synthesis. Because all of the types of mutation described in this chapter have been observed in the hemoglobin disorders, these disorders serve as an important illustration of the clinical consequences of mutation.

The hemoglobin molecule is a tetramer composed of four polypeptide chains, two of which are labeled α and two of which are labeled β. The β chains are encoded by a gene on chromosome 11, and the α chains are encoded by two genes on chromosome 16 that are similar to one another. A normal individual would thus have two normal β genes and four normal α genes (Fig. 3-4). Ordinarily, tight regulation of these genes ensures that roughly equal numbers of α and β chains are produced. Each of these **globin** chains is associated with a **heme** group, which contains an iron atom and binds with oxygen. This property allows hemoglobin to perform the vital function of transporting oxygen in red blood cells.

The hemoglobin disorders can be classified into two broad categories: structural abnormalities, in which the hemoglobin molecule is altered, and thalassemias, a group of conditions in which the hemoglobin is structurally normal but reduced in quantity. Another condition, hereditary persistence of fetal hemoglobin (HPFH), occurs when fetal hemoglobin, encoded by the α-globin genes and by two β-globin-like genes called $^A\gamma$ and $^G\gamma$ (Fig. 3-4), continues to be produced after birth (normally, γ-chain production ceases and β-chain production begins at the time of birth). HPFH does not cause disease but instead can compensate for a lack of normal adult hemoglobin. It is not discussed further here.

Sickle Cell Disease

A large array of different hemoglobin disorders have been identified. The discussion that follows is

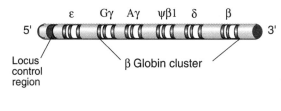

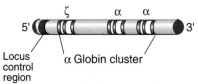

Figure 3-4 ■ **The α-globin gene cluster on chromosome 16 and the β-globin gene cluster on chromosome 11. The β-globin cluster includes the ϵ-globin gene that encodes embryonic globin and the γ-globin genes that encode fetal globin. The $\Psi\beta$I and δ genes are not expressed. The α-globin cluster includes the ζ-globin gene, which encodes embryonic α-globin.**

a greatly simplified presentation of the major forms of these disorders. The hemoglobin disorders, the mutations that cause them, and their major features are summarized in Table 3-1.

The most important of the structural hemoglobin abnormalities is sickle cell disease, a disorder that affects approximately 1 in 400 to 600 African-American births (*SOL* 5-8). It is even more common in parts of Africa, where it can affect up to one in 50 births, and it is also seen occasionally in Mediterranean and Mideastern populations. Sickle cell disease is caused by a single missense mutation that effects a substitution of valine for glutamic acid at position six of the β-globin chain. In homozygous form this amino acid substitution alters the characteristics of the hemoglobin molecule such that the **erythrocytes** (red blood cells) assume a characteristic "sickle" shape (Fig. 3-5,*A*) under conditions of low oxygen tension. These conditions are experienced in capillaries, the tiny vessels whose diameter is smaller than that of the erythrocyte. Normal erythrocytes (Fig. 3-5,*B*) can squeeze through capillaries, but sickled erythrocytes are less flexible and are unable to do so. The resultant vascular obstruction produces localized **hypoxia** (lack of oxygen), painful sickling "crises," and **infarctions** of various tissues, including bone, spleen, kidneys, and lungs (an infarction is a destruction of tissue). Premature destruction of the sickled erythrocytes decreases the number of circulating erythrocytes and the hemoglobin level, producing **anemia**. The spleen becomes enlarged (**splenomegaly**), but infarctions eventually destroy this organ, producing some loss of immune function. This contributes to the recurrent bacterial infections (especially pneumonia) that are commonly seen in individuals with sickle cell disease

and that frequently cause death. In North America it is estimated that about 15% of children with sickle cell disease die before the age of 5.

Sickle cell disease, which causes anemia, tissue infarctions, and multiple infections, is the result of a single missense mutation that produces an amino acid substitution in the β-globin chain.

Thalassemia

The term thalassemia is derived from the Greek word for "sea," *thalassa.* This refers to the fact that thalassemia was first described in populations living near the Mediterranean Sea, although it is also common in portions of Africa, the Mideast, India, and Southeast Asia. Thalassemia can be divided into two major groups, α-thalassemia and β-thalassemia, depending on the chain that is reduced in quantity. When one type of chain is decreased in number, the other chain type, unable to participate in normal tetramer formation, tends to form molecules consisting of four chains of the excess type only (these are termed **homotetramers**, in contrast to the **heterotetramers** normally formed by α and β chains). In α-thalassemia the α-globin chains are deficient, so the β chains (or γ chains in the fetus) are found in excess. They form homotetramers that have a greatly reduced oxygen-binding capacity, producing anemia. In β-thalassemia the excess α-chains form homotetramers that precipitate and damage the cell membranes of red cell precursors (i.e., the cells that form circulating erythrocytes). This leads to premature erythrocyte destruction and anemia.

Most cases of α-thalassemia are caused by deletions of the α-globin genes. A loss of one or two of

Table 3-1 ■ Summary of the hemoglobin disorders

Disease	Mutation type	Major disease features
Sickle cell disease	β-globin missense mutation	Anemia, tissue infarctions, infections
Hb H disease	Deletion or abnormality of 3 of the 4 α-globin genes	Moderately severe anemia, splenomegaly
Hydrops fetalis	Deletion or abnormality of all 4 α-globin genes	Severe hypoxia, congestive heart failure; stillbirth or neonatal death
β^{0}-thalassemia	Usually nonsense, frameshift, or splice site donor or acceptor mutations; no β-globin produced	Severe anemia, splenomegaly, skeletal abnormalities, infections; often fatal during first decade if untreated
β^{+}-thalassemia	Usually missense, regulatory, or splice site consensus sequence or cryptic splice site mutations; small amount of β-globin produced	Features similar to those of β^{0} thalassemia but often somewhat milder

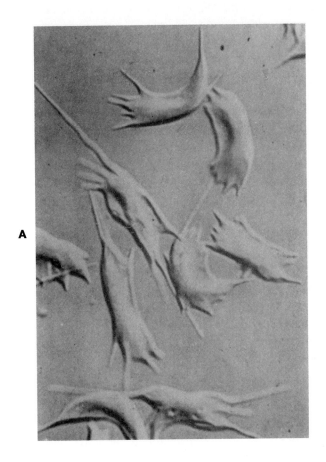

A

these genes has no clinical effect. The loss or abnormality of three of the α genes produces moderately severe anemia and splenomegaly (Hb H disease). Loss of all four α genes, a condition seen primarily among Southeast Asians, produces hypoxia in the fetus and hydrops fetalis (a condition in which there is a massive buildup of fluid; *SOL* 52). Severe hypoxia invariably causes stillbirth or neonatal death.

The α-thalassemia conditions are usually caused by deletions of α-globin genes. The loss of three of these genes leads to moderately severe anemia, and the loss of all four is fatal.

Individuals with a β-globin mutation on one copy of chromosome 11 (heterozygotes) are said to have β-thalassemia minor, a condition that involves little or no anemia and does not ordinarily require clinical management. Those in whom both copies of the chromosome carry a β-globin mutation develop β-thalassemia major (also called Cooley's anemia) or the less serious condition, β-thalassemia intermedia. β-globin may be completely absent (β^0-thalassemia) or reduced to about 10% to 30% of the normal amount (β^+-thalassemia).

Because β-globin is not produced until after birth, β-thalassemia major is not seen clinically until the age of 2 to 6 months. These patients develop severe anemia. If untreated, substantial

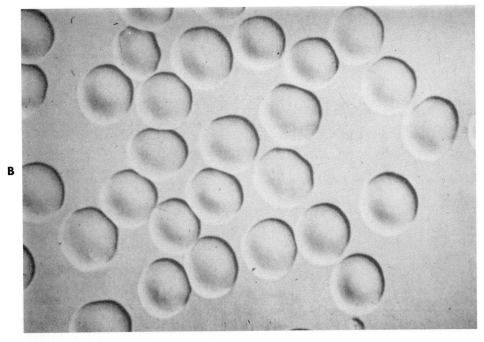

B

Figure 3-5 ▪ Erythrocytes from sickle cell patients assume a characteristic shape under conditions of low oxygen tension (A). Compare with normal erythrocytes (B).

growth retardation can occur. The anemia causes bone marrow expansion, which in turn produces skeletal changes, including protuberant upper jaws and cheekbones and thinning of the long bones (making them susceptible to fracture). Splenomegaly (Fig. 3-6) and infections are common, and untreated β-thalassemia major patients often die during the first decade of life. β-thalassemia can vary considerably in severity, depending on the precise nature of the responsible mutation.

In contrast to α-thalassemia, gene deletions are relatively rare in β-thalassemia. Instead most cases are caused by single-base mutations. Nonsense mutations, which result in premature termination of translation of the β chain, usually produce β^0-thalassemia. Frameshift mutations also typically produce the β^0 form. In addition to mutations in the β-globin gene itself, alterations in regulatory sequences are often seen. β-globin transcription is regulated by a promoter, two enhancers, and an upstream region known as the **locus control region (LCR,** Fig. 3-4). Mutations in these regulatory regions usually result in reduced synthesis of mRNA and a reduction, but not complete absence, of β-globin (β^+-thalassemia). Several types of splice site mutations have also been observed. When a point mutation occurs at the donor or acceptor sites, normal splicing is destroyed completely, producing β^0-thalassemia. Mutations in the surrounding consensus sequences usually produce

β^+-thalassemia. Mutations also occur in the cryptic splice sites found in introns or exons of the β-globin gene, causing these sites to be available to the splicing mechanism. These additional splice sites then compete with the normal splice sites, producing some normal and some abnormal β-globin chains. The result is usually β^+-thalassemia.

Many different types of mutations can produce β-thalassemia conditions. Nonsense, frameshift, and splice site donor and acceptor mutations tend to produce more severe disease. Regulatory mutations and those involving splice site consensus sequences and cryptic splice sites tend to produce less severe disease.

More than 100 different β-globin mutations have been reported. Consequently most β-thalassemia patients are not "homozygotes" in the strict sense: they usually have a different β-globin mutation on each copy of chromosome 11 and are termed **compound heterozygotes.** Even though the mutations differ, each of the two β-globin genes is altered, producing a disease state. It is common to apply the term "homozygote" loosely to compound heterozygotes.

Sickle cell and β-thalassemia major patients are sometimes treated with blood transfusions and with chelating agents that remove excess iron introduced by the transfusions. Prophylactic administration of antibiotics and antipneumococcal vaccination are now being advocated as ways to diminish bacterial infections in sickle cell disease patients, and analgesics are administered for pain relief during sickling crises. Bone marrow transplants, which provide donor stem cells that produce genetically normal erythrocytes, have been performed on patients with severe β-thalassemia and sickle cell disease. However, the mortality rate from these transplants is still fairly high (approximately 10% to 20%). The hemoglobin disorders are a possible candidate for gene therapy (see Chapter 11).

Causes of Mutation

A large number of agents are known to cause **induced mutations.** These mutations, which can be attributed to a known environmental cause, can be contrasted with **spontaneous mutations,** which arise naturally during the process of DNA replication. Agents that cause induced mutations are known collectively as **mutagens.** Animal studies have shown that **radiation** is an important class of mutagen (see Clinical Commentary 3-1).

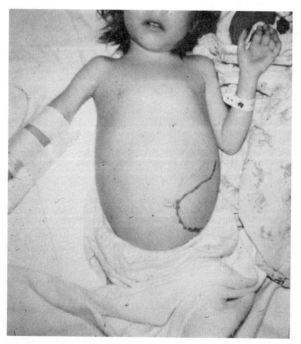

Figure 3-6 ■ A child with β-thalassemia major who has severe splenomegaly.

Because mutation is a rare event, occurring less than once per 10,000 genes per generation, it is difficult to measure directly in humans. The relationship between radiation exposure and mutation is similarly difficult to assess. For a person living in a developed country, a typical lifetime exposure to ionizing radiation is about 6 to 7 rem.* About one third of this amount is thought to originate from medical and dental x-rays.

Certain unfortunate situations have arisen in which specific human populations have received much larger radiation doses. The most thoroughly studied such population consists of the survivors of the atomic bomb blasts that occurred in Hiroshima and Nagasaki, Japan, at the close of World War II. Many of those who were exposed to high doses of radiation died of radiation sickness. Others, however, survived, and many produced offspring.

To study the effects of radiation exposure in this population, a large team of Japanese and American scientists conducted medical and genetic investigations of many of the survivors. A significant number of those exposed developed cancers and chromosome abnormalities in their somatic cells, probably as a consequence of radiation exposure. To assess the effects of radiation exposure on the subjects' germ lines, the scientists compared the offspring of those who suffered substantial radiation exposures with the offspring of those who did not. Although it is difficult to establish radiation doses with precision, there is no doubt that, in general, those who were situated closer to the blasts suffered much greater exposure levels. It is estimated that the exposed group received roughly 30 to 60 rem of radiation, many times the average lifetime radiation exposure.

In a series of more than 76,000 offspring of these individuals, a large number of factors were assessed. These included stillbirths, chromosome abnormali-

*A rem is a standard unit for measuring radiation exposure. It is roughly equal to 0.01 joule of absorbed energy per kilogram of tissue.

ties, birth defects, cancer before age 20, death before age 26, and various measures of growth and development, including intelligence quotients (IQ). There were no statistically significant differences between the offspring of individuals who were exposed to radiation and those who were not. In addition, a genetic study of mutations was conducted using protein electrophoresis, a technique that detects mutations that lead to amino acid changes (see text). Parents and offspring were compared to determine whether mutations had occurred. The numbers of mutations detected in the exposed and unexposed groups were virtually identical.

It is remarkable that, even though there was substantial evidence for radiation effects on somatic cells, no detectable effect could be seen for germ cells. What could account for this? It is likely that DNA repair is at least in part responsible. Also, however, we must recognize that, even with a large sample of individuals who received relatively high doses of radiation, increased mutation levels are difficult to detect.

A number of other studies of the effects of radiation on humans have been reported, including investigations of individuals who live near nuclear power plants. The radiation doses received by these individuals are substantially smaller than those discussed above, and the results of these studies are even more equivocal.

These results do not support the argument, however, that radiation danger should be taken lightly. Recent studies indicate increased rates of leukemia and thyroid cancer among those exposed to above-ground nuclear testing in the American Southwest. Radon, a radioactive gas that is produced by the decay of naturally occurring uranium, can be found at dangerously high levels in some homes and poses a risk for lung cancer. Any unnecessary exposure to radiation, particularly to the gonads or to developing fetuses, should be avoided if at all possible.

Ionizing radiation, such as that produced by x-rays and nuclear fallout, can eject electrons from atoms, forming electrically charged ions. When these ions are situated within or near the DNA molecule, they can promote chemical reactions that change DNA bases. Ionizing radiation can also break double-stranded DNA. This form of radiation can reach all cells of the body, including the germ line.

Nonionizing radiation does not form charged ions but can move electrons from inner to outer orbits in the atom. The atom becomes chemically unstable. Ultraviolet (UV) radiation, which occurs naturally in sunlight, is an example of nonionizing radiation. UV radiation causes the formation of covalent bonds between adjacent pyrimidine bases (i.e., cytosine or thymine). These **pyrimidine dimers** (a dimer is a molecule having two subunits) cannot pair properly with purines during DNA replication, resulting in a base pair substitution (Fig. 3-7). Because UV radiation is absorbed by the epidermis, it does not reach the germ line but can cause skin cancer (Clinical Commentary 3-2, page 39).

A variety of chemicals can also induce mutations, sometimes because of their chemical similarity to

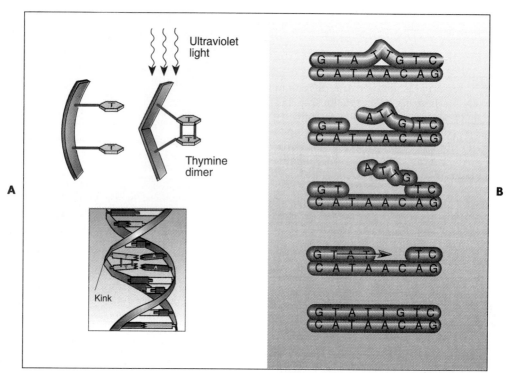

Figure 3-7 ■ Pyrimidine dimers originate when covalent bonds form between adjacent pyrimidine (cytosine or thymine) bases. This deforms the DNA, interfering with normal base pairing (A). The dimer and bases on either side of it are removed and replaced, using the complementary DNA strand as a template (B).

DNA bases. Because of this similarity, these **base analogs**, such as 5-bromouracil, can be substituted for a true DNA base during replication. The analog is not exactly the same as the base it replaces, so it can cause pairing errors during subsequent replications. Other chemical mutagens, such as acridine dyes, can physically insert themselves between existing bases, distorting the DNA helix and causing frameshift mutations. Still other mutagens can directly alter DNA bases, causing replication errors. An example of the latter is nitrous acid, which removes an amino group from cytosine, converting it to uracil. Although uracil is normally found in RNA, it mimics the pairing action of thymine. Thus it pairs with adenine, instead of pairing with guanine, as the original cytosine would have done. The end result is a base pair substitution.

Hundreds of chemicals are now known to be mutagenic in laboratory animals. Among these are nitrogen mustard, vinyl chloride, alkylating agents, formaldehyde, sodium nitrite, and saccharine. It should be emphasized that some of these chemicals are much more potent mutagens than others. Nitrogen mustard, for example, is a powerful mutagen, whereas saccharine is a relatively weak one. Although caffeine (a purine analog) is mutagenic in

some lower organisms such as yeast and fungi, there is no convincing evidence that it is mutagenic in humans. This is probably due in part to the fact that DNA repair, to be discussed next, is highly developed in higher organisms.

> **There are many substances in our environment that are known to be mutagenic. These include ionizing and nonionizing radiation, as well as hundreds of different chemicals. Some mutagens occur naturally, whereas others are generated by humans.**

DNA Repair

Considering that 3 billion DNA bases must be replicated in each cell division and considering the large number of mutagens to which we are exposed, DNA replication is surprisingly accurate. A primary reason for this accuracy is the process of **DNA repair**, which takes place in all normal cells of higher organisms. Several dozen different enzymes are involved in repairing damaged DNA. They collectively recognize an altered base, excise it by cutting the DNA strand, replace it with the correct base (determined from the complementary

Clinical Commentary 3-2: Xeroderma Pigmentosum, a Disease of Faulty DNA Repair

An inevitable consequence of exposure to UV radiation is the formation of potentially dangerous pyrimidine dimers in the DNA of skin cells. Fortunately a highly efficient system of enzymes usually repairs these dimers in normal individuals. Among those affected with the rare disease xeroderma pigmentosum (XP), this system does not work properly, and the resulting replication errors lead to base pair substitutions in skin cells. Varying substantially in severity, XP usually begins within the first 10 years of life. Extensive freckling is followed by numerous skin tumors (Fig. 3-8) and, in some cases, neurologic abnormalities. The tumors are concentrated primarily in sun-exposed parts of the body. Patients are advised to avoid UV light sources (such as sunlight), and cancerous growths are removed surgically. XP patients can develop severe malignancies, sometimes causing death before age 20.

Several different repair enzymes are involved in correcting pyrimidine dimers. They include an endonuclease that cuts the DNA at the site of the dimer, an exonuclease that removes the dimer and nearby nucleotides, a polymerase that fills the gap with DNA bases (using the complementary DNA strand as a template), and a ligase that rejoins the corrected portion of DNA to the original strand. At least seven different genes code for these repair enzymes. An inherited mutation in any one of them can produce XP.

It must be emphasized that our discussion involves two distinct classes of mutations. The repair-enzyme mutations occur in the germ line and can thus can be transmitted from one generation to the next. Because they result in deficient DNA repair, they in turn permit skin cell mutations to persist, resulting in tumors. The skin cell mutations themselves cannot, of course, be inherited.

Although XP is probably the best-known disease that results from deficient DNA repair, it is not the only one. Other diseases that probably result from defects in DNA repair mechanisms include Bloom syndrome, Cockayne syndrome, ataxia telangiectasia, and Fanconi anemia.

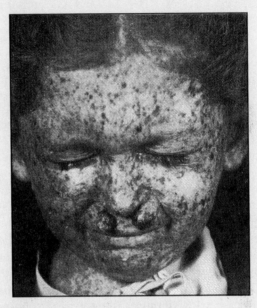

Figure 3-8 ■ A child with xeroderma pigmentosum, showing the multiple skin tumors characteristic of this disease.

strand), and reseal the DNA. It is estimated that these repair mechanisms correct 99.9% of initial errors.

DNA repair is an important mechanism operating in mammalian systems to correct errors that occur in the replication process.

Mutation Rates

How often do spontaneous mutations occur? At the nucleotide level the mutation rate is usually estimated to be about 10^{-10} per base pair per cell division (these represent mutations that have escaped the process of DNA repair). At the level of the gene the mutation rate is variable, ranging from 10^{-4} to 10^{-7} per locus per cell division. There are at least two reasons for this large range of variation.

1. Genes vary tremendously in size. The somatostatin gene, for example, is small, containing 1480 bp. In contrast, the gene responsible for Duchenne muscular dystrophy (DMD) spans more than 2 million bp. As might be expected, larger genes present larger "targets" for mutation and usually experience mutation more often than do smaller genes. The DMD gene and the genes for hemophilia A and type 1 neurofibromatosis are all large and have high mutation rates on a per gene basis.

2. It is well established that certain nucleotide sequences are especially susceptible to mutation. These are termed **mutation hot spots**. The best-known example is the two-base (dinucleotide) sequence CG. In mammals about 80% of CG dinucleotides are **methylated**: a methyl group is attached to the cytosine base. The methylated cytosine, 5-methylcytosine, easily loses an amino group, converting it to thymine. The end result is a mutation from cytosine to thymine (Fig. 3-9). Surveys of mutations in human genetic diseases have shown that the mutation rate at CG dinucleotides is about 12

Figure 3-9 ■ Cytosine methylation. The addition of a methyl group to a cytosine base forms 5-methylcytosine. The subsequent loss of an amino group (deamination) forms thymine, thus resulting in a cytosine → thymine substitution.

times higher than at other dinucleotide sequences. Mutation hot spots, in the form of CG dinucleotides, have been identified in a number of important human disease genes, including the procollagen genes responsible for osteogenesis imperfecta (Chapter 2). Other disease examples are discussed in Chapters 4 and 5.

Mutation rates also vary considerably with the age of the parent. Some chromosome abnormalities increase dramatically with elevated maternal age (see Chapter 6). In addition, single-gene mutations can increase with elevated paternal age. This increase is seen in several single-gene disorders, including Marfan syndrome and achondroplasia. As Figure 3-10 shows, the risk of producing a child with Marfan syndrome is approximately five times higher for a male over age 40 than for a male in his 20s. This paternal age effect is usually attributed to the fact that the stem cells giving rise to sperm cells continue to divide throughout the life of males, allowing a progressive buildup of DNA replication errors to occur.

> **Mutation rates vary substantially in different parts of the genome. Large genes, because of their size, are generally more likely to experience mutations than are small genes. Mutation hot spots, particularly in the form of CG dinucleotides, are also known to occur. For some single-gene disorders, there is a substantial increase in mutation risk with advanced paternal age.**

■ DETECTION AND MEASUREMENT OF GENETIC VARIATION

For centuries humans have been intrigued by the differences that can be seen among individuals. Attention was focused upon observable differences,

such as skin coloration and body shape and size. Only in this century has it been possible to examine variation in genes, the consequence of mutations accumulated through time. The evaluation and measurement of this variation in populations and families are important in mapping genes to specific locations on chromosomes, a key step in determining gene function (Chapter 7). The evaluation of genetic variation also provides the basis for much of genetic diagnosis, and it is highly useful in medical forensics. In this section we discuss several key approaches to detecting genetic variation in humans.

Blood Groups

Several dozen **blood group** systems have been defined on the basis of antigens located on the surfaces of erythrocytes. Some are involved in determining whether a given individual can receive a blood transfusion from a given donor. Because individuals differ extensively in terms of blood groups, these systems provided an important early means of assessing genetic variation.

Each of the blood group systems is determined by a different gene or set of genes. The various antigens that can be expressed within a system are the result of different DNA sequences in these genes. Two blood group systems that have special medical significance, the ABO and Rh systems, are discussed here.

ABO System

Human blood transfusions were carried out as early as 1818, but they were often unsuccessful. After transfusions some recipients would suffer a massive, sometimes fatal, hemolytic reaction. In 1900 Karl Landsteiner discovered that this reaction was due to the ABO antigens located on erythrocyte

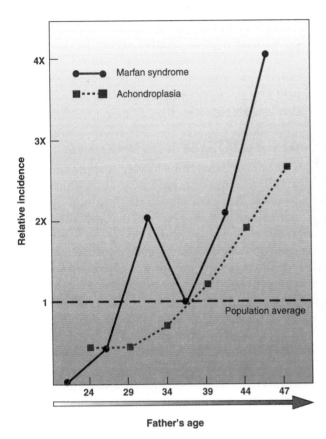

Figure 3-10 ▪ The risk of producing a child with the single-gene diseases achondroplasia and Marfan syndrome (Y-axis) increases with the father's age (X-axis). (From Vogel and Rathenberg, Adv Hum Genet 5:223-318, 1975.)

surfaces. The ABO system consists of two major antigens, labeled A and B. Individuals can have one of four blood types: blood type A individuals carry the A antigen on their erythrocytes, type B individuals carry the B antigen, type AB individuals carry both A and B, and type O individuals carry neither antigen. A person who has one of these antigens on their red blood cell surfaces will have antibodies that react against any other antigens. Thus a person with type A blood has anti-B antibodies, and transfusing type B blood into this individual would provoke a severe antibody reaction. It is straightforward to determine ABO blood type in the laboratory by mixing a small sample of a person's blood with solutions containing different antibodies and then observing which combinations cause the clumping characteristic of an antibody–antigen interaction.

The ABO system, which is encoded by a single gene on chromosome 9, consists of three primary alleles, labeled I^A, I^B, and I^O. In addition, there are subtypes of both the I^A and I^B alleles, but they are not addressed here. Individuals who have the I^A allele have the A antigen on their erythrocyte surfaces (blood type A), whereas those with I^B have the B antigen on their cell surfaces (blood type B). Those with both alleles express both antigens (blood type AB), and those having only two copies of the I^O allele have neither antigen (type O blood). Because the I^O allele produces no antigen, those who are I^AI^O or I^BI^O heterozygotes have blood types A and B, respectively (Table 3-2).

Because populations vary substantially in terms of the frequency with which the *ABO* alleles occur, the *ABO* locus was the first blood group system used extensively in studies of genetic variation among individuals. For example, early studies showed that the A antigen is relatively common in western European populations, and the B antigen is especially common among Asians. Neither antigen is common among Native South American populations, the great majority of whom have blood type O.

Rh System

Like the ABO system, the Rh system is defined on the basis of antigens that are present on erythrocyte surfaces. This system is named after the Rhesus monkey, the experimental animal in which it was first isolated by Landsteiner in the late 1930s. It is typed in the laboratory using a procedure similar to the one described for the ABO system. The Rh system varies considerably among individuals and populations and thus has been another highly useful tool for assessing genetic variation. Recently, the molecular basis of variation in both the ABO system, encoded on chromosome 9, and the Rh system, encoded on chromosome 1, has been elucidated (for further details, see the additional readings at the end of this chapter).

The ABO and Rh systems are both of key importance in determining the compatibility of blood transfusions and tissue grafts. Certain combinations of these systems can produce maternal–fetal incompatibility, sometimes with serious results for the fetus. These issues are discussed in detail in Chapter 9.

Table 3-2 ▪ The relationship between ABO genotype and blood type

Genotype	Blood type	Antibodies present
I^AI^A	A	Anti-B
I^AI^O	A	Anti-B
I^BI^B	B	Anti-A
I^BI^O	B	Anti-A
I^AI^B	AB	None
I^OI^O	O	Anti-A and anti-B

The blood groups, of which the ABO and Rh systems are examples, have provided an important means of studying human genetic variation. Blood group variation is the result of antigens that occur on the surfaces of erythrocytes.

Protein Electrophoresis

Although the blood group systems have been a useful means of measuring genetic variation, their number is limited. **Protein electrophoresis**, developed first in the 1930s and applied widely to humans in the 1950s and 1960s, increased the number of detectable polymorphic systems considerably. This technique makes use of the fact that a single amino acid difference in a protein (the result of a mutation in the corresponding DNA sequence) can cause a slight difference in the electrical charge of the protein. An example is the common sickle cell disease mutation discussed earlier. The replacement of glutamic acid with valine in the β-globin chain produces a difference in electrical charge because glutamic acid has two carboxyl groups, whereas valine has only one carboxyl group.

Electrophoresis can be used to determine whether an individual has normal hemoglobin (HbA) or the mutation that causes sickle cell disease (HbS). The hemoglobin is placed in an electrically charged gel composed of starch, agarose, or polyacrylamide (Fig. 3-11, *A*). The slight difference in charge resulting from the amino acid difference will cause the HbA and HbS forms to migrate at different rates through the gel. After allowing the protein molecules to migrate through the gel for several hours, they can be stained with chemical solutions so that their positions can be seen (Fig. 3-11, *B*). It can then be determined whether an individual is an HbA homozygote, an HbS homozygote, or a heterozygote having HbA on one chromosome and HbS on the other.

Protein electrophoresis has been used to detect amino acid variation in hundreds of human proteins. However, silent substitutions, which do not alter amino acids, cannot be detected using this approach. In addition, some amino acid substitutions do not alter the electrical charge of the protein molecule. Thus it is estimated that protein electrophoresis detects only about one third of mutations occurring in coding DNA. Single-base substitutions in noncoding DNA are not usually detected by protein electrophoresis.

Protein electrophoresis detects variation in genes that encode certain serum proteins. This variation is observable because proteins with slight variations in their amino acid sequence will migrate at different rates through electrically charged gels.

Detection of Variation at the DNA Level

It is estimated that humans vary at approximately 1 in 300 bp. Thus approximately 10 million polymorphisms may exist among the 3 billion bp that compose the human genome. Because there are only about 100 blood group and protein electrophoretic polymorphisms, these approaches have detected only a tiny proportion of our DNA variation. Yet the assessment of this variation is critical to gene mapping and genetic diagnosis, as shown in Chapters 7 and 11. Fortunately new molecular techniques have evolved during the past 15 years that have enabled the detection of thousands of new polymorphisms at the DNA level. These techniques, which have revolutionized both the practice and the potential of medical genetics, are discussed next.

Restriction Fragment Length Polymorphisms (RFLPs)

The earliest major approach to detecting genetic variation at the DNA level took advantage of the existence of bacterial enzymes known as **restriction endonucleases**, or **restriction enzymes**. These enzymes are produced by various bacteria species to "restrict" the entry of foreign DNA into the bacterium by cutting, or cleaving, the DNA at specific recognized sequences. These sequences are referred to as **restriction sites**, or **recognition sites**. For example, the intestinal bacterium, *Escherichia coli,* produces a restriction enzyme, *Eco*RI, which recognizes the DNA sequence GAATTC. Each time this sequence is encountered, the enzyme cleaves the sequence between the G and the A. This produces DNA **restriction fragments**.

Imagine a region of DNA that is several thousand bases in length and includes three recognition sites for *Eco*RI. Suppose that a polymorphism exists within the middle restriction site (e.g., some individuals might have the sequence GAATTT instead of the GAATTC sequence recognized by *Eco*RI). The enzyme will not cleave the GAATTT sequence, although it will cleave the normal restriction sites that are located on either side of the polymorphic sequence. This specific DNA fragment will be longer in the individual who lacks the restriction site

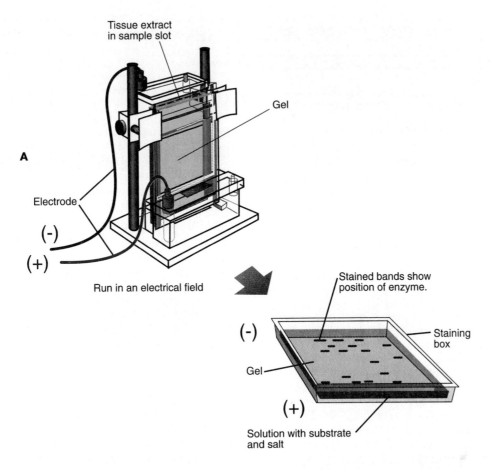

Tissue extract
in sample slot

Gel

A

Electrode

(-)

(+)

Run in an electrical field

Stained bands show
position of enzyme.

(-)

Staining
box

Gel

(+)

Solution with substrate
and salt

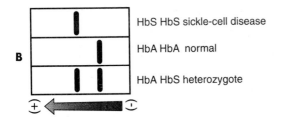

HbS HbS sickle-cell disease

HbA HbA normal

HbA HbS heterozygote

B

Figure 3-11 ■ **The process of protein electrophoresis. A, A tissue sample is loaded in the slot at the top of the gel, and an electrical current is run though the gel. After staining, distinct bands, representing molecules with different electrical charges and thus different amino acid sequences, are visible. HbA homozygotes show a single band closer to the negative pole, whereas HbS homozygotes show a single band closer to the positive pole (B). Heterozygotes, having both alleles, show two bands.**

than in the individual who has it (Fig. 3-12). If these differing lengths could be visualized directly, it would be possible to observe DNA sequence differences among individuals (i.e., DNA polymorphism).

A series of steps has been devised that permits this visualization (Fig. 3-13). First, DNA is extracted from a tissue sample, usually blood. Then the DNA is exposed to a restriction enzyme such as *Eco*RI. This process is termed a **restriction digest**. The digest produces more than 1 million DNA fragments. To assess length variation, these fragments are subjected to gel electrophoresis. This procedure is similar to the protein electrophoresis described above, except that the DNA fragments migrate down the gel according to size rather than electrical charge. The smaller fragments migrate more quickly than the larger ones. The DNA is denatured (i.e., converted from double-stranded to single-stranded form) by exposing it to alkaline chemical solutions. To fix the positions of the DNA fragments permanently, they are transferred from the gel to a solid membrane, such as nitrocellulose (this is termed a **Southern transfer**, after the man who invented the process in the mid-1970s). At this point, the solid membrane, often called a

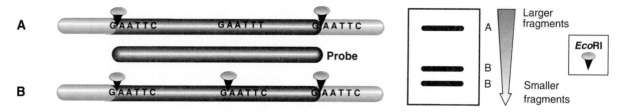

Figure 3-12 ■ Cleavage of DNA by the *EcoRI* restriction enzyme. The enzyme cleaves the 3 GAATTC recognition sequences in B, producing two smaller fragments. In A, the middle sequence is GAATTT instead of GAATTC, so it cannot be cleaved by the enzyme. The result is a single, longer fragment.

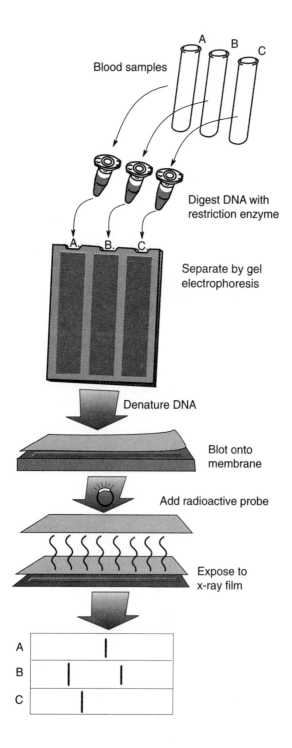

Figure 3-13 ■ The RFLP process. DNA is extracted from blood samples from subjects A, B, and C, digested by a restriction enzyme, and loaded on a gel. Electrophoresis separates the DNA fragments according to their size. The DNA is denatured and transferred to a solid membrane, where it is hybridized with a radioactive probe. Exposure to x-ray film (autoradiography) reveals specific DNA fragments (bands) of different sizes in individuals A, B, and C.

''Southern blot,'' contains many thousands of fragments arrayed according to their size. If one looked at all of these fragments at once, it would be impossible to distinguish one from another because of their large number. How do we pick out specific DNA fragments?

Here it is possible to exploit the principle of complementary DNA base pairing. A **probe** is constructed using recombinant DNA techniques (see Box 3-1; pg. 46). This probe consists of a small piece of single-stranded human DNA (a few kilobases in length) that has been inserted into a vector, such as a phage, plasmid, or cosmid. The probe is labeled typically with a radioactive isotope. The blot is exposed to thousands of copies of the labeled probe, which under proper conditions will then undergo complementary base pairing with the appropriate single-stranded DNA fragments on the blot. Because it is only a few kilobases in size, the probe identifies a specific portion of the DNA, usually just one or two fragments. To visualize the position of the hybridized probe, the blot is exposed to x-ray film, which darkens at the probe's position due to the emission of radioactive particles from the labeled probe. These darkened positions are usually referred to as ''bands,'' and the film is termed an **autoradiogram** (Fig. 3-14).

Having thought through this sequence of steps, the RFLP should now be self-explanatory. These are *polymorphisms* revealed by variation in the *lengths* of *restriction fragments*.

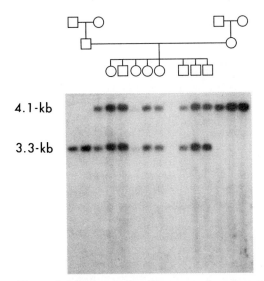

Figure 3-14■ An autoradiogram, showing the positions of a 4.1-kb band and a 3.3-kb band. Each lane represents DNA from a subject in the family shown above the autoradiogram.

4.1-kb

3.3-kb

RFLPs result from variations in DNA sequence at specific restriction sites. These produce variations in DNA fragment lengths, which are sorted by electrophoresis and visualized through the use of labeled probes.

The process can be illustrated using the example of sickle cell disease. As discussed, normal individuals have glutamic acid at position 6 of the β-globin polypeptide. This is encoded by the DNA sequence GAG. If the DNA sequence is instead GTG, valine is

substituted for glutamic acid. The restriction enzyme *Mst*II recognizes the DNA sequence CCTNAGG (the N signifies that the enzyme will recognize any DNA base in this position). Thus it cleaves the DNA sequence of the "normal" chromosome at this site, as well as at the restriction sites on either side of it (Fig. 3-15). This produces two fragments of DNA: one that is 1100 bp long and another that is only 200 bp long. In chromosomes with the valine substitution, *Mst*II can no longer recognize this particular site, so the DNA is not cleaved. The result is a longer DNA fragment, now 1300 bp in size instead of 1100. (The restriction sites flanking the site of interest do not vary, so they are always cut by the enzyme.) The shorter fragment will migrate further on a gel, so the two different sizes can easily be distinguished after hybridizing the blot with a probe containing DNA from the β-globin gene. In this case the RFLP approach permits direct detection of the mutation causing the disease.

There are several hundred known restriction enzymes, each of which recognizes a different DNA sequence; only about a dozen of these are ordinarily used when looking for new polymorphisms, however. In addition, thousands of different probes have been cloned, each representing a different small piece of the total human DNA sequence. By combining these different probes and enzymes, thousands of polymorphic sites have been revealed in human chromosomes. These polymorphisms have been instrumental in localizing many important disease genes, including cystic fibrosis, Huntington disease, and type 1 neurofibromatosis (see Chapter 7).

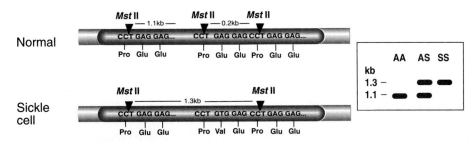

Figure 3-15■ Cleavage of β-globin DNA by the *Mst*II restriction enzyme. The sickle cell mutation removes an MstII recognition site, producing a longer 1.3-kb fragment. The normal DNA sequence includes the restriction site (i.e., CCTGAG becomes CCTGTG), so a shorter 1.1-kb fragment is produced. Sickle cell homozygotes thus have a single 1.3-kb band, whereas normal homozygotes have a single 1.1-kb band. Heterozygotes have both the 1.1-kb and 1.3-kb bands. Note that the banding pattern here, based on DNA sequence differences, resembles the banding pattern shown in Fig. 3-11, which is based on amino acid sequence detected by protein electrophoresis.

Box 3-1. Genetic Engineering, Recombinant DNA, and Cloning

In the last two decades, most of the lay public has acquired at least a passing familiarity with the terms recombinant DNA, cloning, and genetic engineering. Indeed, these techniques lie at the heart of what is often called the "new genetics."

Genetic engineering refers to the laboratory alteration of genes. A number of various alterations can be made. Here we discuss one that is of special importance in medical genetics, the manufacturing of **clones**. Briefly, a clone is an identical copy of a DNA sequence. We outline one approach to the artificial cloning of human genes.

Our goal is to insert human DNA into a rapidly reproducing organism so that copies (clones) of the DNA can be made quickly. One system commonly used for this purpose is the **plasmid**, which is a small, circular, self-replicating piece of DNA that resides in many bacteria. Plasmids can be removed from bacteria or inserted into them without seriously disrupting bacterial growth or reproduction.

To insert human DNA into the plasmid, we need a way to cut DNA into pieces so that it can be manipulated. Restriction enzymes, discussed in the text, perform this function efficiently. The DNA sequence recognized by the restriction enzyme *Eco*RI, GAATTC, has the convenient property that its complementary sequence, CTTAAG, is the same sequence, except backwards. Such sequences are called **palindromes**. When plasmid or human DNA is cleaved with *Eco*RI, the DNA fragments have "sticky ends," as shown in Figure 3-16. This means that if we cut both human and plasmid DNA with this enzyme, both of them will have exposed ends that can undergo complementary base pairing with one another. Then, when the human and plasmid DNA are mixed together, they recombine

(hence the term **recombinant DNA**). The plasmids now contain human DNA **inserts**. They are then inserted back into bacteria, where they can reproduce rapidly through natural cell division. The human DNA sequence, which is reproduced along with the other plasmid DNA, is thus cloned.

The plasmid is referred to as a **vector**. Several other types of vectors may also be used as cloning vehicles. These include **bacteriophages** (viruses that infect bacteria), **cosmids** (a phage–plasmid hybrid that is capable of carrying relatively large DNA inserts), and **yeast artificial chromosomes** (vectors that are inserted into yeast cells and behave much like ordinary yeast chromosomes). Whereas plasmids and bacteriophages can accommodate only relatively small inserts (about 10 and 20 kb, respectively), cosmids can carry inserts of approximately 50 kb and yeast artificial chromosomes can carry inserts up to 1000 kb in length.

Cloning is typically used to create the thousands of copies of human DNA used in Southern blotting and other experimental applications. In addition, this approach is now being used to produce genetically engineered therapeutic products, such as insulin, interferon, human growth hormone, clotting factor VIII (used in the treatment of hemophilia A, a coagulation disorder), and tissue plasminogen activator (a blood clot-dissolving protein that helps to prevent heart attacks and strokes). When these genes are cloned into bacteria or other organisms, the organism produces the human gene product along with its own gene products. In the past these products were obtained from donor blood or from other animals. Obtaining and purifying them was slow and costly. Genetically engineered gene products are rapidly becoming a cheaper and more efficient alternative.

There are thousands of possible combinations of probes and restriction enzymes that can reveal polymorphism at the DNA level. Consequently, RFLPs have been a very useful system for studying genetic variation and diagnosing genetic disease.

Variable Number of Tandem Repeat Polymorphisms (VNTRs)

The approach just described usually detects the presence or absence of a restriction site; these polymorphisms are often termed **restriction site polymorphisms (RSPs)**. In this case a polymorphism has only two possible alleles, placing a limit on the amount of genetic diversity that can be seen. More diversity could be observed if a polymorphic

system had many alleles, rather than just two. A variation on the RFLP approach has provided just such a system. This particular variation exploits the **minisatellites** that exist throughout the genome. Recall from Chapter 2 that minisatellites are regions in which the same DNA sequence is repeated over and over again (in tandem). The genetic variation measured here is in the number of repeats in a region (hence the term **variable number of tandem repeats**, or **VNTRs**).

VNTRs are detected using an approach similar to that used for conventional RFLPs. DNA is digested with a restriction enzyme, and the fragments are electrophoresed, denatured, and transferred to a solid medium. The principal difference is that special probes are used that hybridize only to a given minisatellite region. Whereas RSPs reveal

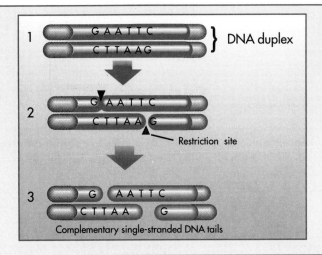

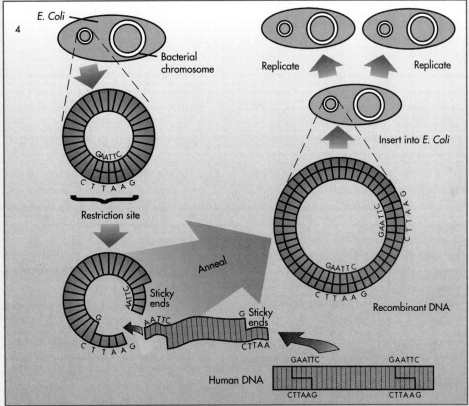

Figure 3-16 ■ Recombinant DNA technology. Human and circular plasmid DNA are both cleaved by a restriction enzyme, producing sticky ends (1-3). This allows the human DNA to anneal and recombine with the plasmid DNA. Inserted into the plasmid DNA, the human DNA is now replicated when the plasmid is inserted into a bacterium, such as *Escherichia coli* (4).

polymorphisms because of the presence or absence of a restriction site, VNTRs reveal polymorphisms because of different numbers of repeats located between two restriction sites (Fig. 3-17). The number of these repeats can vary considerably in populations: a minisatellite region could have as few as two or three repeats or as many as 20 or more. These polymorphisms can therefore reveal a high degree of genetic variation. This is especially useful

for mapping genes using the technique of linkage analysis, to be discussed in Chapter 7.

VNTRs are a form of RFLP that arise from variation in the numbers of tandem repeats in a DNA region. Because VNTR loci can have many different alleles, they are especially useful in medical genetic and other applications.

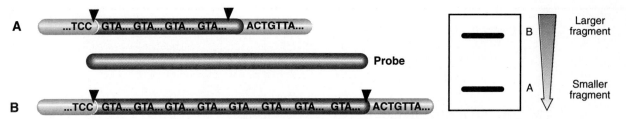

Figure 3-17 ■VNTR polymorphisms. Bands of differing lengths, A and B, are created by different numbers of tandem repeats in the DNA on two different chromosomes. Restriction sites are found on either side of the repeat region, and a radioactively labeled probe hybridizes to the DNA, allowing the different fragment lengths to be visualized on an autoradiogram.

Just as minisatellite regions can vary in length, microsatellites can also vary in length as a result of differing numbers of repeats (see Chapter 2). Each microsatellite repeat is substantially smaller than a minisatellite repeat (2, 3, or 4 bp in length). These are referred to as **dinucleotide, trinucleotide,** and **tetranucleotide repeats**, respectively. A given microsatellite repeat may occur in tandem as many as several hundred times, and this number varies considerably among individuals (and usually between the two homologous chromosomes of an individual). These **microsatellite repeat polymorphisms** differ from the VNTRs just discussed in terms of their size and also in that they are not defined by restriction sites that flank the repeat region. Instead, the polymerase chain reaction technique, discussed next, is used to isolate them. Like VNTRs, microsatellite repeat polymorphisms are highly useful for gene mapping. Both types of polymorphisms are also useful in forensic applications, such as paternity testing and the identification of criminal suspects (Box 3-2).

DNA Amplification Using the Polymerase Chain Reaction (PCR)

The RFLP and VNTR approaches, which typically depend on Southern blotting and cloning procedures, have been useful in many applications; however, they suffer from certain limitations. Cloning is time-consuming, often requiring a week or more of laboratory time. In addition, the standard Southern blotting approach requires relatively large amounts of purified DNA, usually several micrograms (up to 1 ml of fresh blood would be needed to produce this much DNA). A newer approach to making copies of DNA, the **polymerase chain reaction (PCR),** has made the detection of genetic variation at the DNA level much more efficient. Essentially PCR is an artificial means of replicating a short DNA sequence (several kilobases or less) quickly, so that millions of copies of the sequence are made.

The PCR process, summarized in Figure 3-19, on page 50, requires four components:
1. Two **primers**, consisting of 15 to 20 bases of DNA each. These small DNA sequences are termed **oligonucleotides**, oligo meaning "a few." The primers correspond to the DNA sequences immediately adjacent to the sequence of interest (e.g., this sequence may contain a mutation that causes disease or it could contain a microsatellite repeat polymorphism). These oligonucleotide primers are usually synthesized using a laboratory instrument.
2. DNA polymerase. This enzyme, usually derived from the bacterium *Thermus aquaticus,* performs the vital process of DNA replication (here termed **primer extension**).
3. A large number of free DNA bases.
4. Genomic DNA from an individual. Because of the extreme sensitivity of PCR, the quantity of this DNA can be very small.

The genomic DNA is first heated to a relatively high temperature (approximately 95° C) so that it denatures and becomes single-stranded. This DNA is then exposed to large quantities of primers, which hybridize, or anneal, to the appropriate complementary bases in the genomic DNA as it is cooled to an annealing temperature of approximately 35 to 65° C. The DNA is then heated to an intermediate temperature (70 to 75° C). In the presence of a large number of free DNA bases, a new DNA strand is synthesized by the DNA polymerase at this temperature, extending from the primer sequence. The newly synthesized DNA consists of a double strand that has the 5′ end of the primer at one end, followed by the bases added through primer extension by DNA polymerase. The double-stranded DNA is then heated to a high temperature again, causing it to denature. The heating–cooling cycle is then repeated. Now the newly synthesized DNA serves as the template for synthesis. As the cooling–heating cycles are

Box 3-2. DNA Fingerprints

Because of the large number of polymorphisms observed in the human, it is virtually certain that each of us is genetically unique (with the exception of identical twins). It follows that genetic variation could be used to identify individuals, much as a conventional fingerprint does. Since DNA can be found in any tissue sample, including blood, semen, and even hair, genetic variation could have substantial potential in forensic applications (criminal cases, paternity suits, identification of accident victims, and so forth). VNTR and microsatellite repeat polymorphisms, with their many alleles, are useful in this regard. Because of their potential for precise individual identification, they have come to be known as **DNA fingerprints**.

The principle underlying a DNA fingerprint is simple. If we examine enough polymorphisms in a given individual, the probability that any other individual in the population would have the same alleles at every locus becomes extremely small. DNA left at the scene of a crime in the form of blood or hair, for example, can be typed for a series of VNTRs and/or microsatellite polymorphisms. Because of the extreme sensitivity of the PCR approach, even a tiny, several-year-old sample can yield enough DNA for laboratory analysis. These alleles are then compared with the alleles of a suspect (Fig. 3-18). If the alleles in the two samples match, then the suspect is implicated.

A key question arising in this context is whether another person in the general population might have the same alleles as the suspect. Could the DNA fingerprint then falsely implicate the wrong person? In criminal cases the probability of obtaining an allele match with a random member of the population is calculated. Because of the high degree of allelic variation in VNTRs and microsatellite polymorphisms, these probabilities are usually small. Some of the early estimates were as small as 10^{-19}. However, various considerations have led to more conservative probability estimates. Yet, provided that a large enough number of loci are used under well-controlled laboratory conditions and provided that the data are evaluated carefully, these DNA fingerprints can furnish highly useful forensic evidence.

Although we tend to think of such evidence in terms of identifying the guilty party, it should also be pointed out that when a match is not obtained, a suspect may be exonerated. It has been reported that, among approximately one third of the criminal cases in which DNA fingerprints were used, the suspect was freed because his or her DNA did not match that of the evidentiary sample. Thus DNA fingerprints can also benefit those who are falsely accused.

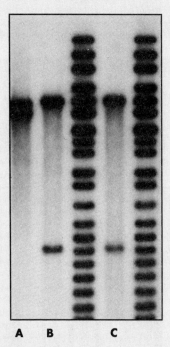

Figure 3-18 ■ DNA fingerprints. The autoradiogram shows that the band pattern of suspect A's DNA does not match the DNA taken from the crime scene (C), whereas the band pattern of suspect B's DNA does match. In practice, several such VNTR systems are assayed to reduce the possibility of a false match. (Courtesy of Jay Henry, Criminalistics Laboratory, Department of Public Safety, State of Utah.)

repeated, the primer-bounded DNA products are amplified geometrically: the number of copies doubles in each cycle (i.e., 2, 4, 8, 16, and so on). This is why the process is termed a "chain reaction." Typically, the cycles are repeated 20 to 30 times, producing millions of copies of the original DNA. In summary, the PCR process consists of three basic steps: DNA denaturing at high temperature, primer hybridization at a low temperature, and primer extension at an intermediate temperature.

Since each heating–cooling cycle requires only a few minutes, a single molecule of DNA can be amplified to make millions of copies in only a few hours. Because the procedure is simple and entirely self-contained, inexpensive machines have been developed to automate it completely. Once the DNA is amplified, it can be analyzed in a variety of ways.

PCR has a number of advantages over older techniques. First, it can be used with extremely small quantities of DNA (nanogram or even picogram amounts, as opposed to the micrograms required for cloning). The amount of DNA in a several-year-old blood stain, or even in a single

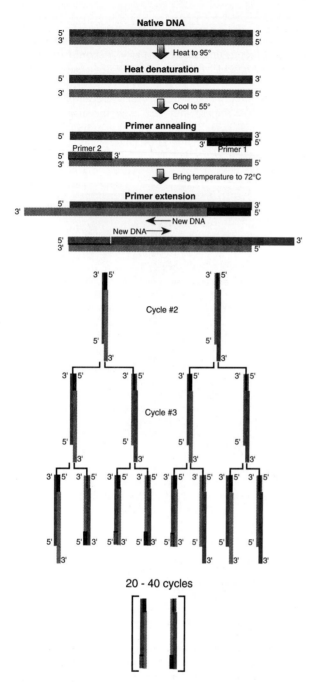

Figure 3-19 ■ **The PCR process. Genomic DNA is first heated and denatured to form single strands. In the annealing phase, the DNA is cooled, allowing hybridization with primer sequences that flank the region of interest. Then the reaction is heated to an intermediate primer extension temperature, in which DNA polymerase adds free bases in the 3′ direction along each single strand, starting at the primer. Blunt-ended DNA fragments are formed, and these provide a template for the next cycle of heating and cooling. Repeated cycling produces a large number of DNA fragments bounded on each end by the primer sequence.**

hair, is often sufficient for analysis. Second, because it does not require gene cloning, the procedure is much faster than older techniques. The genetic diagnosis of sickle cell disease, which required a week or more using older techniques, can be done in a single day with PCR. Finally, because PCR can make large quantities of very pure DNA, it is not usually necessary to use radioactive probes to detect specific DNA sequences or mutations. Instead safer nonradioactive labeling substances, such as biotin, can be used.

PCR entails two primary disadvantages. First, primer synthesis obviously requires knowledge of the DNA sequence flanking the DNA of interest. When no sequence information is available, other techniques must be used. Second, the extreme sensitivity of PCR makes it susceptible to contamination in the laboratory. A number of precautions are commonly taken to guard against contamination.

Because PCR is such a powerful and versatile technique, it is now used extensively in genetic disease diagnosis, forensic medicine, and evolutionary genetics. It has supplanted the Southern blotting technique in many applications and is now sometimes used to generate RFLPs and VNTRs.

PCR provides a convenient and efficient means of making millions of copies of a short DNA sequence. Heating–cooling cycles are used to denature DNA and then build new copies of a specific, primer-bounded sequence. Because of its speed and ease of use, this technique is now widely used for assessing genetic variation, diagnosing genetic diseases, and for forensic purposes.

DNA Sequencing

In many genetic studies a primary goal is to determine the actual array of DNA bases that composes a gene or part of a gene. This **DNA sequence** can indicate a great deal about the nature of a specific mutation, the function of a gene, and the gene's degree of similarity to other known genes. We discuss one technique that is widely used to determine DNA sequences.

The **dideoxy method** of DNA sequencing, invented by Frederick Sanger, makes use of chain-terminating dideoxynucleotides. These are chemically similar to ordinary deoxynucleotides, except that they are missing one hydroxyl group. This prevents the subsequent formation of phospho-diester bonds with free DNA bases. Thus, although dideoxynucleotides can be incorporated into a growing DNA helix, no additional nucleotides can be added once they are included. There are four different dideoxynucleotides, each one corresponding to one of the four nucleotides (A, C, G, and T). The single-stranded DNA whose sequence we wish to determine is mixed with radioactively labeled primers, DNA polymerase, ordinary nucleotides, and one type of dideoxynucleotide (Fig. 3-20). The primer hybridizes to the appropriate

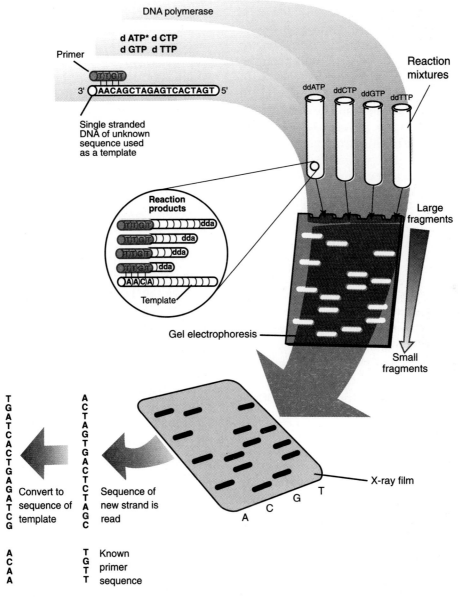

Figure 3-20 ■DNA sequencing using the dideoxy method. The labeled primer is added to the single-stranded DNA, the sequence of which is unknown. DNA polymerase adds free bases to the single strand, using complementary base pairing. Four different reactions are carried out, corresponding to the four different dideoxynucleotides (ddATP, ddCTP, ddGTP, and ddTTP). These terminate the DNA sequence whenever they are incorporated instead of the normal deoxynucleotide (dATP, dCTP, dGTP, and dTTP, corresponding to the bases A, C, G, and T, respectively). This produces fragments of varying length, which can be separated by electrophoresis. The position of each fragment is indicated by the emission of radioactive particles from the label. This then allows the DNA sequence to be read directly.

complementary position in the single-stranded DNA, and DNA polymerase adds free bases to the growing DNA molecule, as in the PCR process. The dideoxynucleotides are incorporated into the chain just as a corresponding nucleotide is. However, once the dideoxynucleotide is incorporated, the chain is terminated. At any given position, either an ordinary nucleotide or the corresponding dideoxynucleotide may be added; this is a random process. This procedure thus yields DNA fragments of varying lengths, each ending with the same dideoxynucleotide. The DNA fragments can be separated according to length by electrophoresis, as discussed previously. Four different sequencing reactions are run, one for each base. The fragments obtained from each reaction are electrophoresed side by side on the same gel, so that the position of each fragment can be compared. Because each band corresponds to a DNA chain terminating with a unique base, the DNA sequence can be read by observing the order of the bands on the gel after autoradiography (the radioactive primer indicates the position of the fragment on the film). Several hundred base pairs can usually be sequenced in one reaction series.

DNA sequencing is commonly accomplished using the dideoxy method. This method depends on the fact that dideoxynucleotides behave in a fashion similar to ordinary deoxynucleotides, except that, once incorporated into the DNA chain, they terminate it. They thus mark the positions of specific bases.

It should be apparent that sequencing DNA in this way is a relatively slow, laborious, and error-prone process. Using computers and other instruments, DNA sequencing is becoming much more rapid and efficient. Eventually it will permit the sequencing of the entire 3 billion-base human genome.

Detection of Mutation at the DNA Level

The detection of mutations in DNA sequences is often a critical step in understanding how a gene causes a specific disease. The molecular methods developed during the past decade have spawned a number of new techniques for detecting mutation at the DNA level. The Southern blotting approach permits the detection of relatively large deletions.

Those smaller than 50 bp cannot be seen on Southern blots because of the limited resolution of this technique. Mutations that alter a restriction site can also be recognized using the Southern blotting approach, but most mutations do not occur at known restriction sites. After using PCR to amplify a specific region of DNA, it can be sequenced directly using the technique described above. Mutations are then detected by comparing the DNA sequence of a patient with that of an unaffected individual.

Although direct sequencing is a useful and accurate means of detecting mutations, it can be time-consuming. Other techniques provide a more rapid approach to surveying large numbers of patients for mutations. These techniques can indicate the existence and location of a mutation, after which the DNA in the indicated region can be sequenced.

Two approaches to be mentioned here make use of the fact that under certain conditions mutations alter the mobility of denatured DNA in gel electrophoresis. **Denaturing gradient gel electrophoresis (DGGE)** employs a gel in which there is an increasing gradient of a denaturing factor, such as temperature. **Single-strand conformation polymorphism (SSCP)** analysis makes use of the fact that the secondary structure of a DNA segment can be altered by a mutation in DNA sequence. This will change the rate of migration of a single-stranded DNA segment in a nondenaturing gel. Using either of these two techniques, sequence differences between a patient's DNA and that of a normal control can be identified. Once a difference is detected, the patient's DNA can be sequenced to determine the precise nature of the mutation. Tests for specific mutations, an important aspect of genetic diagnosis, are discussed further in Chapter 11.

Many techniques can be used to detect mutations at the DNA sequence level. These include Southern blotting, direct DNA sequencing, and electrophoretic techniques, such as denaturing gradient gel electrophoresis and single-strand conformation polymorphism analysis. The detection and characterization of mutations at disease loci are of fundamental importance in understanding the genetic basis of disease.

Box 3-3. The Causes of Genetic Variation

Although mutation is the ultimate source of genetic variation, it cannot alone account for the substantial differences in the incidence of many genetic diseases among different ethnic groups. Why, for example, is sickle cell disease seen in approximately 1 in 600 African-Americans but almost never in northern Europeans? Why is cystic fibrosis 40 times more common in whites than in Asians? Although mutation is the process that introduces diseases into populations, several evolutionary factors determine how common the disease genes become in a population. These include natural selection, genetic drift, and gene flow. These forces change **gene frequencies** in populations (gene frequencies are defined as the proportion of chromosomes having a specific allele; this is discussed further in Chapter 4).

Natural selection is often described as the "editor" of genetic variation. It increases the population frequency of favorable mutations (i.e., those who carry the mutation will produce more surviving offspring), and it decreases the frequency of genes that are unfavorable in a given environment (gene carriers produce fewer surviving offspring). Typically, disease mutations are continually introduced into a population through the error processes described above, while natural selection removes the mutations. Certain environments, however, may result in a selective advantage for a disease mutation. We can turn again to sickle cell disease for an example. As discussed, those who are homozygotes for the sickle cell mutation are much more likely to die early. Heterozygotes ordinarily have no particular advantage or disadvantage. However, it has been shown that sickle cell hetero-

zygotes have a distinct survival advantage in environments in which the *Plasmodium falciparum* malaria is common (as in west-central Africa) (Fig. 3-21). This is because the malaria parasite does not survive well in the erythrocytes of sickle cell heterozygotes. Thus, heterozygotes are less likely to succumb to malaria than are the normal homozygotes. This confers a selective advantage on the sickle cell gene in this environment. Whereas there is selection *against* the gene in sickle cell homozygotes, there is selection *for* the gene in heterozygotes. The result is that the disease gene persists at a relatively high frequency in African populations. In nonmalarial environments (such as northern Europe), the gene has no advantage, so natural selection acts strongly against it. This example illustrates the concept that variation in genetic disease incidence among populations can be caused by natural selection operating differentially in different environments.

Genetic drift is another force that can cause disease genes to vary in frequency among populations. To understand the process of genetic drift, consider a coin-tossing exercise in which 10 coins are tossed. Because heads and tails are equally likely, the expected number of heads and tails in this exercise would be 5 each. However, it is intuitively clear that, by chance, we could observe a substantial departure from this expectation. We would not be surprised to see seven heads and three tails, for example. If, however, we tossed 1000 coins, the degree of departure from the expected proportion of 50% heads and 50% tails is much smaller. A reasonable outcome might be 470 heads and 530 tails, but it would be unlikely to obtain 700 heads and 300 tails. Thus, we see less random fluctuation in larger samples. The

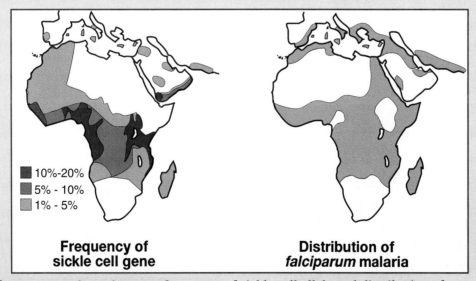

■ 10%-20%
■ 5% - 10%
■ 1% - 5%

Frequency of sickle cell gene

Distribution of *falciparum* malaria

Figure 3-21 ■ Correspondence between frequency of sickle cell allele and distribution of *Falciparum* malaria.

Continued

Box 3-3. The Causes of Genetic Variation—*cont'd*

same principle applies to gene frequencies in populations. In a very small population, a gene frequency can deviate substantially from one generation to the next, but this is unlikely in a large population. Thus, genetic drift is greater in smaller populations. This means that genetic diseases that are otherwise uncommon may be seen fairly frequently in a small population. For example, the Ellis-van Creveld syndrome (*SOL* 51), a rare disorder that involves reduced stature, polydactyly (extra fingers), and congenital heart disease, is seen with greatly elevated frequency among the Old Order Amish population of Pennsylvania. The Amish population was founded in the United States by only about 50 couples. There was thus great potential for genetic drift, resulting in the elevation of certain disease gene frequencies. It is common to observe the effect of genetic drift in small, isolated populations throughout the world.

Gene flow occurs when populations exchange migrants who mate with one another. Through time, gene flow between populations tends to make them genetically more similar to one another. One reason why sickle cell disease is less common among African-Americans than among many African populations is because of gene flow with whites in North America. In addition, because falciparum malaria is not found in North America, the African-American population does not experience selection in favor of the sickle cell mutation.

The forces of mutation, natural selection, genetic drift, and gene flow interact in complex and sometimes unexpected ways to influence the distribution and prevalence of genetic diseases in populations. The study of the ways in which these processes influence genetic evolution is referred to as **population genetics**.

■ STUDY QUESTIONS

1. In the following amino acid sequences, the normal sequence is given first, followed by sequences that are produced by different types of mutations. Identify the type of mutation most likely to cause each altered amino acid sequence:
   Normal, Phe-Asn-Pro-Thr-Arg;
   Mutation 1, Phe-Asn-Pro;
   Mutation 2, Phe-Asn-Ala-His-Thr;
   Mutation 3, Phe-His-Pro-Thr-Arg
2. Missense and transcription (promoter and enhancer) mutations often tend to produce milder disease conditions than do frameshift, donor–acceptor site, and nonsense mutations. Using the globin genes as examples, explain why this is so.
3. Individuals who have mutations that lower their production of both α-globin and β-globin often present with milder disease symptoms than do

those who have mutations lowering only the production of one type of chain. Why?
4. Outline the major differences between restriction site polymorphisms, VNTRs, and microsatellite repeat polymorphisms. Which of these three types of polymorphisms is represented in the accompanying autoradiogram?
5. α_1-Antitrypsin deficiency is a disease that arises when both copies of the α_1-antitrypsin gene are altered by a mutation. Chronic emphysema and pulmonary failure can result. One of the mutations that causes α_1-antitrypsin deficiency occurs in exon 3 of the gene and destroys a recognition site for the restriction enzyme *Bst*EII. RFLP analysis was performed on three members of a family, producing the accompanying autoradiogram. Determine the disease status of each individual.

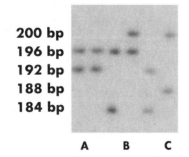

Figure 3-22 ■ Autoradiogram for study question 4.

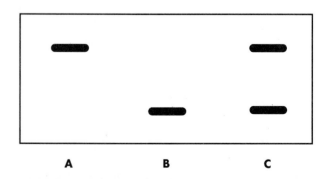

Figure 3-23 ■ Autoradiogram for study question 5.

■ ADDITIONAL READING

Armour JA and Jeffreys AJ: Biology and applications of human minisatellite loci, Curr Opin Genet Dev 2:850–856, 1992.

Clark SJ, Harrison J, Frommer M: CpNpG methylation in mammalian cells. Nature Genet 10:20–27, 1995.

Cooper DN, Krawczak M: Human gene mutation. Oxford, 1993, Bios Scientific.

Cooper DN, Krawczak M, Antonarakis SE: The nature and mechanisms of human mutation. In Scriver CR, Beaudet AL, Sly WS, and Valle D, editors: The Metabolic and Molecular Bases of Inherited Disease ed. 7, New York, 1995, McGraw-Hill.

Crossley M and Orkin SH: Regulation of the β-globin locus, Curr Opin Genet Dev 3:232–237, 1993.

Erlich HA and Arnheim N: Genetic analysis using the polymerase chain reaction, Annu Rev Genet 26:479–506, 1992.

Hearne CM, Ghosh S, and Todd JA: Microsatellites for linkage analysis of genetic traits, Trends Genet 8:288–294, 1992.

Housman D: Human DNA polymorphism, N Eng J Med 332:318–320, 1995.

Jorde LB: Population specific genetic markers and disease. In R. A. Meyers, editor: Molecular biology and biotechnology, New York, VCH Publishers 1995.

Krontiris TG: Minisatellites and human disease, Science 269:1682–1683, 1995.

Lukens JN: The thalassemias and related disorders: quantitative disorders of hemoglobin synthesis. In Lee GR, Bithell TC, Foerster J, Athens JW, and Lukens JN, editors: Wintrobe's clinical hematology, ed 9, Philadelphia, 1993, Lea & Febiger.

Mouro I, Colin Y, Chérif-Zahar B, Cartron J, and Le Van Kim C: Molecular genetic basis of the human Rhesus blood group system, Nature Genet 5:62–65, 1993.

Mullis KB, Ferré F, Gibbs RA: PCR—the polymerase chain reaction, 1994, Birkhauser Verlag AG.

Neel JV: Update on the genetic effects of ionizing radiation, JAMA 266:698–701, 1991.

Neel JV: New approaches to evaluating the genetic effects of the atomic bombs, Am J Hum Genet 57:1263–1266, 1995.

Risch N, Reich EW, Wishnick MM, and McCarthy JG: Spontaneous mutation and parental age in humans, Am J Hum Genet 41:218–248, 1987.

Rosenthal N: Tools of the trade—recombinant DNA, N Eng J Med 331:315–317, 1994.

Rosenthal N: Fine structure of a gene—DNA sequencing, N Eng J Med 332:589–591, 1995.

Sankaranarayanan K: Ionizing radiation, genetic risk estimation and molecular biology: impact and inferences, Trends Genet 9:79–84, 1993.

Schwartz RS: Jumping genes, N Eng J Med 332:941–944, 1995

Vogel F: Mutation in man. In Emery AEH and Rimoin DL, editors: Principles and practice of medical genetics, vol. 1, ed 2, Edinburgh, 1990, Churchill Livingstone.

Weatherall DJ, Clegg JB, Higgs DR, and Wood WG: The hemoglobinopathies. In Scriver CR, Beaudet AL, Sly WS, and Valle D, editors: The metabolic basis of inherited disease, ed 7, New York, 1995, McGraw-Hill.

Yamamoto F, Clausen H, White T, Marken J, and Hakomori S: Molecular genetic basis of the histo-blood group ABO system, Nature 345:229–233, 1990.

4 Autosomal Dominant and Recessive Inheritance

Many important and well-understood genetic diseases are the result of a mutation at a single gene. The 1994 edition of McKusick's *Mendelian Inheritance in Man* lists 6678 known **single-gene** or **monogenic** traits defined thus far in the human. Of these, 6188 are located on autosomes, and 412 are located on the X chromosome. Single-gene traits are the focus of much of the rapid progress now being made in medical genetics. In many cases these genes have been mapped to specific chromosome locations, cloned, and sequenced. This leads to new and exciting insights not only in genetics but also in the basic pathophysiology of disease.

In this chapter we focus on single-gene disorders caused by mutations on the autosomes. Single-gene disorders caused by mutations on the sex chromosomes are the subject of Chapter 5. We discuss the patterns of inheritance of these diseases in families, as well as factors that complicate these patterns. When appropriate, the molecular basis for genetic disease processes is addressed. We also discuss the risks of transmitting single-gene diseases to one's offspring, since this is usually an important concern for at-risk couples.

■ BASIC CONCEPTS OF FORMAL GENETICS

Gregor Mendel's Contributions

Monogenic traits are also known as **mendelian** traits, after Gregor Mendel, a nineteenth century Austrian monk who deduced several important genetic principles from his well-designed experiments with garden peas. Mendel studied seven traits in the pea, each of which is determined by a single gene. These traits included attributes such as height (tall plants vs. short plants) and seed shape (rounded vs. wrinkled). The variation in each of these traits is caused by different alleles at individual loci.

Two central principles emerged from Mendel's work. The first is the **principle of segregation**, which states that sexually reproducing organisms possess genes that occur in pairs and that only one member of this pair is transmitted to the offspring (i.e., it segregates). The prevalent thinking during Mendel's time was that hereditary factors from the two parents are "blended" in the offspring. In contrast, the principle of segregation states that genes remain intact and distinct. An allele for "rounded" seed shape can be transmitted to an offspring who can, in turn, transmit the same allele to its own offspring. If, instead of remaining distinct, genes were somehow blended in offspring, it would be impossible to trace genetic inheritance from one generation to the next. Thus the principle of segregation was a key development in modern genetics.

Mendel's **principle of independent assortment** is his second great contribution to genetics. This principle states that genes at different loci are transmitted independently. Consider the two loci mentioned above. One locus can have either the "rounded" or "wrinkled" allele, and the other can have either the "tall" or the "short" allele. In a reproductive event a parent will transmit one allele from each locus to its offspring. The principle of independent assortment dictates that the allele transmitted at one locus ("rounded" or "wrinkled") has no effect on which allele is transmitted at the other locus ("tall" or "short").

Mendel's experiments also showed that the effects of one allele may mask those of another. He performed **crosses** (matings) between pea plants homozygous for the "tall" gene (i.e., they had two identical copies of an allele we label *H*) and plants homozygous for the "short" gene (having two copies of an allele labeled *h*). This cross, which can only produce heterozygous *(Hh)* offspring, is illustrated in the **Punnett square** shown in Figure 4-1.

Parent

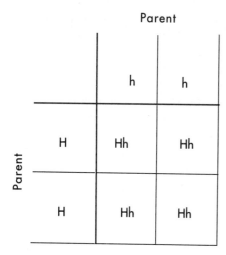

Figure 4-1 ■ **Punnett square illustrating a cross between HH and hh homozygote parents.**

Parent

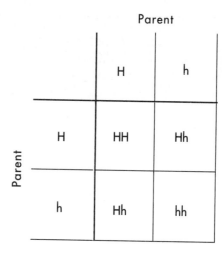

Figure 4-2 ■ **Punnett square illustrating a cross between two Hh heterozygotes.**

Mendel found that the offspring of these crosses, even though they were heterozygotes, were all tall. This reflects the fact that the *H* allele is **dominant**, whereas the *h* allele is **recessive** (it is conventional to label the dominant allele in upper case and the recessive allele in lower case). The term recessive comes from a Latin root meaning "to hide." This describes the behavior of recessive alleles well: in heterozygotes the consequences of a recessive allele are hidden. Whereas a dominant allele exerts its effect both in the homozygote *(HH)* and heterozygote *(Hh)*, the presence of the recessive allele is detected only when it occurs in homozygous form *(hh)*. Thus short pea plants could be created only by crossing parent plants that each carry at least one *h* allele. An example would be a heterozygote × heterozygote cross, shown in Figure 4-2.

The principle of segregation describes the behavior of chromosomes in meiosis. The genes on chromosomes segregate during meiosis, and they are transmitted as distinct entities from one generation to the next. When Mendel performed his critical experiments, he had no knowledge of chromosomes, meiosis, or genes (indeed, the latter term was not coined until 1909, long after Mendel's death). Although his work was published in 1865 and cited occasionally, its fundamental significance was unrecognized for several decades. Yet Mendel's research, which was eventually replicated by other researchers at the turn of the twentieth century, forms the foundation of much of modern genetics.

Mendel's key contributions were the principles of segregation and independent assortment, and his definition of dominance and recessiveness.

Basic Concepts of Probability

Risk assessment is an important part of medical genetics. For example, the physician or genetic counselor routinely informs couples of their risk of producing a child with a genetic disorder. To understand how such risks are estimated, some basic concepts of probability must be presented. A **probability** is defined as the proportion of times that a specific outcome occurs in a series of events. Thus we may speak of the probability of obtaining a 4 when a die is tossed, or the probability that a couple will produce a son versus a daughter. Because probabilities are proportions, they lie between zero and one, inclusive.

During meiosis, one member of a chromosome pair is transmitted to a given sperm or egg cell. The probability that one member of the pair is transmitted is 1/2, and the probability that the other member of the pair is transmitted is also 1/2 (note that for any given experiment the probabilities of all possible events must add to 1). Because this is directly analogous to coin tossing, in which the probabilities of obtaining heads or tails are each 1/2, we use coin tossing as our illustrative example.

When a coin is tossed repeatedly, the outcome of each toss has no effect on subsequent outcomes. The events are thus said to be **independent**. Even if we have obtained 10 heads in a row, the probability of obtaining heads or tails on the next toss remains 1/2. Similarly, the probability that a parent will transmit one of the two alleles at a locus is independent from one reproductive event to the next.

The independence principle allows us to deduce two fundamental concepts of probability: the **multiplication rule** and the **addition rule**. The multiplication rule states that if two trials are independent, then the probability of obtaining a given outcome in both trials is the product of the probabilities of each outcome. For example, we may wish to know the probability that an individual will obtain heads on both tosses of a fair coin. Because the tosses are independent events, this probability is given by the product of the probabilities of obtaining heads in each individual toss: $1/2 \times 1/2 = 1/4$. Similarly, the probability of obtaining two tails in a row is $1/2 \times 1/2 = 1/4$.

The multiplication rule can be extended for any number of trials. Suppose that a couple wants to know the probability that all three of their planned children will be girls. Because the probability of producing a girl is approximately 1/2 and because these are essentially independent events (although there may be rare exceptions), the probability of producing three girls is $1/2 \times 1/2 \times 1/2 = 1/8$. However, if the couple has already produced two girls and *then* wants to know the probability of producing a third girl, it is simply 1/2. This is because the previous two events are no longer probabilities; they have actually occurred. Because of independence, these events have no effect on the outcome of the third event.

The addition rule states that if we want to know the probability of either one outcome *or* another, we can simply add the respective probabilities together. For example, the probability of getting two heads in a row ($1/2 \times 1/2$, or $1/4$) *or* the probability of getting two tails in a row ($1/4$) is given by adding the two probabilities together: $1/4 + 1/4 = 1/2$. As another example, imagine that a couple plans to have three children, and they have a strong aversion to having three children all of the same sex. They can be reassured somewhat by knowing that the probability of producing three girls (1/8) or three boys (1/8) is only 1/4 ($1/8 + 1/8$). The probability that they will have some combination of boys and girls is thus 3/4 because the sum of the probabilities of all possible outcomes must add to 1.

> **Basic probability enables us to understand and estimate genetic risks. The multiplication rule is used to estimate the probability that two events will occur together. The addition rule is used to estimate the probability that one event or another occurs.**

Gene and Genotype Frequencies

The prevalence of many genetic diseases can vary considerably from one population to another. For example, cystic fibrosis (CF), a severe respiratory disorder (see Clinical Commentary 4-1), is common among whites, affecting approximately 1 in 2500 births. It is rare in Asian populations, affecting only 1 in 90,000 births. As discussed in Chapter 3, sickle cell disease is common among African-Americans, affecting approximately 1 in 600 births. Yet it is almost never seen among individuals of northern European descent. The concepts of **genotype frequency** and **gene frequency** help us to measure and understand population variation in disease genes.

Imagine that we have typed 200 individuals in a population for the MN blood group. This blood group, which is encoded by a locus on chromosome two, has two major alleles, labeled *M* and *N*. This is a system in which the effects of both alleles can be observed in the heterozygote. *M* and *N* are thus said to be **codominant**; the heterozygote can be distinguished from both homozygotes. Any individual in the population can have one of three possible genotypes (recall from Chapter 3 that the genotype is one's genetic makeup at a locus). The individual could be homozygous for *M* (genotype *MM*), heterozygous *(MN)*, or homozygous for *N (NN)*. After typing each person in our sample, we find the following distribution of genotypes: *MM,* 64; *MN,* 120; *NN* 16. Then the genotype frequency is obtained simply by dividing each genotype count by the total number of subjects. The frequency of *MM* is 64/200 (= 0.32), the frequency of *MN* is 120/200 (= 0.60), and the frequency of *NN* is 16/200 (= 0.08). The sum of these frequencies must, of course, equal one.

The gene frequency for each allele, *M* and *N*, can be obtained here by the process of **gene counting**. Each *MM* homozygote has two *M* alleles, whereas each heterozygote has one *M* allele. Similarly, *NN* homozygotes have two *N* alleles, and heterozygotes have one *N* allele. In the sample measured here, there are:

$$(64 \times 2) + 120 = 248 \ M \text{ genes}$$
$$(16 \times 2) + 120 = 152 \ N \text{ genes}$$

In total, there are 400 genes at the *MN* locus (i.e., twice the number of subjects, because each has two alleles). To obtain the frequency of *M,* we then take 248/400 = 0.62. The frequency of *N,* 152/400, is 0.38. The sum of the two frequencies must equal one.

Clinical Commentary 4-1. Cystic Fibrosis

Cystic fibrosis (CF) is one of the most common single-gene disorders in North America, affecting approximately 1 in 2500 white newborns (SOL 29, 30). It is less common in other ethnic groups. The prevalence among African-Americans is about 1 in 17,000, and it is seen in only 1 in 90,000 Asians. Approximately 30,000 Americans suffer from this disease.

CF was first identified as a distinct disease entity in 1938, and its earlier name was "cystic fibrosis of the pancreas." This refers to the fibrotic lesions that develop in the pancreas, one of the principal organs affected by this disorder. Approximately 85% of CF patients have pancreatic insufficiency (i.e., the pancreas is unable to secrete digestive enzymes, resulting in chronic malnutrition). The gut is also affected, and approximately 10% of newborns with CF have **meconium ileus** (a thick plug of fecal material that blocks the colon). The sweat glands of CF patients are abnormal, resulting in high levels of chloride in the sweat. This is the basis for the **sweat chloride test**, commonly used in the diagnosis of this disease. More than 95% of males with CF are sterile due to absence or obstruction of the vas deferens. The most serious problem facing CF patients is obstruction of the lungs by heavy, thick mucus. Because this mucus cannot be cleared effectively, the lungs are highly susceptible to infection by bacteria such as *Staphylococcus aureus* and (most seriously) *Pseudomonas aeruginosa*. Chronic infection leads to destruction of the lung tissue, resulting eventually in death from respiratory failure.

As a result of improved antibiotics, aggressive chest physical therapy, and pancreatic enzyme replacement therapy, the survival rates of CF patients have improved substantially during the past three decades. Median survival is now 29 years of age. This disease has highly variable expression, with some patients experiencing relatively little respiratory difficulty and nearly normal survival. Others may have much more severe respiratory problems and survive for only a few years.

The CF gene was mapped to chromosome 7q in 1985 by investigators in London, Toronto, and Salt Lake City, and it was cloned 4 years later by investigators in Michigan and Toronto. It is a large gene, spanning 250 kb and including 27 exons. Much research has been devoted to understanding this gene and its protein product. The protein product, labeled the "cystic fibrosis transmembrane regulator" (CFTR) is clearly involved in the transport of chloride ions across the membranes of specialized epithelial cells (such as those that line the gut and lung). There is good evidence that CFTR is the chloride ion channel itself. The similarity of CFTR to membrane transport proteins suggests that it may also be involved in the transport of ions across the cell membrane.

The fact that CFTR is involved in chloride transport helps us to understand the multiple effects of mutations at the CF locus. Defective chloride transport results in salt imbalances, producing the obstructive mucus seen in the lungs and pancreas. It also explains the abnormally high concentrations of chloride in the sweat secretions of CF patients.

DNA sequence analysis has revealed more than 400 different mutations at the CF locus. The most common of these is a 3-base deletion resulting in a loss of a phenylalanine at position 508 of the CFTR protein. This mutation is labeled "ΔF508" (i.e., deletion of phenylalanine at position 508). Although there are many different CF mutations, ΔF508 accounts for 70% of the mutations seen among those of northern European ancestry. This mutation, along with several other relatively common ones, is useful for genetic diagnosis of CF (see Chapter 11).

Identification of the specific mutation(s) responsible for CF in a patient can be useful in predicting the course of the disease. For example, patients homozygous for the ΔF508 mutation nearly always have pancreatic insufficiency, and they often have a relatively severe degree of respiratory involvement. There are, however, exceptions, indicating that additional factors (possibly genes at other loci) must influence the expression of the disease.

In addition to enhancing our understanding of the pathophysiology of CF, cloning the CF gene has opened the possibility of gene therapy (see Chapter 11). Research in experimental systems has shown that insertion of normal CF genes into cells with defective chloride ion transport can correct the defect. This and other research have led to the initiation of clinical trials in which normal CF genes are inserted into adenoviruses, which then are introduced into the lungs of CF patients. It is hoped that the adenoviruses will insert the normal gene into airway epithelial cells, inducing normal chloride channel function in these cells. This could eventually lead to a cure for this usually fatal disease.

Gene and genotype frequencies specify the proportions of each allele and each genotype, respectively, in a population. Under simple conditions these frequencies can be estimated by direct counting.

The Hardy-Weinberg Principle

The example given above for the *MN* locus presents an ideal situation for gene frequency estimation; because of codominance, the three genotypes can easily be distinguished and counted. What happens when one of the homozygotes is indistinguishable from the heterozygote (i.e., when there is dominance)? Here the basic concepts of probability can be used to specify a predictable relationship between gene frequencies and genotype frequencies.

Imagine a locus having two alleles, labeled *A* and *a*. Suppose that, in a population, we know the frequency of allele *A*, which we call *p*, and the frequency of allele *a*, which we call *q*. From this we wish to determine the expected population frequencies of each genotype, *AA*, *Aa*, and *aa*. We assume that individuals in the population mate at random with regard to their genotype at this locus (**random mating** is also referred to as **panmixia**). Thus the genotype has no effect on mate selection. If men and women mate at random, then the assumption of independence is fulfilled. This allows us to apply the addition and multiplication rules to estimate genotype frequencies.

Suppose that the frequency, *p*, of allele *A* in our population is 0.7. Then 70% of the sperm cells in the population must have allele *A*, and 70% of the egg cells must have allele *A*. Since *p* and *q* must sum to 1, 30% of the egg and sperm cells must carry allele *a* (i.e., *q* = 0.30). Under panmixia, the probability that a sperm cell carrying *A* unites with an egg cell carrying *A* is given by the product of the gene frequencies: $p \times p = p^2 = 0.49$ (multiplication rule). This is the probability of producing an offspring with the *AA* genotype. Using the same reasoning, the probability of producing an offspring with the *aa* genotype is given by $q \times q = q^2 = 0.09$.

What about the frequency of heterozygotes in the population? There are two ways a heterozygote can be formed. Either a sperm cell carrying *A* can unite with an egg carrying *a*, or a sperm cell carrying *a* can unite with an egg carrying *A*. The probability of each of these two outcomes is given by the product of the gene frequencies, *pq*. Because we want to know the overall probability of obtaining a heterozygote (i.e., the first event *or* the second), we can

apply the addition rule, adding the probabilities to obtain a heterozygote frequency of 2*pq*. These operations are summarized in Figure 4-3. This relationship between gene frequencies and genotype frequencies was established independently by two men, Godfrey Hardy and Wilhelm Weinberg, and is termed the **Hardy-Weinberg principle**.

As already mentioned, we can use this principle to estimate gene and genotype frequencies when dominant homozygotes and heterozygotes are indistinguishable. This is often the case for recessive diseases such as CF. Only the affected homozygotes, with genotype *aa*, are distinguishable. The Hardy-Weinberg principle tells us that the frequency of *aa* should be q^2. For CF in the white population, $q^2 = 1/2500$ (i.e., the prevalence of the disorder among newborns). To estimate *q*, we take the square root of both sides of this equation: $q = \sqrt{1/2,500} = 1/50 = 0.02$. Since $p + q = 1$, $p = 0.98$. We can then estimate the genotype frequencies of *AA* and *Aa*. The latter genotype, which represents heterozygous **carriers** of the disease allele, is of particular interest. We find that $2pq = 1/25$ (note that, since *p* is nearly 1.0, we can simplify this calculation by rounding *p* up to 1.0; then without a significant loss of accuracy, $2q = 2/50 = 1/25$). This tells us something rather remarkable about CF and about recessive diseases in general. Whereas the incidence of affected homozygotes is only 1 in 2500, heterozygous carriers of the disease gene are much more common (one

Male population

	A (p)	a (q)
A (p)	AA (p^2)	Aa (pq)
a (q)	Aa (pq)	aa (q^2)

Female population

Figure 4-3 ■ The Hardy-Weinberg principle. The population frequencies of genotypes *AA*, *Aa*, and *aa* are predicted on the basis of gene frequencies (*p* and *q*). It is usually assumed that the gene frequencies are the same in males and females.

in 25 individuals). The vast majority of recessive disease alleles then are effectively "hidden" in the genomes of heterozygotes.

> **Under panmixia, the Hardy-Weinberg principle specifies the relationship between gene frequencies and genotype frequencies. It is useful in estimating gene frequencies from disease prevalence data and in estimating the incidence of heterozygous carriers of recessive disease genes.**

The Concept of Phenotype

The term genotype has been defined as an individual's genetic constitution at a locus. The **phenotype** is what we actually observe physically or clinically. Genotypes do not uniquely correspond to phenotypes. Two different genotypes, a dominant homozygote and a heterozygote, may have the same phenotype. An example would be CF. Conversely, the same genotype may produce different phenotypes in different environments. An example of this is the recessive disease phenylketonuria (PKU), seen in approximately 1 in 10,000 white births. Mutations at the locus encoding the metabolic enzyme phenylalanine hydroxylase render the homozygote unable to metabolize the amino acid phenylalanine. Although PKU babies are normal at birth, their metabolic deficiency produces a buildup of phenylalanine and various toxic metabolites. This is highly destructive to the central nervous system, and it eventually produces severe mental retardation. It has been estimated that untreated PKU babies lose, on average, one to two IQ points per week during the first year of life. Thus the PKU genotype can produce a severe disease phenotype. However, it is easy to screen for PKU at birth (see Chapter 11), and the disease can be avoided by initiating a low phenylalanine diet within 1 month after birth. The individual still has the PKU genotype, but the phenotype of mental retardation has been profoundly altered by environmental modification.

This example shows that the phenotype is the result of the interaction of genotype and environmental factors. It should be emphasized that "environment" can include the genetic environment (i.e., genes at other loci, the products of which may interact with a specific gene or its product).

> **The phenotype, which is physically observable, results from the interaction of genotype and environment.**

Basic Pedigree Structure

The **pedigree** is one of the most commonly used tools in medical genetics. It illustrates the relationships among family members, and it shows which family members are affected with a genetic disease and which members are unaffected. Typically an arrow denotes the **proband**, the first individual diagnosed in the pedigree. The proband is sometimes also referred to as the **index case** or **propositus** (**proposita** for females). Figure 4-4 describes the features of pedigree notation.

When discussing relatives in families, one often refers to degrees of relationship. First-degree relatives are those who are related at the parent—

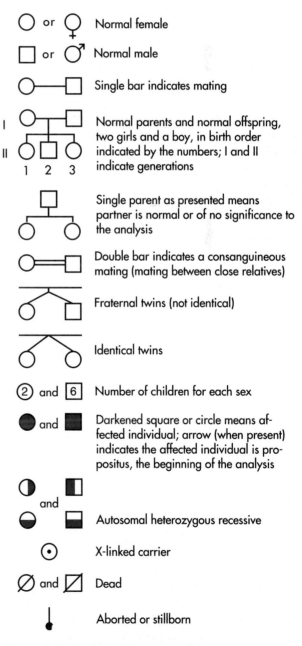

Figure 4-4 ▪ Basic pedigree notation.

offspring or sibling (brother and sister) level. Second-degree relatives are those who removed by one extra "step" (e.g., grandparents and grand-children, uncles/aunts, and nieces/nephews). Continuing this logic, third-degree relatives would include, for example, first cousins, great-grand-children, and so on.

■ AUTOSOMAL DOMINANT INHERITANCE

Characteristics of Autosomal Dominant Inheritance

Currently, there are more than 3700 known autosomal dominant traits, most of which are diseases. Individually, each autosomal dominant disease is rather rare in populations, with the most common ones having gene frequencies of about 0.001. Matings between two individuals both affected by the same autosomal dominant disease are thus uncommon. Most often, affected offspring are produced by the union of a normal parent with an affected heterozygote. The Punnett square in Figure 4-5 illustrates this mating. The affected parent can pass either a disease gene or a normal gene to his or her children. Each event has a probability of 0.5. Thus on the average, half of the children will be heterozygotes and will express the disease, and half will not.

Postaxial polydactyly, the presence of an extra digit next to the fifth digit (Fig. 4-6), can be inherited as an autosomal dominant trait. Let *A* symbolize the gene for polydactyly, and let *a*

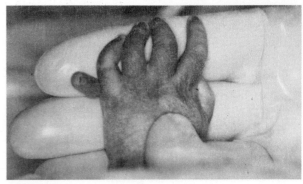

Figure 4-6 ■ **Postaxial polydactyly. An extra digit is located next to the fifth digit.**

symbolize the normal allele. An idealized pedigree for this disease is shown in Figure 4-7. This pedigree illustrates several important characteristics of autosomal dominant inheritance. First, the two sexes exhibit the trait in approximately equal proportions, and males and females are equally likely to transmit the trait to their offspring. This reflects the fact that this is an *autosomal* disease (as opposed to a disease caused by an X chromosome mutation, in which these proportions typically differ). Second, there is no skipping of generations: if an individual has polydactyly, one parent must also have it. This leads to a vertical transmission pattern, in which the disease phenotype is usually seen in one generation after another. Also, if neither parent has the trait, none of the children has it. Third, father–son transmission of the disease gene

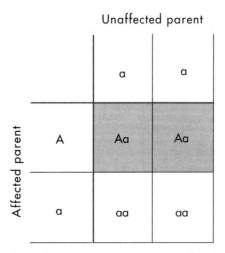

Figure 4-5 ■ **Punnett square illustrating the mating of an unaffected individual (*aa*) with an individual who is heterozygous for an autosomal dominant disease gene (*Aa*). The genotypes of affected offspring are shaded.**

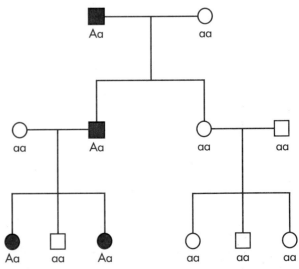

Figure 4-7 ■ **A pedigree illustrating the inheritance pattern of postaxial polydactyly, an autosomal dominant disorder. Affected individuals are represented by shading.**

is observed. Although father–son transmission is not *required* to establish autosomal dominant inheritance, its presence in a pedigree excludes certain other modes of inheritance (particularly X-linked inheritance; see Chapter 5). Finally, as we have already seen, an affected (heterozygote) individual transmits the trait to approximately half of his or her children. However, because gamete transmission, like coin tossing, is subject to chance fluctuations, it is possible that all or none of the children of an affected parent will have the trait. When large numbers of matings of this type are studied, the proportion of affected children will closely approach one half.

Autosomal dominant inheritance is characterized by vertical transmission of the disease phenotype, a lack of skipped generations, and roughly equal numbers of affected males and females. Father–son transmission may be observed.

Recurrence Risks

Parents at risk for producing children with a genetic disease are often concerned with the question: What is the chance that our future children will have this disease? When one or more children have already been born with a genetic disease, the parents are given a **recurrence risk**. This is the probability that subsequent children will also have the disease. If the parents have not yet had children but are known to be at risk for having children with a genetic disease, an **occurrence risk** can be given. When one parent is affected by an autosomal dominant disease (heterozygote) and the other is normal, the occurrence and recurrence risks for each child are one half. It is important to keep in mind that each birth is an *independent event,* as in the coin-tossing examples. Thus, even though parents may have already had a child with the disease, their recurrence risk remains one half. Even if they have had several children, all affected (or all unaffected) with the disease, the law of independence dictates that the probability that their next child will have the disease is still one half. Although this concept may seem intuitively obvious, it is frequently misunderstood by the lay population. Further aspects of communicating risks to families will be discussed in Chapter 12.

The recurrence risk for autosomal dominant disorders is 50%. Because of independence, this risk remains constant no matter how many affected or unaffected children are born.

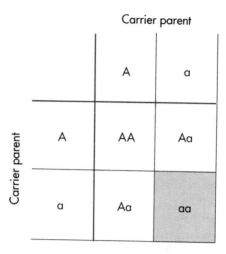

Figure 4-8 ■ Punnett square illustrating the mating of two heterozygous carriers of an autosomal recessive gene. The genotype of affected offspring is shaded.

■ AUTOSOMAL RECESSIVE INHERITANCE

Like autosomal dominant diseases, autosomal recessive diseases are fairly rare in populations. As shown previously, heterozygous carriers for recessive disease genes are much more common than affected homozygotes. Consequently, the parents of individuals affected with autosomal recessive diseases are usually both heterozygous carriers. As the Punnett square in Figure 4-8 demonstrates, one fourth of their offspring will be normal homozygotes, half will be phenotypically normal carrier heterozygotes, and one fourth will be homozygotes affected with the disease (on average).

Characteristics of Autosomal Recessive Inheritance

Figure 4-9 is a pedigree showing the inheritance of Hurler syndrome, a rare autosomal recessive disorder resulting from a deficiency of the lysosomal enzyme, α-L-iduronidase. This enzyme deficiency results in a buildup of mucopolysaccharides in the lysosomes, leading to skeletal abnormalities, short stature, mental retardation, and coarse facial features (Fig. 4-10).* The pedigree demonstrates most of the important criteria for distinguishing autosomal recessive inheritance (these criteria, along with those of autosomal dominant inheritance, are summarized in Table 4-1). First, unlike autosomal dominant diseases, in which the disease phenotype is seen in one generation after another,

---

*Diseases in which metabolic products accumulate in lysosomes are termed **lysosomal storage disorders**.

autosomal recessive diseases are usually seen in one or more siblings but not in earlier generations. Second, as in autosomal dominant inheritance, males and females are affected in equal proportions. Third, on average, one fourth of the offspring of two heterozygous carriers will be affected with the disorder. Finally, **consanguinity** is present more often in pedigrees involving autosomal recessive diseases than in those involving other types of inheritance (Fig. 4-9). The term consanguinity (Latin, "with blood") refers to the mating of related individuals. It is often a factor in recessive disease because related individuals are more likely to share the same disease genes. Consanguinity will be discussed in greater detail below.

Autosomal recessive inheritance is characterized by clustering of the disease phenotype among siblings, but the disease is not usually seen among parents or other ancestors. Equal numbers of affected males and females are usually seen, and consanguinity may be present.

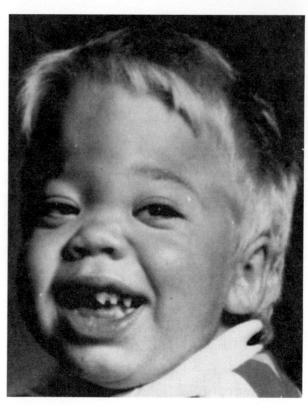

Figure 4-10 ■ A child with Hurler syndrome. Note the low, flat nasal root, thickened lips, widely spaced teeth, and facial fullness.

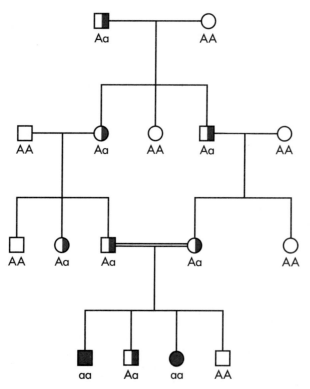

Figure 4-9 ■ **Pedigree showing the inheritance pattern of Hurler syndrome, an autosomal recessive disease. Consanguinity in this pedigree is denoted by a double bar connecting the related parents of the affected individuals.**

Recurrence Risks

As already mentioned the most common mating type seen in recessive disease involves two heterozygous carrier parents. This reflects the relative commonness of heterozygous carriers and the fact that many autosomal recessive diseases are severe enough so that affected individuals are less likely to become parents.

The Punnett square (Fig. 4-8) demonstrated that one fourth of the offspring from this mating will be homozygous for the disease gene and thus affected. The recurrence risk for the offspring of carrier parents is then 25%. As before, these are average figures. In any given family there will likely be chance fluctuations, but a study of a large number of families would yield a figure close to this proportion.

Occasionally a carrier of a recessive disease gene mates with an individual homozygous for the disease gene. In this case roughly half of their children will be affected, and half will be heterozygous carriers. The recurrence risk is 50%. Because this

Table 4-1 ■ A comparison of the major attributes of autosomal dominant and autosomal recessive inheritance patterns

	Autosomal dominant	Autosomal recessive
Usual recurrence risk	50%	25%
Transmission pattern	Vertical; disease phenotype seen in generation after generation	Horizontal; disease phenotype seen in multiple siblings but usually no earlier generations affected
Sex ratio	Equal number of affected males and females (usually)	Equal number of affected males and females (usually)
Other	Father–son transmission of disease gene is possible	Consanguinity is sometimes seen, especially for rare recessive diseases

pattern of inheritance mimics that of an autosomal dominant trait, it is sometimes referred to as **quasidominant** inheritance. With extended studies of pedigrees, in which carrier matings are observed, it can be distinguished from true dominant inheritance.

When two individuals affected by a recessive disease mate, all of their children must also be affected. This observation helps to distinguish recessive from dominant inheritance because two parents both affected by a dominant disease will nearly always both be heterozygotes and thus one fourth of their children will be unaffected.

The recurrence risk for autosomal recessive diseases is usually 25%. Quasidominant inheritance, with a recurrence risk of 50%, is seen when an affected homozygote mates with a heterozygote.

"Dominant" versus "Recessive": Some Cautions

The preceding discussion has treated dominant and recessive disorders as though they belong in rigid categories. However, these distinctions are becoming less strict as our understanding of these diseases increases. Many (perhaps most) "dominant" diseases are actually more severe in affected homozygotes than in heterozygotes. An example is given by achondroplasia, an autosomal dominant disorder in which heterozygotes have reduced stature (Fig. 4-11). Heterozygotes enjoy a nearly normal life span, estimated to be only about 10 years less than average. Affected homozygotes are much more severely affected and usually die in infancy of respiratory failure.

Although heterozygous carriers of recessive disease genes are clinically normal, the effects of recessive genes can often be detected in heterozy-

gotes because they result in reduced levels of enzyme activity. This is usually the basis for biochemical carrier detection tests (see Chapter 11). A

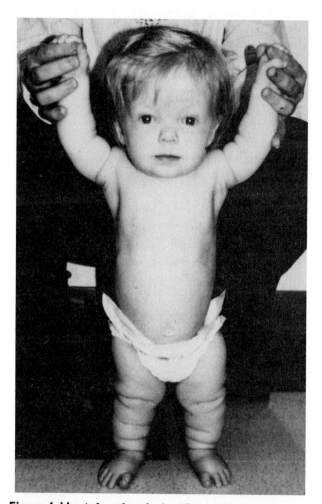

Figure 4-11 ■ Achondroplasia. This girl has short limbs relative to trunk length. Note also the prominent forehead, low nasal root, and redundant skin folds in the arms and legs (*SOL* 24).

useful and valid way to distinguish dominant and recessive disorders is that heterozygotes are clinically affected in most cases of dominant disorders, whereas they are nearly always clinically normal in recessive disorders.

> **Although the distinction between dominant and recessive diseases is not rigid, a dominant disease allele will produce disease in a heterozygote, whereas a recessive disease allele will not do so.**

Another caution is that a disease may be inherited in autosomal dominant fashion in some cases and autosomal recessive fashion in others. Familial isolated growth hormone deficiency (IGHD), another reduced stature disorder, is an example of one such disease. DNA sequencing of a pituitary growth hormone gene on chromosome 17 *(GH1)* has revealed a number of different mutations that can produce IGHD. Recessive IGHD can be caused by nonsense and splice site mutations that apparently alter the protein product (pituitary growth hormone) such that it cannot proceed to the secretory granules of the cell (cytoplasmic structures that secrete growth hormone and other products from the cell). Because they have one normal chromosome, heterozygotes still produce half of the normal amount of growth hormone. This is sufficient for normal stature. Homozygotes for these mutations produce no *GH1* product and have reduced stature.

How then can a mutation at this locus produce dominant inheritance? In one form of dominantly inherited IGHD, a splice site mutation deletes the third exon of the *GH1* gene, producing a protein product that does proceed to the secretory granules. Here the abnormal *GH1* product encoded by the mutated chromosome forms disulfide bonds with the normal product encoded by the normal chromosome. This *disables* the normal growth hormone molecules, resulting in little or no production of GH1 product and thus reduced stature. (This type of mutation, in which the abnormal product can suppress or destroy the normal product, is termed a **dominant negative**.) This example illustrates some of the difficulties in applying the terms "dominant" and "recessive," and it also shows how molecular analysis of a gene can help to explain important disease features.

> **In a few cases, a disease may be inherited in either autosomal dominant or autosomal recessive fashion, depending on the nature of the mutation that alters the gene product.**

A final caution is that the terms dominant and recessive, strictly speaking, apply to traits, not genes. To see why, consider the sickle cell mutation, discussed in Chapter 3. Homozygotes for this mutation develop sickle cell disease. Heterozygotes, said to have sickle cell trait, are usually clinically normal. However, a heterozygote has an increased risk for splenic infarctions at high altitude. Is the mutant gene then dominant or recessive? Clearly, it makes more sense to refer to sickle cell *disease* as recessive and sickle cell *trait* as dominant. Nonetheless, it is common (and often convenient) to apply the terms dominant and recessive to genes.

■ FACTORS THAT MAY COMPLICATE INHERITANCE PATTERNS

The inheritance patterns described for postaxial polydactyly and Hurler syndrome are straightforward. However, many autosomal diseases display more complex patterns. Some of these complexities are described next.

New Mutation

If a child has been born with a genetic disease and there is no history of the disease in the family, it is possible that the child is the product of a **new mutation** (this is especially likely if the disease in question is an autosomal dominant). That is, the gene transmitted by one of the parents underwent a change in DNA resulting in a mutation from a normal to a disease-causing allele. The genes at this locus in the parent's other germ cells would still be normal. In this case the recurrence risk for the parents' subsequent offspring is not elevated above that of the general population. However, the offspring of the affected child may have a substantially elevated occurrence risk (e.g., it would be 50% for an autosomal dominant disease). A large proportion of the observed cases of many autosomal dominant diseases are the result of new mutations. For example, it is estimated that seven eighths of all cases of achondroplasia are due to new mutations, whereas only one eighth are transmitted by achondroplastic parents. This is primarily because the disease tends to limit the potential for reproduction. To provide accurate risk estimates, it is essential to know whether an observed case is due to an inherited disease gene or a new mutation. This can be done only if an adequate family history has been taken.

> **New mutations are a frequent cause of the appearance of a genetic disease in an**

individual with no previous family history of the disorder. The recurrence risk for the individual's siblings is very low, but it may be substantially elevated for the individual's offspring.

Germline Mosaicism

Occasionally, two or more offspring will present with an autosomal dominant disease when there is no family history of the disease. Because mutation is a rare event, it is unlikely that this would be due to multiple mutations in the same family. The mechanism most likely to be responsible is termed **germline mosaicism** (a **mosaic** is an individual who has more than one genetically distinct cell line in his or her body). During the embryonic development of one of the parents, a mutation occurred that affected all or part of the germline but few or none of the somatic cells of the embryo. Thus the parent carries the mutation in his or her germ line but does not actually express the disease. As a result, he or she can transmit the mutation to multiple offspring. This phenomenon, although relatively rare, can have significant effects on recurrence risks when it occurs.

Germline mosaicism has been studied extensively in the lethal perinatal form of osteogenesis imperfecta (OI type II, see Chapter 2), which is caused by mutations in the type 1 procollagen genes. The fact that unaffected parents sometimes produced multiple offspring affected with this disease led to the conclusion that type II OI was an autosomal recessive trait. This has been disputed by recent studies in which the polymerase chain reaction (PCR) technique was used to amplify DNA from the sperm of a father of two type II OI cases. This DNA was compared with DNA extracted from his somatic cells (skin fibroblasts). Although procollagen mutations were not detected in the fibroblast DNA, they were found in approximately one in eight sperm cells. This is a direct demonstration of germline mosaicism in this individual. Although germline mosaicism has thus been demonstrated for type II OI, most cases are thought to be caused by isolated new mutations, and a few cases of true autosomal recessive inheritance have also been documented.

Other diseases in which germline mosaicism has been observed include achondroplasia, Duchenne muscular dystrophy, and hemophilia A (see Chapter 5 for further discussion of the latter two diseases).

Germline mosaicism occurs when all or part of a parents' germline is affected by a disease mutation but the somatic cells are not. It elevates the recurrence risk for future offspring of the mosaic parent.

Delayed Age of Onset

While some genetic diseases are expressed at birth or shortly afterward, many others do not become apparent until well into adulthood. This is known as **delayed age of onset**. One of the best-known examples is Huntington disease, a neurologic disorder whose main features are progressive dementia and increasingly uncontrollable movements of the limbs (see Clinical Commentary 4-2 for further details). The latter feature is known as **chorea** (from the Greek word for dance, *khoreia*), and the disease is sometimes called Huntington's chorea. This autosomal dominant disorder is named after Dr. George Huntington, who first described the disease in 1872. Symptoms are not usually seen until age 30 or later (Fig. 4-12). Thus, those who develop the disease have often had children before they are aware that they carry the gene. If the disease were present at birth, nearly all affected persons would die before reaching reproductive age, and the frequency of the gene in the population would be much lower. Delaying the age of onset thus reduces natural selection against a disease gene, increasing its frequency in a population. Delayed age of onset can cause difficulties in deducing the mode of inheritance of a disease because it is not possible to determine until later in life whether an individual carries the disease gene.

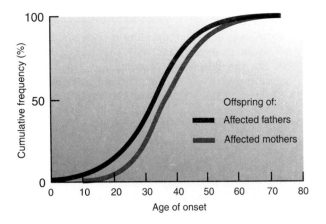

Figure 4-12 ■ Distribution of the age of onset for Huntington disease. Note that age of onset tends to be somewhat earlier when the affected parent is male. (Redrawn from Conneally: Am J Hum Genet 36:520, 1984.)

Clinical Commentary 4-2: Huntington Disease

Huntington disease affects approximately 1 in 20,000 persons of European descent. It is substantially less common among Japanese, and it may be less common among Africans. The disorder usually presents between ages 30 and 50, although it has been observed as early as 2 years of age and as late as 80 years of age.

Huntington disease is characterized by a progressive loss of motor control ("chorea") and by psychiatric problems, including dementia and affective disorder. There is a substantial loss of neurons in the brain, detectable by scanning techniques such as magnetic resonance imaging. Although many parts of the brain are affected, the area most seriously damaged is the corpus striatum. In some patients the disease leads to a loss of 25% or more of total brain weight (Fig. 4-13).

The clinical course of Huntington disease is protracted. Typically the interval from initial diagnosis to death is approximately 15 years. As in many neurologic disorders, patients with Huntington disease experience difficulties in swallowing; aspiration pneumonia is the most common cause of death. Cardiorespiratory failure and subdural hematoma (due to head trauma) are other frequent causes of death. The suicide rate among Huntington disease patients is several times higher than in the general population. Treatment includes the use of drugs such as benzodiazepines to help control the choreic movements. Affective disturbances are sometimes controlled with antipsychotic drugs and tricyclic antidepressants. Although these drugs help to control some of the symptoms of Huntington disease, there is currently no way to alter the course of the disease.

Huntington disease has one of the lowest known mutation rates of all human disease genes, estimated at approximately 1 per 1 million (per locus per generation). There are currently only a few well-documented examples of individuals in whom the disease arose as a new mutation. This disorder is also notable in that affected homozygotes appear to display exactly the same clinical course as heterozygotes (in contrast to many or most dominant disorders, in which homozygotes are more severely affected). Huntington disease also has the distinction of being the first genetic disease mapped to a specific chromosome using an RFLP marker. James Gusella and colleagues mapped the disease gene to a region on the distal tip of chromosome 4p in 1983.

After 10 years of work by a large number of investigators, the disease gene itself was cloned. DNA sequence analysis shows that the mutation is a CAG expanded repeat (Chapter 3) located within the coding portion of the gene. Unaffected individuals typically have 11 to 34 copies of this repeat; those with Huntington disease may have from 36 to more than 100 copies of the repeat. This discovery has already begun to reveal insights about the disease. It has been shown, for example, that a larger number of repeats is correlated with earlier age of onset of the disorder. Also there is a tendency for greater repeat expansion when the parent transmitting the disease gene is a male. This helps to explain the difference in ages of onset for maternally and paternally transmitted disease seen in Figure 4-12. In particular, 80% of cases with onset prior to 20 years (termed juvenile Huntington disease) are paternally transmitted, and these cases are accompanied by especially large repeat expansions. It remains to be seen why the degree of repeat instability in the Huntington gene is greater in paternal transmission than in maternal transmission.

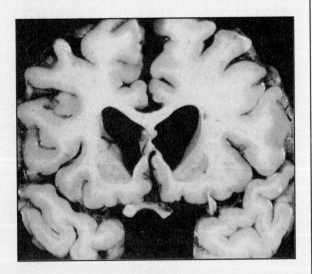

Figure 4-13 ■ Cross section of a brain of an adult with Huntington disease, illustrating marked striatal atrophy (*SOL* 20–23). (Courtesy of Dr. Jeanette Townsend, University of Utah Health Sciences Center.)

A person whose parent has Huntington disease has a 50% chance of inheriting the disease gene. Until fairly recently, this individual would be confronted with a torturous question: should I have children, knowing that there is a 50–50 chance that I might have this disease gene and then pass it to half of my children? With the identification of the mutation responsible for Huntington disease, it is now possible for at-risk individuals to know with a high degree of certainty whether or not they carry the disease allele.

As mentioned above, a number of important genetic diseases have a delayed age of onset. These include polycystic kidney disease (*SOL* 49, 50), a disorder in which the formation of renal cysts leads eventually to kidney failure; hemochromatosis, a potentially fatal recessive disorder of iron storage; familial Alzheimer disease (Chapter 10); and an autosomal dominant form of breast cancer.*

Delayed age of onset is observed in many genetic diseases. It complicates the interpretation of inheritance patterns in families.

Reduced Penetrance

Another important characteristic of many genetic diseases is reduced **penetrance**: an individual who has the genotype for a disease may not exhibit the disease phenotype at all, even though he or she can transmit the disease gene to the next generation. Retinoblastoma, a malignant eye tumor (see Clinical Commentary 4-3), is a good example of an autosomal dominant disorder in which reduced penetrance is seen. The transmission pattern of this disorder is illustrated in Figure 4-15. Family studies have shown that about 10% of the **obligate carriers** of the retinoblastoma susceptibility gene (i.e., those who have an affected parent and affected children and therefore must themselves carry the gene) do not have the disease. The penetrance of the gene is then said to be 90%. Penetrance rates are usually estimated by examining a large number of families and determining what proportion of the obligate carriers or obligate homozygotes (in the case of recessive disorders) develop the disease phenotype.

Disease genes in which an individual may have the disease genotype without expressing the disease phenotype are said to have reduced penetrance.

Variable Expression

A similar complication is **variable expression**. Here the penetrance may be complete, but the severity of the disease can vary greatly. A well-studied example of variable expression in an autosomal dominant disease is neurofibromatosis type 1, or von Recklinghausen disease (named after the German physician who described the disorder in 1882). Clinical Commentary 4-4 provides further discussion of this disorder. A parent with mild expression of the disease, so mild that he or she is not aware of it, can transmit the gene to a child who can have severe expression. As with delayed age of onset and reduced penetrance, variable expression provides a mechanism for disease genes to survive at higher frequencies in populations.

---

*Epidemiologic studies indicate that about 5% of breast cancer cases in the United States are due to autosomal dominant inheritance. See Chapter 10 for further discussion.

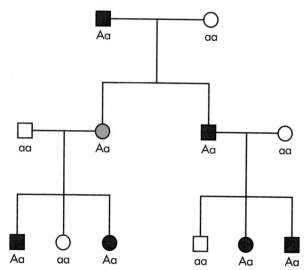

Figure 4-15 ■ Pedigree illustrating the inheritance pattern of retinoblastoma, a disorder with reduced penetrance. The unaffected obligate carrier is lightly shaded.

It should be emphasized that penetrance and expression are distinct entities. Penetrance is an all-or-none phenomenon: one either has the disease phenotype or does not. Variable expression refers to the extent of expression of the disease phenotype.

The causes of variable expression are usually not known. Environmental effects can sometimes be responsible: in the absence of a certain environmental factor, the gene is expressed with diminished severity or not at all. Another possible cause is the interaction of other genes, called **modifier genes**, with the disease gene. Finally as the molecular basis of mutation becomes better understood, it is clear that some cases of variable expression are due to different types of mutations at the same disease locus. This is termed **allelic heterogeneity**. In some cases clinically distinct diseases may be the result of allelic heterogeneity (e.g., as in the β-globin mutations that can cause sickle cell disease or various β-thalassemias).

Osteogenesis imperfecta (OI) is one disease in which genetic studies have helped to explain variable expression. Mutations that affect amino acids near the carboxyl terminal of the procollagen molecule generally cause more severe consequences than do mutations affecting the molecule near its amino terminal. It is also well documented that affected members of the same family, having the same mutation, can manifest large differences in the severity of their OI. This may be due to different genetic "backgrounds" (i.e., modifier loci) in related individuals. And nongenetic events, such as

Clinical Commentary 4-3. Retinoblastoma

Retinoblastoma (Fig. 4-14) is the most common childhood eye tumor, affecting approximately 1 in 20,000 children. The tumor begins during embryonic development, when retinal cells are actively dividing and proliferating. It nearly always presents clinically by age 5.

Approximately 40% of retinoblastoma cases are familial (the remainder are **sporadic** and are not transmitted from one generation to the next). Prior to the mapping of this gene to chromosome 13 and subsequent molecular analyses in the early 1980s, the cause of reduced penetrance in familial retinoblastoma was the subject of much speculation. The ability to examine changes in DNA near the disease gene finally explained the mechanism responsible for reduced penetrance. Briefly, an affected individual will transmit the disease gene to half of his or her children, on average. Thus the offspring has inherited a mutation on one member of the chromosome 13 pair in every cell of his or her body. However, this is not sufficient to cause tumor formation (if it were, every cell in the body would give rise to a tumor). A second event must occur in the same region of the normal, homologous chromosome 13 in a fetus's developing retinal cell to initiate a tumor (this "two-hit" process is discussed further in Chapter 9). The second event, which can be considered a somatic mutation, has a relatively low probability of occurring. However, there are at least 1 million retinal cells in the developing fetus, each representing a potential "target" for the event. Usually, a fetus that has inherited a copy of the retinoblastoma disease gene will experience a second "hit" in several different retinal cells, giving rise to several tumors. Familial retinoblastoma is thus usually multifocal (consisting of several tumor foci) and bilateral (affecting both eyes). Because the second hits are random events, a small proportion of individuals who inherit the disease allele never experience a second hit in any retinal cell. They do not develop a retinoblastoma. The requirement for a second hit thus explains the reduced penetrance seen in this disorder.

The retinoblastoma gene has been cloned and sequenced, and its function has been studied closely. It appears to help to control the cell cycle, thus preventing uncontrolled cell proliferation. It belongs to a class of genes known as **tumor suppressors** (see Chapter 9).

If untreated, retinoblastomas can grow to considerable size. Reports from the 19th century described tumors achieving the size of "two fists." Fortunately these tumors are now usually detected and treated before they become large. If found early enough through ophthalmologic examination, the tumor may be treated successfully with radiation or cryotherapy (freezing). In more advanced cases enucleation (removal) of the eye is necessary. Because individuals with familial retinoblastoma have inherited a chromosome 13 mutation in all cells of their body, they are also susceptible to other types of cancers later in life. In particular, about 15% of those who inherit the mutation later develop osteosarcomas (malignant bone tumors). Careful monitoring for subsequent tumors is thus an important aspect of managing the retinoblastoma patient.

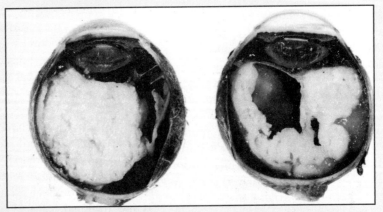

Figure 4-14 ■ **Bilateral retinoblastoma showing presence of neoplastic tissue (*SOL* 15-19).** (From McCance KL and Huether SE: Pathophysiology, ed 2, St Louis, 1994, Mosby.)

Clinical Commentary 4-4. Neurofibromatosis, a Disease with Highly Variable Expression

The von Recklinghausen form of neurofibromatosis (Fig. 4-16A, B) is one of the most common autosomal dominant disorders, affecting approximately one in 3000 individuals. It offers a good example of variable expression in a genetic disease. Some patients will have only a few *café-au-lait* spots (from the French for "coffee with milk," describing the color of the hyperpigmented skin patches), Lisch nodules (benign growths on the iris), and perhaps a few neurofibromas (nonmalignant peripheral nerve tumors). These individuals are often unaware that they have the condition. Other patients may have a much more severe expression of the disorder, including hundreds to thousands of neurofibromas, optic gliomas (benign tumors of the optic nerve), learning disabilities, hypertension, scoliosis (lateral curvature of the spine), and malignancies (e.g., neurofibrosarcomas). Fortunately about two thirds of patients have only a mild cutaneous involvement. Fewer than 10% develop malignancies as a result of the disorder. Expression can vary significantly within the same family. Thus a mildly affected parent can produce severely affected offspring.

A standard set of diagnostic criteria for neurofibromatosis has been developed. The criteria are that two or more of the following must be present: (1) six or more *café-au-lait* spots greater than 5 mm in diameter in prepubertal subjects and greater than 15 mm in postpubertal subjects; (2) freckling in the armpits or groin area; (3) two or more neurofibromas of any type or one plexiform neurofibroma; (4) two or more

Lisch nodules; (5) optic glioma; (6) distinctive bone lesions, particularly an abnormally formed sphenoid bone or tibial pseudarthrosis*; and (7) a first-degree relative diagnosed with neurofibromatosis using the previous six criteria.

There are several forms of neurofibromatosis, of which the von Recklinghausen form (also known as peripheral neurofibromatosis) is the most common. It is now labeled "neurofibromatosis type 1," or NF1. Neurofibromatosis 2 (NF2) is much rarer and is distinguished by the fact that it involves bilateral acoustic neuromas (tumors affecting the eighth cranial nerve; SOL 14). The *NF2* gene has been mapped to chromosome 22 and cloned. These forms of neurofibromatosis can be distinguished from familial *café-au-lait* spots (which involves only *café-au-lait* spots) and segmental neurofibromatosis. In the latter form, the disorder is confined to only one part of the body. This is thought to be the result of a postzygotic mutation leading to somatic mosaicism.

Although NF1 has highly variable expression, the penetrance of this gene is virtually 100%. It has one of the highest known mutation rates, about 1 per 10,000 loci per generation. Approximately 50% of NF1 cases are the result of new mutations. In 1987 the gene was mapped to chromosome 17q by researchers in Salt Lake City, and it was isolated and cloned 3 years later. It is a large gene, spanning approximately 350 kb of

---

*Pseudarthrosis occurs when a weight-bearing long bone, such as the tibia, undergoes a loss of bone cortex, leading to weakening and fracture. Abnormal callus formation causes a "false joint" in the bone, leading to the term ("arthron" = joint).

A

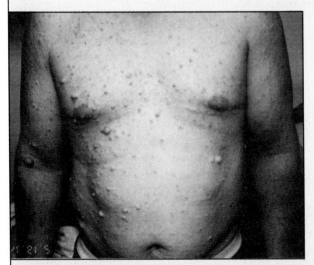

B

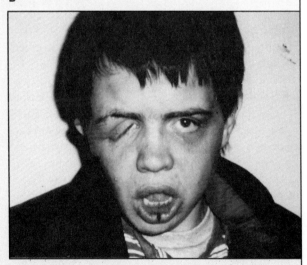

Figure 4-16 ■ Neurofibromatosis type 1. A, A young adult with multiple dermal neurofibromas of the trunk. Note also a *café-au-lait* spot in the right upper abdomen. B, In a second patient with NF1, a plexiform neurofibroma of the right orbit has distorted the eyelid, turning it down and producing facial asymmetry (*SOL* 9-13).

Continued.

an accidental bone fracture, can influence the severity of the disorder. Once a fracture occurs, casting and immobilization lead to a loss of bone mass, which further predisposes the patient to future fractures. Thus a chance environmental event (such as trauma leading to a fracture in a baby during delivery) can cause a significant increase in severity of expression. OI thus provides examples of each factor thought to influence variable expression: environmental events, modifier loci, and different mutations at the disease locus.

> **Variable expression of a genetic disease may be caused by environmental effects, modifier genes, or different mutations at the disease locus.**

Pleiotropy and Heterogeneity

Genes having more than one discernible effect on the body are said to be **pleiotropic**. A good example of a gene with pleiotropic effects is given by Marfan syndrome. First described in 1896 by Antoine Marfan, a French pediatrician, this autosomal dominant disorder affects the eye, the skeleton, and the cardiovascular system (see Clinical Commentary 4-5). All of the observed features of Marfan syndrome are due to unusually stretchable connective tissue. The gene for Marfan syndrome has been mapped to chromosome 15q, and it has been demonstrated that mutations in the gene encoding fibrillin, a component of connective tissue, are responsible for the multiple defects seen in this disorder. We have discussed several other single-gene diseases in which pleiotropy is seen (e.g., cystic fibrosis, in which sweat glands, lungs, and pancreas can be affected; OI, in which bones, teeth, and sclerae can be affected; sickle cell disease, in which erythrocytes, bone, and spleen can be affected).

> **Genes that exert effects on multiple aspects of physiology or anatomy are pleiotropic. Pleiotropy is a common feature of human genes.**

Just as a single gene may have multiple effects, a single disease phenotype may be caused by mutations at different loci in different families. A good example is given by OI. Recall from Chapter 2 that the subunits of the procollagen triple helix are encoded by two genes, one on chromosome 17 and the other on chromosome 7 (Fig. 4-18). A mutation occurring in either of these genes can alter the normal structure of the triple helix, resulting ultimately in OI. In one family the disease may be due to the chromosome 7 mutation, whereas in another family it may be due to the chromosome 17 mutation. The disease states produced by mutations of these two genes are in some cases clinically indistinguishable. The causation of the same disease phenotype by mutations at distinct loci is termed **locus heterogeneity** (compare with allelic heterogeneity, above). Table 4-2 lists some additional examples of diseases in which there is locus heterogeneity.

> **A disease that can be caused by mutations at different loci in different families is said to exhibit locus heterogeneity.**

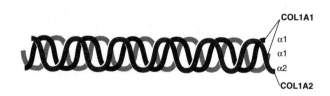

Figure 4-18 ■ Structure of the triple helix type 1 collagen protein. The two α1 chains are encoded by a gene on chromosome 17, and the α2 chain is encoded by a gene on chromosome 7.

Clinical Commentary 4-5. Marfan Syndrome, an Example of Pleiotropy

Marfan syndrome (Fig. 4-17) is seen in approximately 1 in 10,000 to 20,000 North Americans. It is characterized by defects in three major systems: the ocular, skeletal, and cardiovascular. The ocular defects include myopia, present in most Marfan patients, and detached lens (ectopia lentis), observed in about half of Marfan patients. The skeletal defects include dolichostenomelia (unusually long and slender limbs), pectus excavatum ("hollow chest"), pectus carinatum ("pigeon chest"), scoliosis, and arachnodactyly (literally "spider fingers," denoting the characteristically long, slender fingers). Marfan patients also typically exhibit joint hypermobility. The most life-threatening defects are those of the cardiovascular system. Most Marfan patients develop a prolapse of the mitral valve, a condition in which the cusps of the mitral valve protrude upward into the left atrium during systole. This can result in mitral regurgitation (leakage of blood back into the left atrium from the left ventricle). Mitral valve prolapse, however, is seen in 2% to 5% of the general population and is often of little consequence. Much more serious is dilatation (widening) of the ascending aorta, which is seen in 90% of Marfan patients. As dilatation increases, the aorta becomes susceptible to fatal dissection or rupture, particularly when cardiac output is high (as in heavy exercise or pregnancy). As the aorta widens, the left ventricle enlarges, and cardiomyopathy (damage to the heart muscle) ensues. The end result is congestive heart failure, another frequent cause of death among Marfan patients.

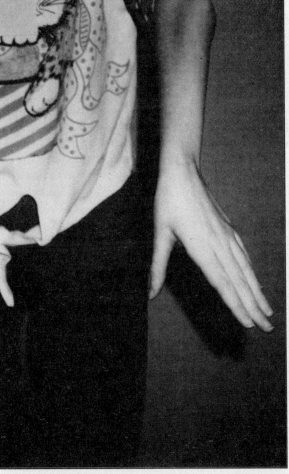

Figure 4-17 ■ *above,* A young man with Marfan syndrome, showing characteristically long limbs and narrow face. *right,* Arachnodactyly in an 8-year-old girl with Marfan syndrome (*SOL* 25, 26).

Continued.

Clinical Commentary 4-5. Marfan Syndrome, an Example of Pleiotropy—*cont'd*

All of these defects involve overly "stretchy" connective tissue. The role of connective tissue may be obvious for defects such as aortic dilatation and detached lens, but it may be less so for the skeletal defects. Normal bone growth is opposed by the periosteum, the connective tissue that covers bone. When the periosteum is more elastic than it should be, overgrowth of bone occurs, resulting in skeletal defects.

What is the basis of the connective tissue disorder? Answers are being provided by the recent discovery that Marfan patients have mutations of the chromosome 15 gene encoding **fibrillin**, a connective tissue protein. Fibrillin, a major component of microfibrils, is found in the aorta, the suspensory ligament of the lens, and the periosteum. The location of the gene product and its role as a component of connective tissue nicely explain the pleiotropic effects causing disturbances in the eye, the skeleton, and the cardiovascular system.

Treatment for Marfan syndrome includes regular ophthalmologic examinations and the avoidance of heavy exercise and contact sports. In addition, β-adrenergic blockers, such as propranolol, can be administered to decrease the abruptness of heart contractions. This reduces stress on the aorta. In some cases the aorta and aortic valve are surgically replaced with a synthetic tube and artificial valve.

A number of historical figures are thought to have possibly had Marfan syndrome, including Niccolo Paganini, the violinist, and Sergei Rachmaninoff, the composer and pianist. Most controversial is the proposal that Abraham Lincoln may have had Marfan syndrome. He had skeletal features consistent with the disorder, and examination of his medical records has shown that he may well have had aortic dilatation. Some have suggested that he was in congestive heart failure at the time of his death and that, had he not been assassinated, he still would not have survived his second term of office. Lincoln has no living descendants that could be evaluated for Marfan syndrome. However, samples of his blood, bone, and hair have been preserved. Once the specific mutations for Marfan syndrome are better characterized, it may be possible, using PCR, to amplify DNA from these specimens. DNA sequencing could then be used to determine whether indeed Lincoln had Marfan syndrome.

Although this may seem like a silly exercise to some, it should be pointed out that genetic diseases, such as Marfan syndrome, are frequently viewed as serious impediments to success. To find that one of the greatest presidents in United States history had this disorder would be an eloquent reply.

Genomic Imprinting

Mendel's experimental work with garden peas established that the phenotype is the same whether a given allele is inherited from the mother or the father. Indeed this principle has been part of the central dogma of genetics. Recently, however, it has become increasingly apparent that this principle does not always hold. A striking example is provided by a deletion on the long arm of chromosome 15. When this deletion is inherited from the father, the offspring manifest a disease known as Prader-Willi syndrome. The disease phenotype includes short stature, obesity, mild to moderate mental retardation, and hypogonadism (Fig. 4-19, *A*). When the deletion is inherited from the mother, the offspring develop Angelman syndrome, which is characterized by severe mental retardation, seizures, and an ataxic gait (Fig. 4-19, *B*). In most cases the deletions inherited from the father and the mother are cytogenetically indistinguishable.

Table 4-2 ■ Examples of diseases in which there is locus heterogeneity

Disease	Description	Chromosomes on which known loci are located
Retinitis pigmentosa	Progressive retinopathy and loss of vision	1, 3, 4, 5, 6, 7, 8, 11, 14, 15, 16, 17, 19, X
Osteogenesis imperfecta	Brittle bone disease	7, 17
Charcot-Marie-Tooth disease	Peripheral neuropathy	1, 3, 8, 17, X
Familial Alzheimer disease	Progressive dementia	14, 19, 21
Familial melanoma	Autosomal dominant melanoma (skin cancer)	1, 9
Hereditary nonpolyposis colorectal cancer	Autosomal dominant colorectal cancer	2, 3
Adult polycystic kidney disease	Accumulation of renal cysts leading to kidney failure	4, 16

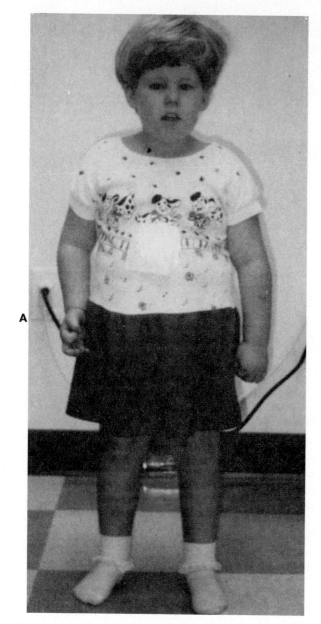
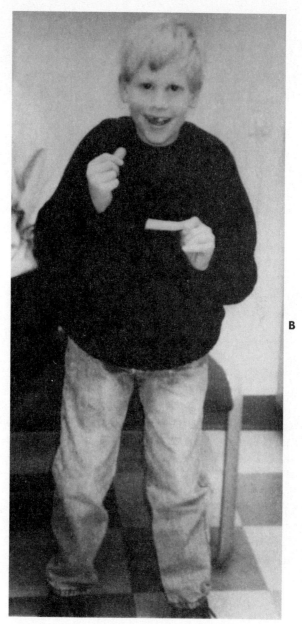

Figure 4-19 ■ Illustration of the possible effect of imprinting on chromosome 15 deletions. A: Inheritance of the deletion from the father produces Prader-Willi syndrome (note the inverted V-shaped upper lip and truncal obesity). B: Inheritance of the deletion from the mother produces Angelman syndrome (note the characteristic posture). C: Pedigrees illustrate the inheritance of this deletion (see page 76).

Continued.

What could cause these differences? It now appears that they involve the phenomenon of **genomic imprinting**. That is, genes inherited from the mother, while identical in DNA sequence to those inherited from the father, differ in some other way (the "imprint"). The imprint alters the activity level of genes, so deletions of paternally and maternally derived chromosomes may produce different phenotypes. The precise nature of genomic imprints is not yet understood. However, research with transgenic mice (mice that have had a single foreign gene, a transgene, placed in their genome using recombinant DNA techniques) indicates that the expression level of these transgenes is influenced by the parental origin of the gene (imprinting) *and* that the activity level is associated with the degree of methylation of the gene. Genes that are more highly methylated are less likely to be transcribed into messenger RNA. Methylation could represent the imprint itself. At this point, however, only an *association* between methylation and imprinting has been established. It is not clear wheth-

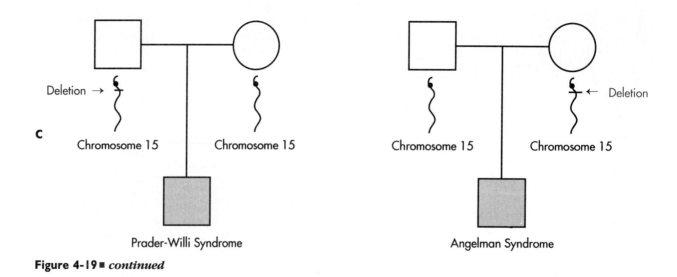

Figure 4-19 ■ *continued*

er methylation is the actual mechanism or merely a secondary consequence of imprinting.

Molecular analysis using many of the tools and techniques outlined in Chapter 3 (RFLPs, microsatellite polymorphisms, cloning, and DNA sequencing) has identified several specific genes in the "critical region" of chromosome 15 that is associated with Prader-Willi and Angelman syndromes. These studies support the imprinting hypothesis at the single-gene level: defects in some genes cause Prader-Willi syndrome only when inherited from the father, whereas defects in one or more other genes cause Angelman syndrome only when inherited from the mother.

> **Some disease genes may be expressed differently when inherited from one sex versus the other. This is genomic imprinting. It is associated with, and possibly caused by, methylation.**

Anticipation

Since the early part of this century, it has been observed that some genetic diseases seem to display an earlier age of onset and/or more severe expression in more recent generations of a pedigree. This pattern was termed **anticipation**, and it has been the subject of considerable controversy and speculation. Many researchers believed that it was an artifact of better observation and clinical diagnosis in more recent times: a disorder that previously may have been undiagnosed until age 60 might now be diagnosed at age 40 simply because of better diagnostic tools. Others, however, believed that anticipation may be a real biological

phenomenon, although evidence for the actual mechanism was elusive.

Recently molecular genetics has provided good evidence that anticipation does in fact have a biological basis. This has come in part from studies of myotonic dystrophy, an autosomal dominant disease that involves progressive muscle deterioration (Fig. 4-20). Seen in approximately 1 in 8000 individuals, myotonic dystrophy is the most common muscular dystrophy that affects adults. In addition to affecting skeletal muscles, this disorder involves cardiac arrhythmia (abnormal heart rhythm) and cataracts. It has been mapped to chromosome 19, and the gene was recently cloned.

Analysis of the gene has produced some surprising results. The disease mutation is an expanded CTG trinucleotide repeat (Chapter 3) that lies in the 3′ untranslated portion of the gene (i.e., a region transcribed into mRNA but not translated into protein). The *number* of these repeats is strongly correlated with severity of the disease. Unaffected individuals typically have 5 to 30 copies of the repeat. Those with 50 to 100 copies may be mildly affected or have no symptoms. Those with full-blown myotonic dystrophy may have anywhere from 100 to several thousand copies of the repeat sequence. The number of repeats often increases with succeeding generations: a mildly affected parent with 80 repeats may produce a severely affected offspring with more than 1000 repeats (Fig. 4-21). Several families have now been documented in which the number of repeats increases through successive generations, accompanied by increasing severity of the disorder. There is thus strong evidence that expansion of this tri-

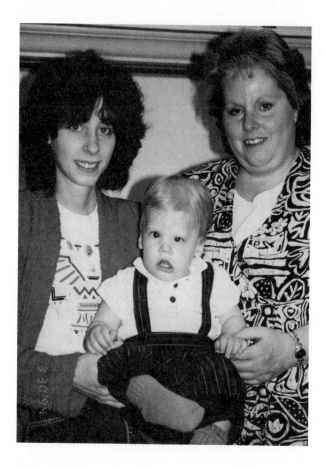

Figure 4-20 ■ **A three-generation family affected with myotonic dystrophy. The degree of severity increases in each generation. The grandmother (*right*) is only slightly affected, but the mother (*left*) has a characteristic narrow face and somewhat limited facial expression. The baby is more severely affected and has the facial features of children with neonatal-onset myotonic dystrophy, including an open, triangular-shaped mouth. The infant has more than 1000 copies of the trinucleotide repeat, whereas the mother and grandmother each have approximately 100 repeats. (*SOL 27, 28*)**

nucleotide repeat is the cause of anticipation in myotonic dystrophy.

Much remains to be discovered about this phenomenon. How does expansion occur? How does it affect the gene product? Why does the severe congenital form of myotonic dystrophy arise only when the disease gene is inherited from the mother? Is imprinting involved? It is especially mystifying that the repeated sequence lies *outside* of the translated portion of the gene. This subject is now the focus of intense investigation, and it promises to reveal further insights into the molecular basis of genetic disease.

As discussed in Clinical Commentary 4-2, repeat expansion is also seen in Huntington disease. It has

also been observed in the fragile X syndrome, a leading genetic cause of mental retardation to be discussed in Chapter 5. It is correlated with forms of anticipation in both of these diseases. In addition, repeat expansion is seen in spinocerebellar ataxia type 1, an autosomal dominant neurodegenerative disease. As in myotonic dystrophy, larger repeat unit expansions are correlated with earlier age of onset of the disorder. Kennedy disease (spinal bulbar muscular atrophy), a disorder that involves progressive muscle weakness secondary to neural degeneration, is also characterized by a repeat expansion. Table 4-3 lists several additional diseases that are caused by trinucleotide repeat expansions.

Anticipation refers to progressively earlier or more severe expression of a disease in more recent times. Expansion of DNA repeats has been shown to cause anticipation in some genetic diseases.

■ CONSANGUINITY IN HUMAN POPULATIONS

Although relatively rare in Western populations, consanguinity is common in many populations of the world. For example, first-cousin marriage is seen in 20% to 50% of marriages in many countries of the Mideast, and uncle-niece and first-cousin marriages are common in some parts of India. Because relatives often share disease genes inherited from a common ancestor, consanguineous unions are more likely to produce offspring affected by autosomal recessive disorders. It is possible to quantify the proportion of genes shared by a pair of relatives by estimating the **coefficient of relationship** (Box 4-1 pg. 80). Estimation of this quantity shows, for example, that siblings share one half of their genes on average, first cousins share one eighth, first cousins once removed share one sixteenth, second cousins share one thirty-second, and so on.*

Consanguinity and the Frequency of Recessive Diseases

Recall that about one in 25 whites is a heterozygous carrier of the CF gene. A man who carries the CF gene thus has a one in 25 chance of meeting

---

*First cousins are the offspring of two siblings and thus share a set of grandparents. A first cousin once removed is the offspring of one's first cousin. Second cousins are the offspring of two different first cousins and thus share a set of great-grandparents.

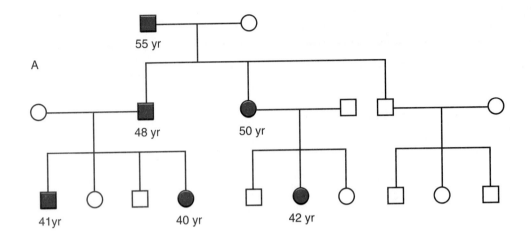

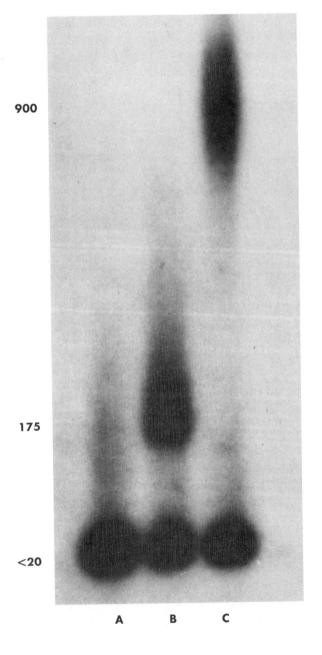

Figure 4-21 ■ *above,* Myotonic dystrophy pedigree illustrating anticipation. In this case the age of onset for family members affected with an autosomal dominant disease is lower in more recent generations. *left,* An autoradiogram from a Southern blot analysis of the myotonic dystrophy gene in three individuals. Individual A is homozygous for two 4-5 repeat alleles and is normal. Individual B has one normal allele and one disease allele (175 repeats); this individual has myotonic dystrophy. Individual C is also affected with myotonic dystrophy and has one normal allele and a disease-causing allele with approximately 900 repeats. (Courtesy of Drs. Kenneth Ward and Elaine Lyon, University of Utah Health Sciences Center).

another carrier if he mates with somebody in the general population. He only triples his chance of meeting another carrier when he mates with a first cousin, who has a 1/8 chance of carrying the same gene. However, a carrier of a relatively rare recessive disease, such as classical galactosemia (a metabolic disorder in which galactose cannot be metabolized), has only a 1/170 chance of meeting another carrier in the general population (*SOL* 57). However, because he shares one eighth of his genes with his first cousin, the chance that his first cousin also has the galactosemia gene is still one eighth. With this rarer disease, a carrier is 21 times more likely to mate with another carrier in a first cousin marriage than in a marriage with an unrelated individual. This illustrates an important principle: the rarer the recessive disease, the more likely that the parents of the case are consanguineous.

This principle has been substantiated empirically. It has been estimated that only about 5% of cases of PKU, in which the carrier frequency is about 1/50 in whites, are due to consanguineous matings.

Table 4-3 ■ Diseases associated with trinucleotide repeat expansions

Disease	Description	Repeat sequence	Normal and abnormal range	Parent in whom expansion usually occurs	Anticipation
Huntington disease	Loss of motor control, dementia, affective disorder	CAG	11–34; 36–100 or more	More often in father	Yes
Myotonic dystrophy	Muscle loss, cardiac arrhythmia, cataracts, frontal balding	CTG	5–30; 100 to several thousand	Either parent but expansion to congenital form through mother	Yes
X-linked spinal and bulbar muscular atrophy	Adult-onset motor neuron disease associated with androgen insensitivity	CAG	17–26; 40–52	More often through father	Yes
Spinocerebellar ataxia type 1	Progressive ataxia, dysarthria, dysmetria	CAG	19–36; 43–81	More often through father	Yes
Fragile X syndrome (FRAXA)	Mental retardation, large ears and jaws, macroorchidism in males	CGG	6–50; >230	Exclusively through mother	Yes
Fragile site FRAXE	Mild mental retardation	CGG	6–35; >200	More often through mother	?
Dentatorubral-pallidoluysian atrophy/Haw River syndrome	Cerebellar atrophy, ataxia, myoclonic epilepsy, choreoathetosis, dementia	CAG	7–25; 49–75	More often through father	Yes
Machado-Joseph disease	dystonia, distal muscular atrophy, ataxia, external ophthalmoplegia	CAG	12–37; 66–84	More often through father	Yes
Friedreich's ataxia	progressive limb ataxia, dysarthria, hypertrophic cardiomyopathy, pyramidal weakness in legs	GAA	7–22; 200–900	Disorder is autosomal recessive, so disease alleles are inherited from both parents	No

However, Wilson disease (a recessive disorder in which excess copper is retained resulting in severe liver damage) is much rarer, with an estimated carrier frequency between 1/110 and 1/160 (*SOL* 58, 59). Here, approximately 50% of cases are the result of consanguineous matings.

Consanguinity increases the chance that a mating couple will both carry the same disease gene. It is seen more frequently in pedigrees involving rare recessive diseases than in those involving common recessive diseases.

Health Consequences of Consanguinity

It has been estimated that each person carries the equivalent of one to five recessive genes that would be lethal to offspring if matched with another copy of the gene. It would therefore be expected that matings between relatives would more often produce offspring with genetic diseases. Most empirical studies show that the mortality rates among the offspring of first-cousin marriages are substantially greater than those of the general population (Table 4-4 page 81). Similarly, the prevalence of genetic disease is roughly twice as high among the offspring of first-cousin marriages as among the offspring of unrelated individuals. First-cousin marriages are illegal in most states of the United States. Marriages between closer relatives (except double first cousins, who share both sets of grandparents) are prohibited throughout the United States.

Box 4-1. Measurement of Consanguinity: The Coefficient of Relationship

To determine the possible consequences of a consanguineous mating, it is useful to know what proportion of genes are shared by two related individuals. The **coefficient of relationship** is a measure of this proportion. Clearly, individuals who are more closely related must share a greater proportion of their genes. To begin with a simple example, an individual receives half of his or her genes from each parent. Thus the coefficient of relationship between a parent and offspring is 1/2. This also means that the probability that the parent and offspring share a given gene (for example, a disease allele) is 1/2.

To continue with a more complex example, suppose that a man is known to be a heterozygous carrier for galactosemia, a relatively rare autosomal recessive metabolic disorder. If he mates with his first cousin, what is the probability that she also carries this disease gene? We know that this probability must be higher than that of the general population, because first cousins share one set of grandparents. There is thus a possibility that the grandparent who transmitted the galactosemia gene to the known carrier also transmitted it to the carrier's cousin. The coefficient of relationship specifies this probability. A pedigree for a first-cousin mating is shown in Figure 4-22, *A*. The carrier is labeled A, and his cousin is labeled E. Because we are interested only in the family members who are related to both the man and his cousin, the pedigree is condensed in Figure 4-22, *B*. The diagram in Figure 4-22, *B* includes only the individuals who form a "path" between the man and his cousin.

To estimate the coefficient of relationship, we begin with the carrier and ascend the pedigree. We know that there is a probability of 1/2 that the known carrier inherited the gene from the parent in the path, labeled B. There is also a probability of 1/2 that he inherited the gene from his other parent, who is not related to his cousin and is thus not included in the diagram. By similar reasoning the probability that individual B inherited the disease gene from his parent, individual C, is also 1/2. The probability that individual C in turn passed on the disease gene to his offspring, D, is 1/2, and the probability that D passed the disease gene to E is also 1/2. Thus, for E to share a disease gene with A, each of these four events must have taken place. The multiplication rule dictates that, to find the probability that all four events have taken place, we take the product of all four probabilities. Because each of these probabilities is 1/2, this gives $(1/2)^4 = 1/16$.

If individuals A and E shared only one grandparent, the coefficient of relationship would be 1/16. But as with most first cousins, they share a common grandfather and grandmother. Thus there are two paths through which the disease gene could have passed. To obtain the probability that the gene passed through the second path, we use the same procedure as in the previous paragraph and obtain a probability of 1/16. Now we need to estimate the probability that the gene went through either the first path *or* the second (i.e., through one grandparent or the other). The addition rule states that we can add these two probabilities together to get the overall probability that A and E share a disease gene: 1/16 + 1/16 = 1/8. The probability that the carrier's cousin shares his disease allele, as a result of their descent from a common set of grandparents, is thus 1/8. This is the coefficient of relationship for first cousins.*

---

*A related quantity, frequently used in population genetics, is the **inbreeding coefficient**. This coefficient is the probability that an individual is homozygous at a locus as a result of consanguinity in his or her parents. For a given type of mating, the inbreeding coefficient of an individual always equals the parents' coefficient of relationship multiplied by one half (e.g., the inbreeding coefficient for the offspring of a first-cousin mating is 1/16).

Continued.

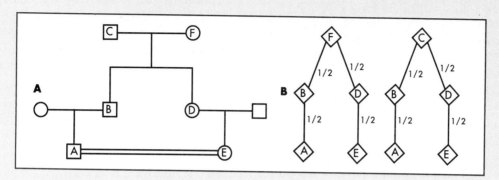

Figure 4-22 ■ A, Pedigree for a first-cousin mating. **B,** this pedigree is condensed to show only those individuals in the pedigree who are related to both of the first cousins.

It should be recognized that individual E could also inherit a disease allele from an ancestor not included in either of these paths. However, for disease alleles, which are relatively rare in populations, this probability is small and can usually be disregarded.

The rules for calculating the coefficient of relationship can be summarized as follows:

1. Each individual can appear in a route only once.

2. Always begin with one individual, proceed up the pedigree to the common ancestor, then down the pedigree to the other individual.

3. The coefficient of relationship for one route is given by $(1/2)^{n-1}$, where n is the number of individuals in the route.

4. If there are multiple routes (i.e., multiple common ancestors), the probabilities estimated for each route are added together.

Table 4-4 ■ Mortality levels among cousin and unrelated control marriages in selected human populations*

Population	Mortality type	1.0 cousin %	1.0 cousin N	1.5 cousin† %	1.5 cousin† N	2.0 cousin %	2.0 cousin N	Unrelated %	Unrelated N
Amish (Old Order)	Prereproductive	14.4	1218‡	—	—	13.3	6064	8.2	17,200
Bombay, India	Perinatal	4.8	3309	2.8	176	0	30	2.8	35,620
France (Loir-et-Cher)	Prereproductive	17.7	282	6.7	105	11.7	240	8.6	1117
Fukuoka, Japan	0–6 years	10.0	3442	8.3	1048	9.2	1066	6.4	5224
Hirado, Japan	Prereproductive	18.9	2301	15.3	764	14.7	1209	14.3	28,569
Kerala, India	Prereproductive	18.6	391	—	—	11.8	34	8.7	770
Punjab, Pakistan	Prereproductive	22.1	3532	22.9	1114	20.1	57	16.4	4731
Sweden	Prereproductive	14.1	185	13.7	227	11.4	79	16.4	625
Utah Mormons	Prereproductive	22.4	1048	15.3	517	12.2	1129	13.2	302,454

*Modified from Jorde LB: In Dulbecco R, editor: Encyclopedia of human biology, vol 4, San Diego, 1991, Academic Press.
†First cousins once removed.
‡Includes 1.5 cousins.

Very few data exist for matings between first-degree relatives (defined as **incest**). The limited data indicate that the proportion of abnormal offspring produced by incestuous matings is very high: between one fourth and one half. Mental retardation is particularly common among these offspring. Because of small sample sizes in these studies, it is difficult to separate the effects of genetics and substandard environment. It is likely that the problems experienced by the offspring of incestuous matings are due to both genetic and environmental influences.

At the population level consanguinity increases the frequency of genetic disease and mortality. The closer the degree of consanguinity, the greater the increase.

■ STUDY QUESTIONS

1. Using protein electrophoresis, 100 members of a population have been studied to determine whether they carry genes for normal hemoglobin (HbA) or sickle hemoglobin (HbS). The following genotypes were observed:

   HbA/HbA, 88; HbA/HbS, 10; HbS/HbS, 2. What are the gene frequencies of HbA and HbS? What are the observed genotype frequencies? Assuming Hardy-Weinberg proportions, what are the *expected* genotype frequencies?

2. Approximately 1 in 10,000 whites is born with PKU. What is the frequency of the disease gene? What is the frequency of heterozygous carriers in the population?

3. A man who has achondroplasia marries a phenotypically normal woman. If they have four children, what is the probability that none of them will be affected with this disorder? What is the probability that all of them will be affected?

4. The estimated penetrance for familial retinoblastoma is approximately 90%. If a man has had familial retinoblastoma and mates with a woman who does not have the retinoblastoma gene, what is the risk that their offspring will develop retinoblastoma?

5. A 30-year-old woman had a sister who died of infantile Tay-Sachs disease, an autosomal recessive disorder that is fatal by age 6. What is the probability that this woman is a heterozygous carrier of the Tay-Sachs gene?

6. It is possible to extract the nucleus from a somatic cell and place it into a mature egg cell. In amphibians the egg cell will then develop and mature into an adult without fertilization by a sperm cell (a process known as parthenogenesis). The same experiment has been attempted in mice, but it always results in early prenatal death. Explain this.

7. Two individuals who share a single great-grandparent mate (they are labeled A and B in the accompanying diagram). What is their coefficient of relationship? Suppose that one member of this couple is a heterozygous carrier for PKU. What is the probability that this couple will produce a child affected with PKU?

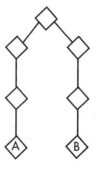

■ ADDITIONAL READING

Barlow DP: Gametic imprinting in mammals. Science 270:1610–1613, 1995.

Bernards A, Gusella JF: The importance of genetic mosaicism in human disease, N Eng J Med 331:1447–1449, 1994.

Buiting K, Saitoh S, Gross S, Dittrich B, Schwartz S, Nicholls RD, Horsthemke B: Inherited microdeletions in the Angelman and Prader-Willi syndromes define an imprinting centre on chromosome 15. Nature Genet 9:395–400, 1995.

Dietz HC, Ramirez F, Sakai LY: Marfan's syndrome and other microfibrillar diseases, Adv Hum Genet 22:153–186, 1994.

Dietz HC, Pyeritz RE: Mutations in the human gene for fibrillin-1 (FBN1) in the Marfan syndrome and related disorders, Hum Molec Genet 4:1799–1809, 1995.

Folstein SE: Huntington's disease: a disorder of families, Baltimore, 1989, Johns Hopkins University Press.

Francomano CA: The genetic basis of dwarfism. N Eng J Med 332:58–59, 1995.

Godfrey M: The Marfan syndrome. In Beighton P., editor: McKusick's heritable disorders of connective tissue, ed 5, St Louis, 1993 Mosby-Year Book.

Harper PS, Harley WG, Reardon W, and Shaw DJ: Anticipation in myotonic dystrophy: new light on an old problem, Am J Hum Genet 51:10–16, 1992.

Harris PC, Ward CJ, Peral B, Hughes J: Autosomal dominant polycystic kidney disease: molecular analysis, Hum Molec Genet 4:1745–1749, 1995.

Huntington's Disease Collaborative Research Group: A novel gene containing a trinucleotide repeat that is expanded and unstable on Huntington's disease chromosomes, Cell, 72:971–983, 1993.

Huson SM, Hughes RAC (editors): The neurofibromatoses: A pathogenetic and clinical overview, London, 1994, Chapman & Hall Medical.

Jorde LB: Inbreeding in human populations. In Dulbecco R, editor: Encyclopedia of Human Biology, vol 4, San Diego, 1991, Academic Press.

Phillips JA and Cogan JD: Genetic basis of endocrine disease, 6, Molecular basis of familial human growth hormone deficiency, J Clin Endocrinol and Metab 78:11–16, 1994.

Shen MH, Harper PS, Upadhyaya M: Molecular genetics of neurofibromatosis type 1 (NF1), J Med Genet 33:2–17, 1996.

Spritz RA: Molecular genetics of oculocutaneous albinism, Hum Molec Genet 3:1469–1475, 1994.

Sutherland GR, Richards RI: Simple tandem DNA repeats and human genetic disease, Proc Natl Acad Sci USA 92:3636–3641, 1995.

Viskochil D, White R, and Cawthon R: The neurofibromatosis type 1 gene, Annu Rev Neurosci 16:183–205, 1993.

Warren ST: The expanding world of trinucleotide repeats, Science 271:1374–1375, 1996.

Weinberg RA: The retinoblastoma protein and cell cycle control, Cell 81:323–330, 1995.

Welsh MJ, Smith AE: Cystic fibrosis, Sci. Amer. 273:52–59, 1995.

Wilkie AOM: The molecular basis of dominance, J. Med. Genet. 31:89–98, 1994.

5 Sex-linked and Mitochondrial Inheritance

The previous chapter dealt with disease genes located on the 22 autosomes. In this chapter we discuss disease genes located on the sex chromosomes and the mitochondria. The human X chromosome is a large chromosome, containing about 5% of the nuclear genome's DNA (approximately 160 million base pairs, or 160 mb). More than 400 coding genes have been localized to the X chromosome. Diseases caused by genes on this chromosome are said to be **X-linked**. The great majority of known X-linked diseases are recessive, although there are also a few X-linked dominant diseases. In contrast to the X chromosome, the Y chromosome is small (70 mb) and contains very few known genes. No genetic diseases are known to be Y-linked. Several diseases are now known to be caused by mutations in mitochondrial DNA; these are discussed at the end of this chapter.

■ X INACTIVATION

It has long been known that females have two X chromosome and males have only one. It has also been known for most of this century that the X chromosome contains many important protein-coding genes. Thus, females have two copies of each X-linked gene, whereas males have only one copy. Yet males and females do not differ in terms of the products (such as enzyme levels) produced by most of these genes. What could account for this?

In the early 1960s Mary Lyon hypothesized that one X chromosome in each somatic cell of the female is inactivated. This would result in **dosage compensation**, an equalization of X-linked gene products in males and females. The **Lyon hypothesis** stated that X inactivation occurs early in female embryonic development and that the X chromosome contributed by the father is inactivated in some cells, whereas in other cells the X chromosome contributed by the mother is inactivated. This

inactivation process is *random,* so the maternally and paternally derived X chromosomes will each be inactivated in about half of the embryo's cells. Thus inactivation, like gamete transmission, is analogous to a coin-tossing experiment. Once an X chromosome is inactivated in a cell, it will remain inactive in all descendants of the cell. X inactivation is therefore said to be randomly determined, but fixed. As a result of X inactivation, all females have two distinct populations of cells: one population has an active paternally derived X chromosome, and the other has an active maternally derived X chromosome (see Fig. 5-1 for a summary of this process). With two populations of cells, females are mosaics (see Chapter 4) for the X chromosome. Males, having only one copy of the X chro-

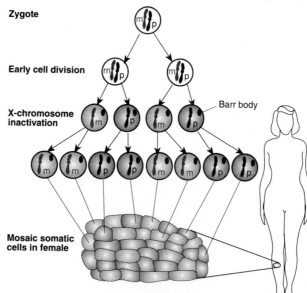

Figure 5-1 ■ The X inactivation process. The maternal (m) and paternal (p) X chromosomes are both active in the zygote and in early embryonic cells. X inactivation then takes place, resulting in cells having *either* an active paternal X or an active maternal X. Females are thus X chromosome mosaics, as shown in the tissue sample at the bottom of the figure.

mosome, are not mosaics and are **hemizygous** for the X chromosome (hemi = "half").

> **The Lyon hypothesis states that one X chromosome in each cell is randomly inactivated early in the embryonic development of females. This ensures that females, who have two copies of the X chromosome, will produce X-linked gene products in quantities roughly similar to males (dosage compensation).**

The Lyon hypothesis relied on several pieces of evidence, most of which were derived from animal studies. First, it was known that females are typically mosaics for some X-linked traits while males are not. For example, female mice heterozygous for certain X-linked coat-color genes exhibit a dappled coloring of their fur, whereas male mice do not. A similar example is given by the "calico cat." These female cats have alternating black and orange patches of fur that correspond to two populations of cells: one that contains X chromosomes in which the "orange" allele is active and one containing X chromosomes in which the "black" allele is active. Male cats of this species do not exhibit alternating colors. A final example, seen in humans, is X-linked ocular albinism. This is an X-linked recessive condition characterized by a lack of melanin production in the retina and ocular problems such as **nystagmus** (rapid involuntary eye movements)

and decreased visual acuity. Males who inherit the mutation show a uniform lack of melanin in their retinas, while female heterozygotes exhibit alternating patches of pigmented and nonpigmented tissue (Fig. 5-2A, B).

The Lyon hypothesis was also supported by biochemical evidence. The enzyme glucose-6-phosphate dehydrogenase (G6PD) is encoded by a gene on the X chromosome and is present in equal quantities in males and females (dosage compensation). In females heterozygous for two common G6PD alleles (labeled *A* and *B*), some skin cells produced only the *A* variant of the enzyme and others produced only the *B* variant. This is further proof of X chromosome mosaicism in females.

Finally, cytogenetic studies in the 1940s had shown that interphase cells of female cats often contained a densely staining chromatin mass in their nuclei (Fig. 5-3). These masses were never seen in males. They were termed **Barr bodies**, after Murray Barr, one of the scientists who described them. Barr and his colleague Ewart Bertram hypothesized that the Barr body, also termed **sex chromatin**, represented a highly condensed X chromosome. It is now known that Barr and Bertram were correct and that the inactive X chromosome is observable as a Barr body in the somatic cells of normal females. Its condensed state reflects the fact that its DNA is replicated later in the S phase than that of other chromosomes.

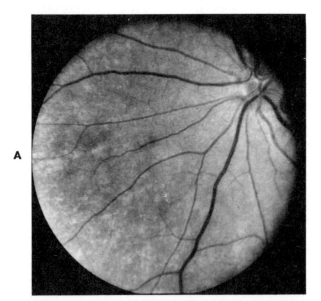 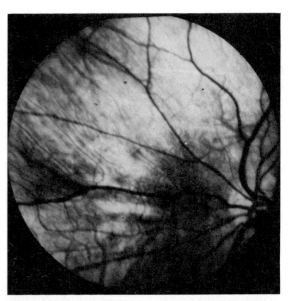

Figure 5-2 ■ A, Fundus photograph of a female heterozygous carrier for X-linked ocular albinism. The pigmented and nonpigmented patches in the retina demonstrate mosaicism. **B,** Fundus photograph of the heterozygous carrier's affected son, showing a distinct lack of melanin pigment. (Courtesy of Dr. Don Creel, University of Utah Health Sciences Center.)

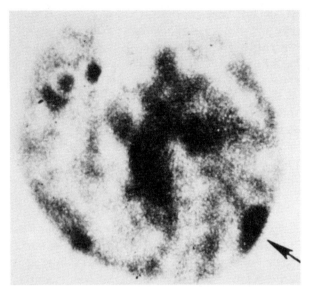

Figure 5-3 ■ A Barr body, which is the inactive X chromosome, is visible as a densely staining chromatin mass in the interphase nucleus of a normal female's somatic cell. DNA-based tools have now supplanted Barr bodies as a means of sex determination.

The Lyon hypothesis is supported by cytogenetic evidence: Barr bodies, which are inactive X chromosomes, are seen only in cells with two or more X chromosomes. It is also supported by biochemical and animal studies showing mosaicism in female heterozygotes.

Further study has largely verified the Lyon hypothesis. mRNA is transcribed from only one X chromosome in each somatic cell of a normal female. The inactivation process takes place within approximately 2 weeks after fertilization, when the embryo consists of several hundred to several thousand cells. Inactivation is initiated at a single location on the X chromosome (the **X inactivation center**) and then spreads along the chromosome. Although inactivation is random among cells that make up the embryo itself, only the paternally derived X chromosome is inactivated in cells that will become extraembryonic tissue (e.g., the placenta). Although X inactivation is permanent for all somatic cells in the female, the inactive X chromosome must become *reactivated* in the female's germ line so that each egg cell will receive one active copy of the chromosome.

An important implication of the Lyon hypothesis is that the number of Barr bodies in somatic cells is always one less than the number of X chromosomes. Normal females have one Barr body in each somatic cell, whereas normal males have

none. Females with Turner syndrome (see Chapter 6), having only one X chromosome, have no Barr bodies. Males with Klinefelter syndrome (two X chromosomes and a Y chromosome), have one Barr body in their somatic cells, and females having three X chromosomes per cell have two Barr bodies in each somatic cell. This pattern leads to another question: if the extra X chromosomes are inactivated, why aren't people with extra (or missing) X chromosomes phenotypically normal?

The answer to this question is that X inactivation is *incomplete.* Several regions of the X chromosome remain active in all copies. In particular, the tip of the short arm of the X chromosome does not undergo inactivation. This is the region that is highly homologous to the distal short arm of the Y chromosome (see Chapter 6). Other regions that escape inactivation include those that contain the genes for steroid sulfatase, the Xg blood group, and Kallman syndrome (a disorder that causes hypogonadism and an inability to perceive odor). Having extra (or missing) copies of active portions of the X chromosome must contribute to phenotypic abnormality.

X inactivation is random, fixed, and incomplete. The latter fact helps to explain why, despite X inactivation, individuals with abnormal numbers of sex chromosomes are not phenotypically normal.

The actual mechanism underlying X inactivation is not well understood. However, it is known that X inactivation is correlated with methylation. Many CG dinucleotides in the 5' regions of genes on the inactive X are heavily methylated, and administration of demethylating agents, such as 5-azacytidine, can partially reactivate an inactive X chromosome in vitro. However, methylation does not appear to be involved in spreading the inactivation signal from the inactivation center to the remainder of the X chromosome. It is thus likely to be an important part of the inactivation process, but not the sole mechanism.

The gene responsible for X inactivation has been isolated. This gene, termed *XIST,* is located on the proximal long arm of the X chromosome. As expected, it is transcribed only on the inactive X chromosome, and its mRNA transcripts are detected in normal females but not in normal males. Further study of this gene and its product will doubtless lead to a much better understanding of the process of X inactivation.

X inactivation is associated with methylation of the inactive X chromosome. The gene responsible for X inactivation, which is expressed only on the inactive X chromosome, has been identified.

■ SEX-LINKED INHERITANCE

Sex-linked genes are those that are located on either the X or the Y chromosomes. Because no disease genes are known to be located on the human Y chromosome, our attention is focused on X-linked diseases.

X-Linked Recessive Inheritance

A number of well-known diseases and traits are caused by X-linked recessive genes. These include hemophilia A (Clinical Commentary 5-1), Duchenne muscular dystrophy (Clinical Commentary 5-2), and red-green color blindness (Box 5-1). The inheritance patterns and recurrence risks for X-linked recessive diseases differ substantially from those of diseases caused by autosomal genes.

Because females inherit two copies of the X chromosome, they can be homozygous for a disease allele at a given locus, heterozygous, or homozygous for the normal allele at the locus. In other words, an X-linked recessive trait behaves much like an autosomal recessive trait in females. However, only one X chromosome is active in any given somatic cell. This means that about half of the cells in a heterozygous female will express a disease allele and half of the cells will express the normal allele. Thus, as with autosomal recessive traits, the heterozygote will produce about 50% of the nor-

mal level of gene product. Ordinarily this is sufficient for a normal phenotype. The situation is different for males, who are hemizygous for the X chromosome. If a male inherits a recessive disease gene on the X chromosome, he will be affected by the disease because the Y chromosome does not carry a normal allele to counteract the effects of the disease gene. Hence, in X-linked inheritance, the terms "dominant" and "recessive" really apply only to females.

An X-linked recessive disease with gene frequency q will be seen in a proportion q of males. This is because of the fact that all males having the mutation will manifest the disease. Females, needing two copies of the mutant allele to express the disease, will have a disease frequency of only q^2, as in autosomal recessive diseases. For example, hemophilia A ("classical" hemophilia; see Clinical Commentary 5-1) is seen in about 1 in 10,000 males ($q = 0.0001$). Affected female homozygotes are almost never seen, since $q^2 = 0.00000001$, or 1 in 100,000,000. This example shows that in general males are more frequently affected with X-linked recessive diseases than females, with this difference becoming more pronounced as the disease becomes rarer.

Because females have two copies of the X chromosome and males have only one (hemizygosity), X-linked recessive diseases are much more common among males than females.

Pedigrees for X-linked recessive diseases display several characteristics that distinguish them from pedigrees for autosomal dominant and recessive

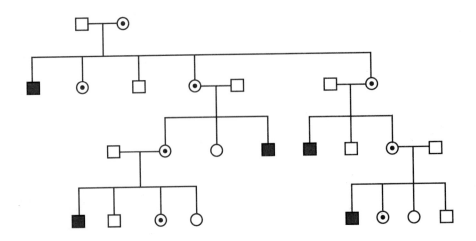

Figure 5-6 ■ A pedigree showing the inheritance of an X-linked recessive trait. Solid symbols represent affected individuals, and dotted symbols represent heterozygous carriers.

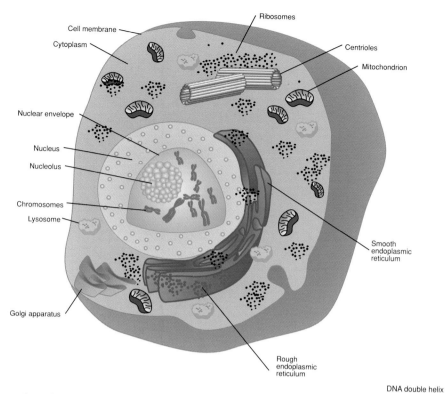

Color Plate 1. The anatomy of the cell. See also Figure 2-1.

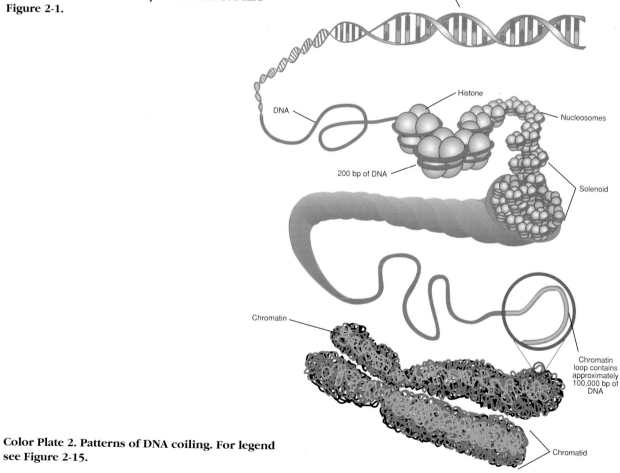

Color Plate 2. Patterns of DNA coiling. For legend see Figure 2-15.

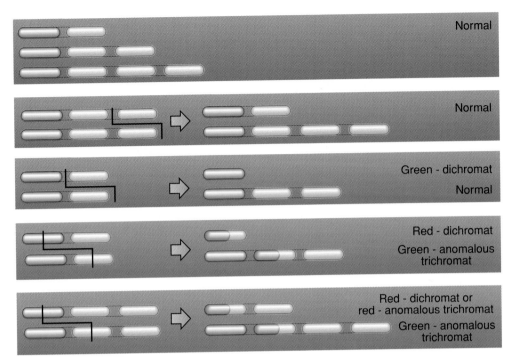

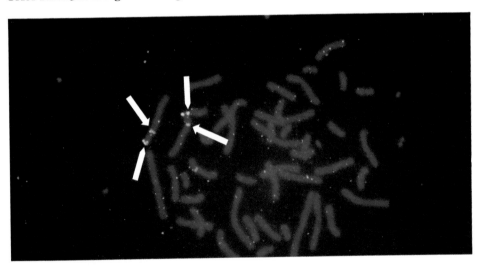

Color Plate 3. For legend see Figure 5-17.

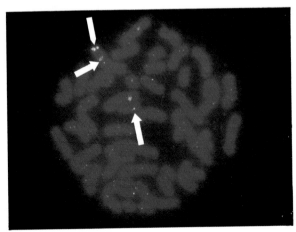

Color Plate 4. For legend see Figure 6-4, *A*.

Color Plate 5. For legend see Figure 6-4, *B*.

Clinical Commentary 5-1. Hemophilia A

Hemophilia A (*SOL* 32, 33), or "classical" hemophilia, affects approximately 1 in 5000 to 10,000 males worldwide. It is the most common of the severe bleeding disorders and has been recognized as a familial disorder for centuries. The Talmud states that boys whose brothers or cousins bled to death during circumcision are exempt from the procedure (this may well be the first recorded example of genetic counseling). Queen Victoria carried the gene for hemophilia A, transmitting it to one son and two carrier daughters. They in turn transmitted the gene to many members of the royal families of Germany, Spain, and Russia (Fig. 5-4, page 88). One of the males affected by the disease was the Tsarevitch Alexis of Russia, the son of Tsar Nicholas II and Alexandra. Grigori Rasputin, the so-called "mad monk," had an unusual ability to calm the Tsarevitch during bleeding episodes, probably through hypnosis. As a result he came to have considerable influence in the royal court, and some historians feel that his destabilizing effect helped to bring about the 1917 Bolshevik Revolution.

Hemophilia A is caused by deficient or defective factor VIII, a key component of the clotting cascade. Fibrin formation is affected, resulting in prolonged and often severe bleeding from wounds and hemorrhages in the joints and muscles. Bruising is frequently seen. **Hemarthroses** (bleeding into the joints) are common in weight-bearing joints, such as the ankles, knees, hips, and elbows (Fig. 5-5). They are often painful, and repeated episodes can lead to destruction of the synovium and loss of joint function. Intracranial bleeding is also common, and prior to effective treatment for bleeding episodes, it was the leading cause of death among hemophiliacs. It should be emphasized that platelet activity is normal in hemophiliacs, so minor lacerations and abrasions do not usually lead to excessive bleeding.

Hemophilia A varies considerably in its severity, and this variation is correlated directly with factor VIII level. About half of hemophilia A patients fall into the "severe" category, with factor VIII levels that are less than 2% of normal. These individuals experience relatively frequent bleeding episodes, often several per month. Moderate hemophiliacs (2% to 5% of normal factor VIII) generally have bleeding episodes only after mild trauma and typically experience one to several episodes per year. Mild hemophiliacs have more than 5% of the normal factor VIII level and usually experience bleeding episodes only after surgery or relatively severe trauma.

Until about 30 years ago, hemophilia A was often fatal by about age 20. Then it became possible to purify factor VIII from donor plasma. Factor VIII is usually administered at the first sign of a bleeding episode and is a highly effective treatment. By the 1970s the median age of death of hemophiliacs had increased to 68 years. The major drawback of donor-

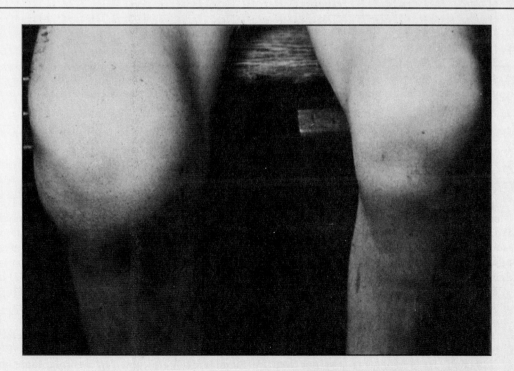

Figure 5-5 ■ The enlarged knee joints of a patient with hemophilia A, demonstrating the effects of hemarthrosis. (Courtesy of Dr. Richard O'Brien, Primary Children's Medical Center, Salt Lake City, Utah.)

Continued

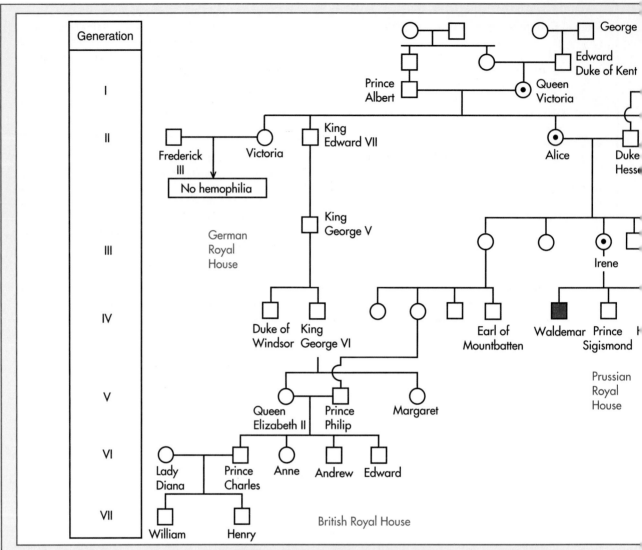

Figure 5-4 ■ **A pedigree showing the inheritance of hemophilia in the European royal families. The first known carrier in the family was Queen Victoria. Note that all of the affected individuals are male.** (Modified from Raven PH, Johnson GB: Biology ed 3, St Louis, 1992, Mosby.)

derived factor VIII is the fact that, because a typical infusion contains plasma products from hundreds of different donors, it is frequently contaminated by viruses. Hemophiliacs often suffer from hepatitis B and C. More seriously, human immunodeficiency virus (HIV) can be transmitted in this manner, and recent surveys show that 50% to 90% of severe hemophiliacs test positively for HIV antibodies. Acquired immune deficiency syndrome (AIDS) is now the most common cause of death among hemophiliacs, and this disease produced a decrease in the median age of death to 49 years in the 1980s. Heat treatment of donor-derived factor VIII kills HIV and hepatitis B virus and has now nearly eliminated the threat of infection. For reasons that are not well understood, approximately 10% to 15% of hemophiliacs develop "inhibitor" antibodies to factor VIII itself, which further complicates treatment.

The factor VIII gene has been mapped to the distal long arm of the X chromosome and cloned. It contains 186 kb of DNA in 26 exons and 25 introns. The 9-kb mRNA transcript encodes a mature protein consisting of 2332 amino acids. Cloning and sequencing the gene have led to a number of insights. Patients with nonsense mutations usually develop severe hemophilia, whereas those with missense mutations usually have relatively mild disease. This is expected because nonsense mutations produce a truncated protein, while missense mutations produce a single amino acid substitution. About 5% of patients have deletions, which usually lead to relatively severe disease. It has recently been shown that about 45% of severe cases of hemophilia A are caused by a chromosome inversion (see Chapter 6) that disrupts the factor VIII gene. Intron 22 of the factor VIII gene contains an embedded gene that is transcribed in the direction opposite

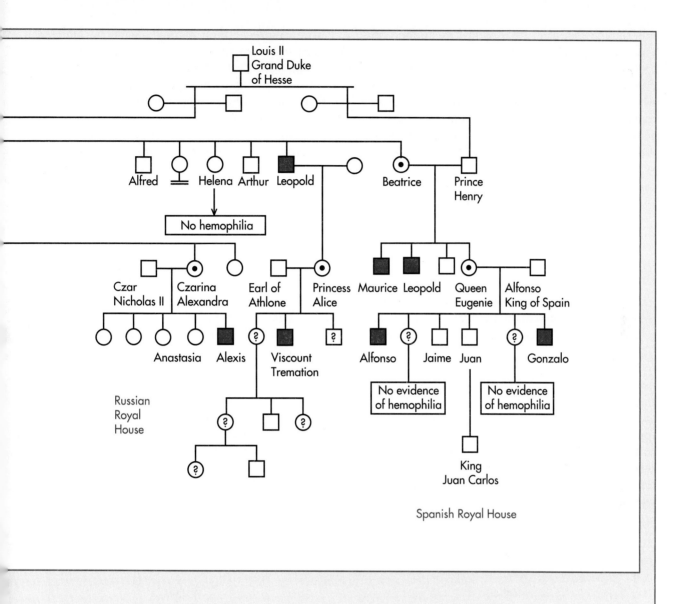

that of the remainder of the gene. A second embedded gene is transcribed in the same direction as the factor VIII gene. Its first exon, located inside intron 22, is spliced to exons 23 to 26 of the factor VIII gene.

Cloning of the factor VIII gene has enabled the production of human factor VIII using recombinant DNA techniques. Recombinant factor VIII has been tested extensively in clinical trials, and it appears to work as effectively as donor-derived factor VIII. It has, of course, the advantage that there is no possibility of viral contamination. However, as with other forms of factor VIII, recombinant factor VIII does generate inhibitor antibody production in a minority of patients.

There are two other major bleeding disorders, hemophilia B and von Willebrand disease. Hemophilia B, sometimes called "Christmas disease,"* is also an X-linked recessive disorder and is caused by a deficiency of clotting factor IX. It is less severe than hemophilia A, and it is only about one fifth as common. The factor IX gene has also been cloned, and it consists of 34 kb of DNA and eight exons. The disorder can be treated with donor-derived factor IX. von Willebrand disease is an autosomal dominant disorder that is highly variable in expression. Although it may affect as many as 1% of whites, it reaches severe expression in fewer than 1 in 10,000. The von Willebrand factor, which is encoded by a gene on chromosome 12, acts as a carrier protein for factor VIII. In addition, it binds to platelets and damaged blood vessel endothelium, thus promoting the adhesion of platelets to damaged vessel walls.

---

*"Christmas" was the name of the affected patient.

inheritance (see Fig. 5-6). As just mentioned, the trait is seen much more frequently in males than in females. Because a father can transmit only a Y chromosome to his son, X-linked genes are not passed from father to son. In contrast, father–son transmission *can* be observed for autosomal disease genes. The disease allele can be transmitted through a series of phenotypically normal heterozygous females, causing the appearance of "skipped" generations. The gene is passed from an affected father to all of his daughters, who, as carriers, transmit it to approximately half of their sons, who are affected.

X-linked recessive inheritance is characterized by an absence of father–son transmission, "skipped" generations when genes are passed through female carriers, and a preponderance of affected males.

The most common mating type involving X-linked recessive genes is the combination of a carrier female and a normal male. The carrier mother will transmit the disease gene to half of her sons and half of her daughters. As Figure 5-7 shows, half of the daughters in such a mating will be carriers and half will be normal (on the average). Half of the sons will be normal and half, on average, will have the disease.

The other common mating type is an affected father and a normal mother (Fig. 5-8). Here all of the sons must be normal because the father can transmit only his Y chromosome to them. Because all of the daughters must receive the father's X chromosome, they will all be heterozygous carriers. None of the children will manifest the disease, however. Because the father *must* transmit his X chromosome to his daughters and cannot transmit it to his sons, these risks, unlike those in the previous paragraph, are exact figures rather than probability estimates.

A much less common mating type is that of an affected father and a carrier mother (Fig. 5-9). Half of the daughters will be heterozygous carriers, while half, on average, will be homozygous for the disease gene and thus affected. Half of the sons will be normal and half will be affected. Note that it may appear that father–son transmission of the disease has occurred, but the affected son has actually received the disease allele from his mother.

Recurrence risks for X-linked recessive disorders are more complex than for autosomal disorders. The risks depend on the genotype of each parent and the sex of the offspring.

Occasionally, females who inherit only a single copy of an X-linked recessive disease gene can be

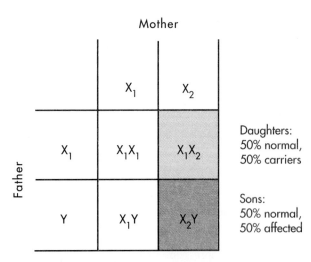

Figure 5-7 ■ Punnett square representation of mating of a heterozygous female who carries an X-linked recessive disease gene with a normal male. In this and the following two figures, X_1 is the chromosome with the normal allele and X_2 is the chromosome with the disease allele.

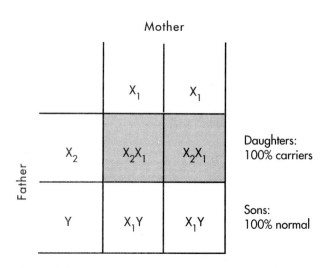

Figure 5-8 ■ Punnett square representation of mating of a normal female with a male who is affected by an X-linked recessive disease.

affected with the disease. Imagine a female embryo that has received a normal factor VIII gene from one parent and a mutated factor VIII gene from the other. Ordinarily X inactivation will result in approximately equal numbers of cells having active paternal and maternal X chromosomes. In this case the female carrier would produce about 50% of the normal level of factor VIII and would be phenotypically normal. However, because X inactivation is a random process, it will occasionally result in a heterozygous female in whom nearly all of the active X chromosomes happen to be the ones carrying the disease mutation. These females exhibit the disorder and are termed **manifesting heterozygotes**. Because such females usually maintain at least a small proportion of active normal X chromosomes, they tend to be relatively mildly affected. For example, approximately 5% of females who are heterozygous for hemophilia A have factor VIII levels low enough to be classified as mild hemophiliacs.

> **Because X inactivation is a random process, some female heterozygotes may experience inactivation of most of the normal X chromosomes in their cells. These manifesting heterozygotes are usually mildly affected.**

Less commonly, females having only a single X chromosome (Turner syndrome) have been seen with X-linked recessive diseases such as hemophilia A. Females can also be affected with X-linked recessive diseases as a result of translocations or deletions of X chromosome material (see Chapter 6). These events are rare.

X-Linked Dominant Inheritance

While there are a number of important and relatively common X-linked recessive diseases, X-linked dominant diseases are, for the most part, much less significant clinically. An example of an X-linked dominant disease is hypophosphatemic rickets, a disease in which the kidneys are impaired in their ability to reabsorb phosphate. This results in abnormal ossification, with bending and distortion of the bones. Another example is incontinentia pigmenti type 1, a disorder characterized by abnormal skin pigmentation, conical or missing teeth, and ocular and neurologic abnormalities. This disorder is seen only in females. It is thought that hemizygous males are so severely affected that they do not survive to term. Heterozygous females, having one normal X chromosome, tend generally to have milder expression of X-linked dominant traits (just as heterozygotes for most autosomal dominant disease genes are less severely affected than are homozygotes).

Figure 5-12 illustrates a pedigree for X-linked dominant inheritance. As with autosomal dominant diseases, an individual need inherit only a single copy of an X-linked dominant disease gene to manifest the disorder. Because females have two X chromosomes, either of which can potentially have

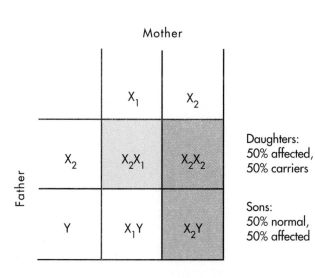

Figure 5-9 ■ Punnett square representation of mating of a carrier female with a male affected with an X-linked recessive disease.

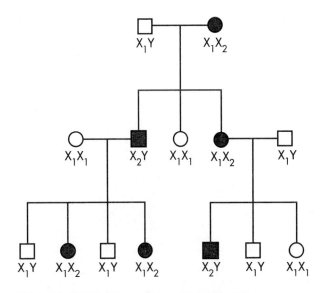

Figure 5-12 ■ Pedigree demonstrating the inheritance of an X-linked dominant trait. X_1 is the normal allele; X_2 is the disease allele.

Clinical Commentary 5-2. Duchenne Muscular Dystrophy

Muscular dystrophy, defined as a progressive weakness and loss of muscle, exists in at least a dozen different forms. Of these, Duchenne muscular dystrophy (DMD), named after the French neurologist who first described the disease in 1868, is the most severe and the most common (*SOL* 34, 35). It affects approximately 1 in 3500 males; this prevalence figure is similar among all ethnic groups studied thus far.

The symptoms of DMD are usually seen before the age of 5, with parents often noticing clumsiness and muscle weakness. Pseudohypertrophy of the calves, the result of infiltration of muscle by fat and connective tissue, is often seen early in the course of the disease. All skeletal muscle degenerates eventually (Fig. 5-10), and most DMD patients are confined to wheelchairs by age 11. The heart and respiratory musculature become impaired, and death usually results from respiratory or cardiac failure. Survival beyond age 25 is uncommon. Despite much effort, there is no effective treatment for this disease.

As muscle cells die, the enzyme creatine kinase (CK) is leaked into the bloodstream. Serum CK assays show that it is elevated at least 20 times above the upper limit of the normal range in DMD patients. This elevation can be observed preclinically (i.e., before clinical symptoms such as muscle wasting are seen). Other diagnostic tools include electromyography, which reveals reduced action potentials, and muscle biopsy (Fig. 5-11).

Female heterozygous carriers of the *DMD* gene are usually free of disease, although 8% to 10% have some degree of muscle weakness. In addition, serum CK exceeds the 95th percentile in approximately two thirds of heterozygotes.

A

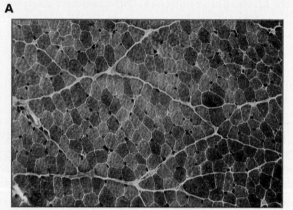

B

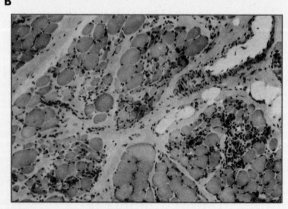

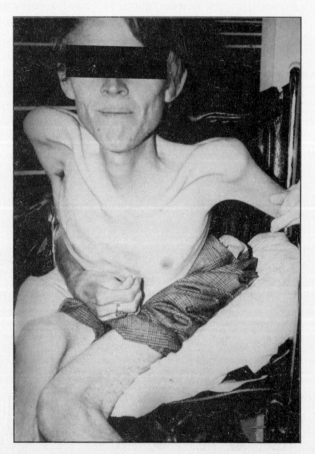

Figure 5-10 ■ A patient with late-stage Duchenne muscular dystrophy, showing severe muscle loss.

Figure 5-11 ■ Transverse section of gastrocnemius muscle from (A), a normal boy and (B), a boy with Duchenne muscular dystrophy. Normal muscle fiber is replaced with fat and connective tissue. (Courtesy of Dr. Jeanette Townsend, University of Utah Health Sciences Center.)

Continued.

Until the *DMD* gene was isolated and cloned in 1986, little was known about the mechanism responsible for muscle deterioration. Cloning of the gene and identification of the gene product have advanced our knowledge tremendously. The *DMD* gene covers approximately 2.4 million base pairs of DNA, making it by far the largest gene known in the human. It contains at least 79 exons that produce a 14-kb mRNA transcript (because of this gene's huge size, transcription of an mRNA molecule may take as long as 24 hours). The mRNA is translated into a mature protein of 3685 amino acids. The protein product, named dystrophin, was unknown prior to the cloning of the *DMD* gene. Dystrophin accounts for only about 0.002% of a striated muscle cell's protein mass and is localized on the cytoplasmic side of the cell membrane. While its function is still being explored, it is likely to be involved in maintaining the structural integrity of the cell's cytoskeleton. The amino terminal of the protein binds actin, a key cytoskeletal protein. The carboxyl terminal of dystrophin binds a complex of glycoproteins that span the cell membrane. It thus appears to link these two cellular components. Dystrophin is completely lacking in the muscle cells of 99% of DMD patients, so a dystrophin assay provides a highly accurate diagnostic tool for this disorder.

The large size of the *DMD* gene helps to explain its high mutation rate, about 10^{-4}. As with neurofibromatosis type 1, the *DMD* gene presents a large target for mutation. A slightly altered form of the *DMD* gene product is normally found in brain cells. Its absence in DMD patients helps to explain why approximately 25% have IQs below 75. In brain cells the transcription initiation site is further downstream in the gene, and a different promoter is used. Thus the mRNA transcript and the resulting gene product differ from the gene product found in muscle cells. A third promoter has been identified for DMD transcripts expressed in cerebellar Purkinje cells. This is an intriguing example of a single gene that can produce different gene products as a result of modified transcription.

Becker muscular dystrophy (BMD) is another X-linked recessive dystrophic condition, the expression of which is milder than that of the Duchenne form (*SOL* 36). The progression is also much slower, with onset at 11 years of age, on average. One study showed that, while 95% of DMD cases are confined to wheelchairs before 11 years of age, 95% of BMD cases become wheelchair bound after 11 years of age. Some never lose their ability to walk. BMD is considerably less common than DMD, affecting only about 1 in 18,000 male births. Earlier studies indicated a much lower prevalence, but dystrophin assays have shown that many previously undiagnosed or misdiagnosed cases actually have BMD.

For some time it was known that the *BMD* gene was located close to *DMD* on the X chromosome. It was unclear, however, whether the two diseases were caused by distinct loci or by different mutations at the same locus. Cloning the gene has shown that the two diseases are indeed allelic forms [i.e., they are caused by different mutations (alleles) at the same locus] and thus represent another example of allelic heterogeneity. Both diseases usually result from deletions (65% of DMD cases and 85% of BMD cases) or duplications (6% to 7% of DMD and BMD cases). Whereas the great majority of DMD deletions and duplications produce frameshifts, the majority of BMD mutations are in-frame alterations (i.e., a multiple of 3 bases is deleted or duplicated). One would expect that a frameshift, which is likely to alter the protein substantially (see Chapter 3), would produce a more severe disease than would an in-frame alteration.

The consequences of these different mutations can be observed in the gene product. While dystrophin is absent in nearly all DMD patients, it is usually present in reduced quantity (or as a shortened form of the protein) in BMD patients. Thus a dystrophin assay can help to distinguish between the two diseases. It also helps to distinguish both diseases from other forms of muscular dystrophy because dystrophin appears to be affected only in these two forms.

Precise identification of the *DMD* gene has led to animal models for the disease (a mouse model and a dog model). Animal research is contributing considerably to our understanding of the human form of the disease. In addition, work is progressing on therapy for DMD, either by injection of normal muscle cells into the muscles of patients or through gene therapy (see Chapter 11). However, because all muscles of the body, including the heart, are affected, professionals involved in this type of therapy face formidable challenges.

the disease gene, they are about twice as commonly affected as males (unless the disorder is lethal in males, as in incontinentia pigmenti). Affected fathers cannot transmit the trait to their sons. All of their daughters must inherit the disease gene, so all are affected. Affected females are usually heterozygotes and thus have a 50% chance of passing the disease allele to their daughters and sons. The characteristics of X-linked dominant and X-linked recessive inheritance are summarized in Table 5-1.

X-linked dominant diseases display characteristic patterns of inheritance. They are about twice as common in females as males, skipped generations are uncommon, and father–son transmission is not seen.

The Fragile X Story: Molecular Genetics Explains a Puzzling Pattern of Inheritance

Since the nineteenth century, it has been observed that there is an approximate 25% excess of males among the institutionalized mentally retarded. This excess is partly explained by several X-linked conditions causing mental retardation. The fragile X syndrome is the most common of these, accounting for approximately 40% of all X-linked mental retardation. Seen in approximately 1 in 1250 males and 1 in 2500 females, the fragile X syndrome is the single most common inherited cause of mental retardation. In addition to mental retardation, fragile X syndrome is characterized by an abnormal facial appearance with large ears and long face (Fig. 5-13), hypermobile joints, and macroorchidism (increased testicular volume) in postpubertal males. The degree of mental retardation tends to be milder and more variable in females than in males. The term "fragile X" is derived from the fact that the X chromosomes of affected individuals, when cultured in a medium that is deficient in folic acid, sometimes exhibit breaks and gaps near the tip of the long arm (Fig. 5-14).

Fragile X syndrome is an X-linked dominant condition with 80% penetrance in males and only 30% penetrance in females. The lower degree of penetrance in females, as well as variability in expression, is thought to be related to X-inactivation. Males who carry the gene but do not express the disease are termed "normal transmitting males." In the mid-1980s, studies of fragile X pedigrees revealed a perplexing pattern: whereas only about 9% of the brothers of transmitting males have the fragile X syndrome, 40% of their grandsons and 50% of their great-grandsons have the syndrome (Fig. 5-15). Daughters of transmitting males are never affected with the disorder, but *their* sons can be affected. This pattern, dubbed the "Sherman paradox," is inconsistent with the rules of X-linked inheritance, which dictate equal penetrance in males who inherit the disease gene.

Many mechanisms were proposed to explain this pattern, including autosomal and mitochondrial modifier loci. Resolution of the Sherman paradox came only with the cloning of the disease gene, labeled *FMR1*. This gene is 38 kb in length, contains 17 exons, and produces a 4.8 kb mRNA

Table 5-1 ■ A comparison of the major attributes of X-linked dominant and X-linked recessive inheritance patterns*

	X-linked dominant	X-linked recessive
Recurrence risk for heterozygous female × normal male mating	50% sons affected; 50 % daughters affected	50% sons affected; 50 % daughters heterozygous carriers
Recurrence risk for affected male × normal female mating	0% sons affected; 100% daughters affected	0% sons affected; 100% daughters heterozygous carriers
Transmission pattern	Vertical; disease phenotype seen in generation after generation	Skipped generations may be seen, representing transmission through carrier females
Sex ratio	Twice as many affected females as affected males (unless disease is lethal in males)	Much greater prevalence of affected males; affected homozygous females rare
Other	Male–male transmission not seen; expression less severe in female heterozygotes than in affected males	Male–male transmission not seen; manifesting heterozygotes may be seen in females

*Compare with the inheritance patterns for autosomal diseases shown in Table 4-1.

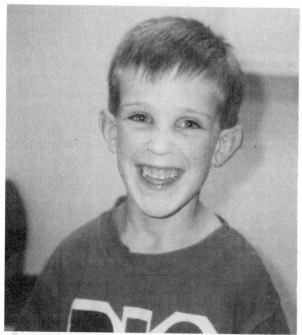

Figure 5-13 ■ A boy with fragile X syndrome. Note the prominent and elongated ears and long face.

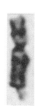

Figure 5-14 ■ An X chromosome from a male with fragile X syndrome, showing an elongated, decondensed region near the tip of the long arm.

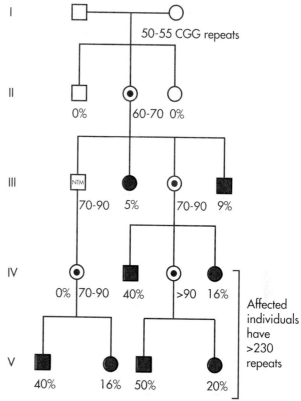

Figure 5-15 ■ A pedigree showing the inheritance of the fragile X syndrome. Females who carry a premutation (50-230 CGG repeats) are dotted. Affected individuals are represented by solid symbols. A normal transmitting male, who carries a premutation of 70-90 repeat units, is designated NTM. Note that the number of repeats increases each time the mutation is passed through another female (anticipation). Note also that only 5% of the NTM's sisters are affected and only 9% of his brothers are affected, whereas 40% of his grandsons and 16% of his granddaughters are affected. This is the Sherman paradox.

transcript. DNA sequence analysis showed that the 5′ untranslated region of the gene contains a CGG repeat unit that is present in 6 to 50 copies in normal individuals. Those with fragile X syndrome have 230 to 1000 or more CGG repeats (a "full mutation"). An intermediate number of repeats, ranging approximately from 50 to 230, is seen in normal transmitting males and their female offspring. When these female offspring transmit the gene to their offspring, there is often an expansion from this "premutation" of 50 to 230 repeats to the full mutation of more than 230 repeats. These expansions do not occur in male transmission. Furthermore, the larger the premutation, the greater is the probability that expansion to the full mutation will occur. These findings explain the

Sherman paradox. They show why males with the premutation cannot transmit the disease to their daughters, and they explain why grandsons and great-grandsons of transmitting males are more likely to be affected with the disorder. Continued repeat expansion through successive generations is an example of anticipation, as in Huntington disease and myotonic dystrophy (see Chapter 4).

Measurement of mRNA transcribed from *FMR1* has shown that the highest mRNA expression levels are in the brain, as might be expected. Individuals with normal and premutation *FMR1* genes have equal levels of expression. However, those with full mutations have no *FMR1* mRNA in their cells, indicating that transcription of the gene has been eliminated. The CGG repeat is heavily methylated among those with the full mutation, as is a CG sequence 5′ of the gene. In addition, the degree of methylation is correlated with severity of expression of the disorder. These correlations indicate that methylation may influence the transcription rate of *FMR1*.

Further study of this region has revealed the presence of another fragile site distal to the fragile X site. This fragile site, termed *FRAXE,* is also associated with mild mental retardation and, like fragile X syndrome, is caused by the expansion of a CGG trinucleotide repeat. Repeat expansion at this locus is also associated with increased methylation. Unlike fragile X syndrome, the CGG repeat at this locus can expand when transmitted either through males or females.

Cloning the *FMR1* gene and identification of a repeat expansion has already explained a great deal about the inheritance and expression of the fragile X syndrome. It has also improved diagnostic accuracy for the condition because cytogenetic analysis of chromosomes often fails to identify fragile X heterozygotes. In contrast, DNA diagnosis of the expanded repeat is very accurate. Many questions remain: What is the role of methylation in gene expression? What is the nature of the gene product and its effects on mental development? When does repeat expansion occur, during meiosis or during early mitosis in the embryo? Further analysis of the fragile X gene and its protein product will help to answer these questions.

Y-Linked Inheritance

At this time no diseases are known to be Y-linked, or **holandric,** and only a few traits are known to be caused by genes on the Y chromosome. These include maleness itself (see Chapter 6) and a minor histocompatibility antigen, termed *Hy.* Transmission of Y-linked traits is strictly father-son (Fig. 5-16).

■ SEX-LIMITED AND SEX-INFLUENCED TRAITS

Confusion sometimes exists regarding traits that are sex-*linked* and those that are **sex-limited** or **sex-influenced.** A sex-limited trait occurs in only one of the sexes, due, for instance, to anatomic differences. Inherited uterine or testicular defects would be examples. A good example of a sex-influenced trait is male-pattern baldness, which occurs in both males and females, but much more commonly in males. Contrary to oft-stated belief, male-pattern baldness is not X-linked. It is thought to be inherited as an autosomal dominant trait in males, whereas in females it is inherited as an autosomal recessive trait. Female heterozygotes can transmit the trait to their offspring but do not manifest it. Females display the trait only when they inherit two copies of the gene. Even then, they are more likely to display marked thinning of the hair, rather than complete baldness.

■ MITOCHONDRIAL INHERITANCE

The great majority of genetic diseases are caused by defects in the nuclear genome. However, a small but significant number of diseases are the result of mitochondrial mutations. Because of the unique properties of the mitochondria, these diseases display characteristic modes of inheritance and a large degree of phenotypic variability.

Each human cell contains several hundred mitochondria in its cytoplasm. Through the complex

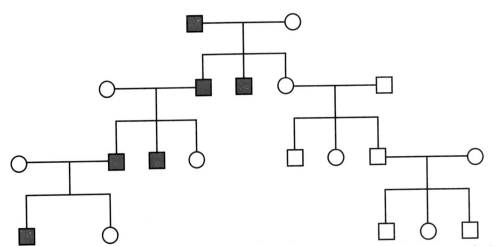

Figure 5-16 ■ **Pedigree demonstrating the inheritance of a Y-linked trait. Transmission is exclusively male–male.**

Box 5-1. Color Vision: Molecular Biology and Evolution

Human vision depends on a system of photoreceptors located in the retina. About 95% of these photoreceptor cells are termed **rod cells**, which contain the light-absorbing protein **rhodopsin** and allow us to see in conditions of dim light. In addition, the retina contains three classes of **cone cells**, which contain light-absorbing proteins (opsins) that react to the three primary colors, red, green, and blue. Color vision depends on the presence of all four of these cell types. Because three major colors are involved, normal color vision is said to be **trichromatic**.

There are many recognized defects of human color vision. The most common of these involve red and green color perception and have been known since 1911 to be inherited in X-linked recessive fashion. Thus they are much more common in males than females. Various forms of "red-green colorblindess" are seen in about 8% of white males, 4% to 5% of Asian males, and 1% to 4% of African and Native American males. Among white males, 2% are **dichromatic**: they are unable to perceive one of the primary colors, usually red or green. The inability to perceive green is termed **deuteranopia**, whereas the inability to perceive red is termed **protanopia**. About 6% of white males can detect green and red, but with altered perception of the relative shades of these colors. These are termed **deuteranomalous** and **protanomalous** conditions, respectively.

It should be apparent that dichromats are not really color*blind* because they can still perceive a fairly large array of different colors. True colorblindness (**monochromacy**, the ability to perceive only one color) is much less common, affecting approximately 1 in 100,000 individuals. There are two major forms of monochromatic vision. Rod monochromacy is an autosomal recessive condition in which all visual function is carried out by rod cells. Blue cone monochromacy is an X-linked recessive condition in which both the red and green cone cells are absent.

Cloning of the genes responsible for color perception has revealed a number of interesting facts about both the biology and evolution of color vision in humans. About 10 years ago, Jeremy Nathans and colleagues reasoned that the opsins in all four types of photoreceptor cells might have similar amino acid sequences because they carry out similar functions. Thus, the DNA sequences of the genes encoding these proteins should also be similar. But none of these genes had been located, and the precise nature of the protein products was unknown. How could they locate these genes? Fortunately, the gene encoding rhodopsin in cattle had been cloned. Even though humans and cattle are separated by millions of years of evolution, their rhodopsin proteins still share about 40% of the same amino acid sequence. Thus the cattle (bovine) rhodopsin gene could be used as a probe to search for a homolog in the human genome. A portion of the bovine rhodopsin gene was converted to single-strand form, radioactively labeled, and hybridized with human DNA (much in the same way that a probe is used in Southern blotting, Chapter 3). "Low stringency" hybridization conditions were used: temperature and other conditions were manipulated so that complementary base pairing would occur despite some sequence differences between the two species. In this way the human rhodopsin gene was identified and mapped to chromosome 3.

The next step was to use the human rhodopsin gene as a probe to identify the cone cell opsin genes. Each of the cone cell opsin amino acid sequences shares 40% to 45% similarity with the human rhodopsin amino acid sequence. By probing with the rhodopsin gene, the gene for blue-sensitive opsin was identified and mapped to chromosome 7. This gene was expected to map to an autosome because variants in blue sensitivity are inherited as an autosomal trait. The genes for the red- and green-sensitive opsins were also identified in this way and, as expected, they were found to be on the X chromosome. The red and green genes are highly similar, sharing 98% of their DNA sequence.

Initially, many investigators expected that people with color vision defects would display the usual array of deletions and missense and nonsense mutations seen in other disorders, but further study revealed some surprises. It was found that the red and green opsin genes are located directly adjacent to one another on the distal long arm of the X chromosome and that normal individuals have one copy of the red gene but could have one to several copies of the green gene. The multiple green genes are 99.9% identical in DNA sequence, and the presence of multiple copies of these genes has no effect on color perception. However, when there are *no* green genes, deuteranopia is produced. Individuals lacking the single red gene have protanopia. The unique aspect of these deletions is that they are the result of **unequal crossover** during meiosis (Fig. 5-17). Unlike ordinary crossover, in which equal segments of chromosomes are exchanged (Chapter 2), unequal crossover results in a loss of chromosome material on one homolog and a gain of material on the other. Unequal crossover seems to be facilitated by the high similarity in DNA sequence among the red and green genes: it is relatively easy for the cellular machinery to make a "mistake" in deciding where the crossover should occur. Thus a female with one red gene and two green genes could produce one gamete containing a red gene with one green gene and another gamete containing a red gene with three green genes. Unequal crossover could also result in gametes with no copies of a gene, producing protanopia or deuteranopia.

Continued.

Box 5-1. Color Vision: Molecular Biology and Evolution—*cont'd*

Unequal crossover also explains protanomalous and deuteranomalous color vision. Here, crossover takes place *within* the red or green genes (Fig. 5-17), resulting in new chromosomes with hybrid genes (e.g., a portion of the red gene fused with a portion of the green gene). The relative proportion of red and green components of these **fusion genes** determines the extent and nature of the red–green anomaly.

Because the opsin genes have DNA sequence similarity and perform similar functions, they are members of a gene family, much like the globin genes (Chapter 3). This suggests that they evolved from a single ancestral gene that, through time, duplicated and diverged to code for different but related proteins. Evidence for this process is provided by comparing these genes in humans and other species.

Because the X-linked red and green opsin genes share the greatest degree of DNA sequence similarity, we would expect that these two genes would be the result of the most recent duplication. Indeed humans share all four of their opsin genes with apes and Old World monkeys, but the less closely related New World monkeys have only a single opsin gene on their X chromosomes. It is thus likely that the red–green duplication occurred sometime after the split of the New and Old World monkeys, which took place about 30 to 40 million years ago. Similar comparisons date the split of the X-linked and autosomal cone opsin genes to approximately 500 million years ago. And finally, comparisons with the fruit fly, *Drosophila melanogaster,* indicate that the split between the rod and cone visual pigment genes may have occurred as much as 1 billion years ago.

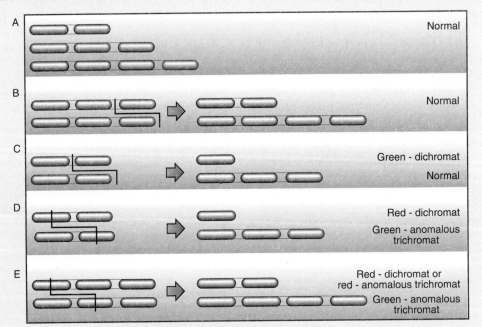

Figure 5-17 ■ **Normal individuals (A) have one red gene and one to several green genes. Unequal crossover causes normal variation in the number of green genes (B). Unequal crossover can produce a green dichromat (C) with no green genes (deuteranopia). Unequal crossover occurring *within* the red and green genes (D) can produce a red dichromat (protanopia) or a green anomalous trichromat (deuteranomaly). Crossovers within the red gene and green genes (E) can also produce red anomalous trichromats (protanomaly). The degree of red and green color perception depends upon where the crossover occurs within the genes.** (Modified from Nathans J, Merbs SL, Sung C, et al: Sci Am 1989.) See color plate 3.

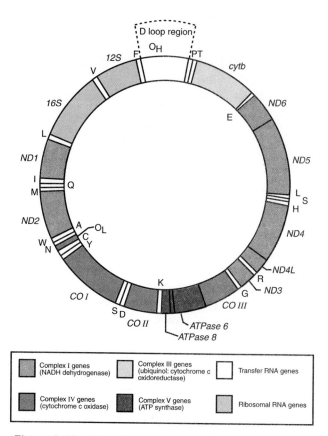

Figure 5-18 ■ The circular mitochondrial DNA
genome. Locations of protein-coding genes
(NADH dehydrogenase, cytochrome c oxidase,
cytochrome c oxidoreductase, and ATP synthase)
are shown, as are the locations of the two
ribosomal RNA genes and 22 transfer RNA genes
(designated by single letters). The replication
origins of the heavy (O_H) and light (O_L) chains
and the noncoding D loop (also known as the
control region) are also shown. (Modified from
Wallace DC: Science 256:628–632, 1992.)

process of oxidative phosphorylation, these organelles produce adenosine triphosphate (ATP), the
energy source essential for cellular metabolism.
Mitochondria are thus critically important for cell
survival.

The mitochondria have their own DNA molecules, occurring in several copies per organelle and
consisting of 16,569 base pairs arranged on a
double-stranded circular molecule (Fig. 5-18). The
mitochondrial genome encodes two ribosomal
RNAs, 22 transfer RNAs, and 13 polypeptides involved in oxidative phosphorylation (another 50
nuclear DNA genes also encode polypeptides involved in this process). Transcription of mitochondrial DNA (mtDNA) takes place in the mitochondrion, independently of the nucleus. Unlike nuclear
DNA, mtDNA contains no introns. Because it is
located in the cytoplasm, mtDNA is inherited exclusively through the maternal line (Fig. 5-19).
Males inherit their mtDNA from their mothers, but
they cannot pass it to their offspring because sperm
cells contain only a few mtDNA molecules that do
not enter the egg. The mutation rate of mtDNA is
about 10 times higher than that of nuclear DNA.
This is caused by a lack of DNA repair mechanisms
in the mtDNA and possibly also by damage from
free radicals released during the oxidative phosphorylation process.

Because each cell contains a *population* of
mtDNA molecules, a single cell can harbor some
molecules that have an mtDNA mutation and other
molecules that do not. This heterogeneity in DNA
composition, termed **heteroplasmy**, is an important cause of variable expression in mitochondrial
diseases. The larger the proportion of mutant

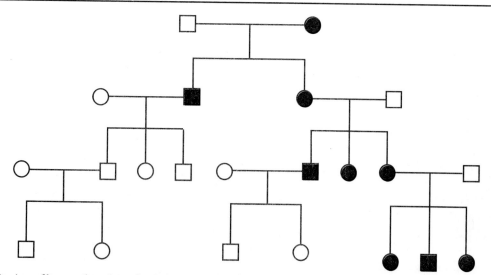

Figure 5-19 ■ A pedigree showing the inheritance of a disease caused by a mitochondrial DNA mutation.
Only females can transmit the disease mutation to their offspring.

mtDNA molecules, the more severe the expression of the disease. The proportion of mutant mtDNA molecules may change through **replicative segregation** as cells divide and as mitochondria proliferate. Changes in the proportion of mutant alleles can occur through chance variation (identical in concept to genetic drift, discussed in Chapter 3) or because of a selective advantage (e.g., deletions produce a shorter mitochondrial DNA molecule that can replicate more quickly than a full-length molecule).

Each tissue type requires a certain amount of mitochondrially produced ATP for normal function. Although some variation in ATP levels may be tolerated, there is typically a threshold level below which cells begin to degenerate and die. Organ systems with large ATP requirements and high thresholds tend to be the ones most seriously affected by mitochondrial diseases. For example, the central nervous system consumes about 20% of the body's ATP production and is thus often affected by mtDNA mutations.

Like the globin disorders, mitochondrial disorders can be classified according to the type of mutation that causes them. Missense mutations in protein-coding mtDNA genes cause one of the best-known mtDNA diseases, Leber hereditary optic neuropathy (LHON) (*SOL* 60). This disease is characterized by rapid loss of vision in the central visual field as a result of optic nerve death. Vision loss typically begins in the early 20s and is usually irreversible. Heteroplasmy is rare in LHON, so expression tends to be relatively uniform and pedigrees for this disorder usually display a clear pattern of mitochondrial inheritance.

Single-base mutations in a tRNA gene can result in myoclonic epilepsy with ragged-red fiber disease (MERRF), a disorder characterized by epilepsy, dementia, ataxia (uncoordinated muscle movement), and myopathy (muscle disease). MERRF is heteroplasmic and thus highly variable in its expression. Another example of a mitochondrial disease caused by a single-base tRNA mutation is mitochondrial encephalomyopathy and strokelike episodes (MELAS). Like MERRF, MELAS is heteroplasmic and highly variable in expression.

The final class of mtDNA mutations consists of duplications and deletions. These can produce Kearns-Sayre disease (muscle weakness, cerebellar damage, and heart failure) and chronic progressive external ophthalmoplegia (CPEO). Mitochondrial deletions have also been associated with rare cases of diabetes and deafness.

> The mitochondria, which produce ATP, have their own unique DNA. Mitochondrial DNA is maternally inherited and has a high mutation rate. Several mitochondrial diseases have been identified.

■ STUDY QUESTIONS

1. Females have been observed with five X chromosomes in each somatic cell. How many Barr bodies would such females have?
2. Explain why 8% to 10% of female carriers of the *DMD* gene have muscle weakness.
3. For X-linked recessive disorders, the ratio of affected males to affected females in populations increases as the disease frequency decreases. Explain this in terms of gene and genotype frequencies.
4. The accompanying pedigree shows the inheritance of hemophilia A in a family. What is the risk that the male in generation IV is affected with hemophilia A? What is the risk that the female in this generation is a heterozygous carrier? What is the risk that she is affected with the disorder?

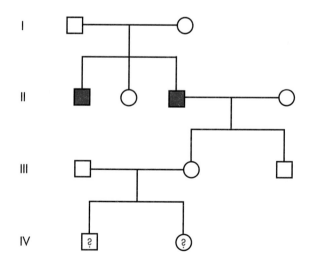

5. Pedigrees for autosomal dominant and X-linked dominant diseases are sometimes difficult to distinguish. Name as many features as you can that would help to tell them apart.
6. How would you distinguish mitochondrial inheritance from other modes of inheritance?

■ ADDITIONAL READING

Brown CJ, Ballabio A, Rupert JL, Lafreniere RG, Grompe M, Tonloren T, and Willard HF: A gene from the region of the human X inactivation centre is expressed exclusively from the inactive X chromosome, Nature 349:38–44, 1991.

Disteche CM: Escape from X inactivation in human and mouse, Trends Genet 11:17–22, 1995.

Emery AEH: Duchenne muscular dystrophy, ed 2. Oxford, 1993, Oxford University Press.

Fu Y, Kuhl DPA, Pizzuti A, Pieretti M, Sutcliffe JS, Richards S, Verkerk AJMH, Holden JJA, Fenwick RG, Warren ST, Oostra BA, Nelson DL, and Caskey CT: Variation of the CGG repeat at the Fragile X site results in genetic instability: resolution of the Sherman paradox, Cell 67:1047–1058, 1991.

Gitschier J: The molecular basis of hemophilia A, Ann NY Acad Sci 614:89–96, 1991.

Heard E, Avner P: Role play in X-inactivation, Hum Molec Genet 3:1481–1485, 1994.

Hoyer LW: Hemophilia A, N Engl J Med 330:38–47, 1994.

Lakich D, Kazazian HH, Antonarakis SE, and Gitshcier J: Inversions disrupting the factor VIII gene are a common cause of severe hemophilia A, Nature Genet 5:236–241, 1993.

Lusher JM, Arkin S, Abildgaard CF, and Schwartz RS: Recombinant factor VIII for the treatment of previously untreated patients with hemophilia A, N Engl J Med 328:453-459, 1993.

Nathans J, Merbs SL, Sung C, Weitz CJ, and Wang Y: Molecular genetics of human visual pigments, Annu Rev Genet 26:403–424, 1992.

Ozawa E, Yoshida M, Suzuko A, Mizuno Y, Hagiwara Y, Noguchi S: Dystrophin-associated proteins in muscular dystrophy, Hum Molec Genet 4:1711–1716, 1995.

Wallace DC: Mitochondrial DNA sequence variation in human evolution and disease, Proc Natl Acad Sci USA 91:8739–8746, 1994.

Warren ST, Nelson DL: Advances in molecular analysis of fragile X syndrome, JAMA 271:536–542, 1994.

Worton R: Muscular dystrophies: diseases of the dystrophin glycoprotein complex, Science 270:755–756, 1995.

6 Clinical Cytogenetics: The Chromosomal Basis of Human Disease

The previous two chapters have dealt with single-gene diseases. We turn now to diseases caused by chromosome alterations that are sufficiently large to be observable under a microscope. Such alterations are termed **chromosome abnormalities**. The study of chromosomes and their abnormalities is termed **cytogenetics**.

Chromosome abnormalities are responsible for a significant proportion of genetic diseases, occurring in approximately 1 in 150 live births. They are the leading known cause of both mental retardation and pregnancy loss. Chromosome abnormalities are seen in 50% and 20% of first- and second-trimester spontaneous abortions, respectively. Thus, they are an important cause of morbidity and mortality.

As in other areas of medical genetics, advances in molecular genetics have contributed many new insights in the field of cytogenetics. For example, molecular techniques have permitted the identification of chromosome abnormalities, such as deletions, that affect very small regions. In some cases specific genes responsible for cytogenetic syndromes are being pinpointed. Thus, the distinction between "chromosome abnormalities" and "single gene diseases" is becoming somewhat blurred. In addition, the ability to identify RFLPs and other polymorphisms in parents and offspring has enabled researchers to specify whether an abnormal chromosome is derived from the mother or father. This has increased our understanding of the biologic basis of meiotic errors and chromosome abnormalities.

In this chapter we discuss abnormalities of chromosome number and structure. The chromosomal and genetic basis of sex determination will be reviewed. The role of chromosome alterations in cancer will be examined, and several diseases caused by chromosomal instability will be discussed. Emphasis will be given to the new contributions of molecular genetics to cytogenetics.

■ CYTOGENETIC TECHNOLOGY AND NOMENCLATURE

Although it was possible to visualize chromosomes under microscopes as early as the mid-1800s, it was difficult to observe individual chromosomes. Thus it was hard to count the number of chromosomes in a cell or to examine structural abnormalities. Beginning in the 1950s, several techniques were developed that improved our ability to observe chromosomes. These included (1) the use of spindle poisons, such as colchicine and colcemid, that arrest dividing somatic cells in metaphase, when chromosomes are maximally condensed and easiest to see, (2) the use of a hypotonic (low salt) solution, which causes swelling of cells, rupture of the nucleus, and better separation of individual chromosomes, and (3) the use of staining materials, which are absorbed differentially by different parts of chromosomes (producing the characteristic bands which help to identify individual chromosomes).

> Our ability to study chromosomes has been improved by the visualization of chromosomes in metaphase, by hypotonic solutions that cause nuclear swelling, and by staining techniques that bring out chromosome bands.

Chromosomes are analyzed by collecting a living tissue (usually blood), culturing the tissue for the appropriate amount of time (usually 48 to 72 hours for peripheral lymphocytes), adding colcemid to produce metaphase arrest, harvesting the cells, placing the cell sediment on a slide, rupturing the cell nucleus with a hypotonic solution, staining with a designated nuclear stain, and photographing the metaphase "spreads" of chromosomes on the slide. The chromosome images are then cut out from the photograph, and the 22 pairs of autosomes are arranged according to length, with the sex chromosomes in the right-hand corner. This ordered display of chromosomes is termed a **karyotype** (Fig. 6-1). More recently, computerized image analyzers are sometimes used to display chromosomes.

After classification by size, chromosomes are further classified according to the position of the centromere. When the centromere occurs near the middle of the chromosome, the chromosome is said to be **metacentric** (Fig. 6-2). An **acrocentric** chromosome has its centromere near the tip, and **submetacentric** chromosomes have centromeres somewhere between the middle and the tip. The tip of each chromosome is termed the **telomere**. Note that the short arm of a chromosome is labeled *p* (from *petite*), while the long arm is labeled *q*. In metacentric chromosomes, where the arms are of roughly equal length, the p and q arms are designated by convention.

A karyotype is a display of chromosomes ordered according to length. Depending on the position of the centromere, a chromosome may be acrocentric, submetacentric, or metacentric.

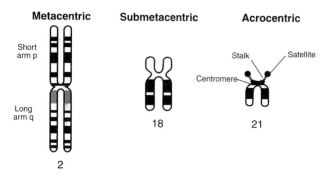

Figure 6-2 ■ Metacentric, submetacentric, and acrocentric chromosomes. Note the stalks and satellites present on the short arms of the acrocentric chromosomes.

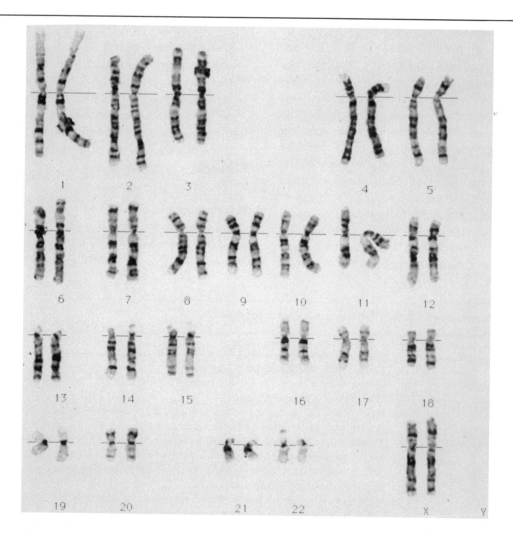

Figure 6-1   A banded karyotype of a normal female. The banded metaphase chromosomes are arranged from largest to smallest in size.

A normal female karyotype is designated 46,XX; a normal male karyotype is designated 46,XY. The nomenclature for various chromosome abnormalities is summarized in Table 6-1 and will be indicated for each condition discussed later.

Chromosome Banding

Early karyotypes were useful in counting the number of chromosomes, but structural abnormalities, such as chromosomal deletions, were often undetectable. Staining techniques were developed in the 1970s that produced the chromosome bands characteristic of modern karyotypes. Chromosome banding helps greatly in the detection of deletions, duplications, and other structural abnormalities, and it facilitates the correct identification of individual chromosomes. The major bands on each chromosome are numbered (Fig. 6-3). Thus 14q32 refers to the second band in the third region of the long arm of chromosome 14. Sub-bands are designated by decimal points following the band (e.g., 14q32.3 is the third sub-band of band 2).

Several chromosome-banding techniques are used in cytogenetics laboratories. **Quinacrine banding** (Q-banding) was the first staining method used to produce specific banding patterns. This method requires a fluorescence microscope and is no longer as widely used as **Giemsa-banding** (G-banding) (a Giemsa stain is applied after the chromosomal proteins are partially digested by trypsin). **Reverse banding** (R-banding) requires heat treatment and reverses the usual white-and-black pattern that is seen in G-bands and Q-bands. This method is particularly helpful in staining the distal ends of chromosomes. Other staining techniques include **C-banding** and **NOR** (nucleolar

organizing region) **stains**. These latter methods specifically stain certain portions of the chromosome. C-banding stains the **constitutive heterochromatin** which lies at and near centromeres, and NOR staining highlights the satellites and stalks of acrocentric chromosomes (Fig. 6-2).

High-resolution banding involves the staining of chromosomes during prophase or early metaphase (prometaphase), before they reach maximal condensation. Because prophase and prometaphase chromosomes are more extended than metaphase chromosomes, the number of bands observable for all chromosomes increases from about 300 (as in Fig. 6-3) to as many as 800. This allows the detection of less obvious abnormalities usually not seen with conventional banding. High- resolution banding is rather tedious and time-consuming, so it is usually used when the clinician is looking for a specific, subtle chromosomal abnormality. An example would be the deletion of the 15q11–13 bands seen in the Prader-Willi syndrome.

> **Chromosome bands help to identify individual chromosomes and structural abnormalities in chromosomes. Banding techniques include quinacrine, Giemsa, reverse, C, and NOR banding. High-resolution banding, using prophase or prometaphase chromosomes, increases the number of observable bands.**

Fluorescence In Situ Hybridization

Fluorescence in situ hybridization (FISH) is a recently developed technique in which a labeled chromosome-specific DNA segment (probe) is hy-

---

Table 6-1 ■ Standard nomenclature for chromosome karyotypes

Karyotype	Description
46,XY	Normal male chromosome constitution
47,XX,+21	Female with trisomy 21, Down syndrome
47,XY,+21/46,XY	Male who is a mosaic of trisomy 21 cells and normal cells
46,XY,del(4)(p14)	Male with distal deletion of the short arm of chromosome 4 band designated 14
46,XX,dup(5p)	Female with duplication of the short arm of chromosome 5
45,XY,−13,−14,t(13q;14q)	A male with a balanced Robertsonian translocation of chromosomes 13 and 14 Karyotype shows that one normal 13 and one normal 14 are missing
46,XY,t(11;22)(q23;q22)	A male with a balanced reciprocal translocation between chromosomes 11 and 22 Breakpoints are at 11q23 and 22q22
46,XX,inv(3)(p21;q13)	An inversion on chromosome 3 that extends from p21 to q13. Because it includes the centromere, this is a pericentric inversion
46,X,r(X)	A female with one normal X chromosome and one ring X chromosome
46,X,i(xq)	A female with one normal X chromosome and an isochromosome of the long arm of the X chromosome

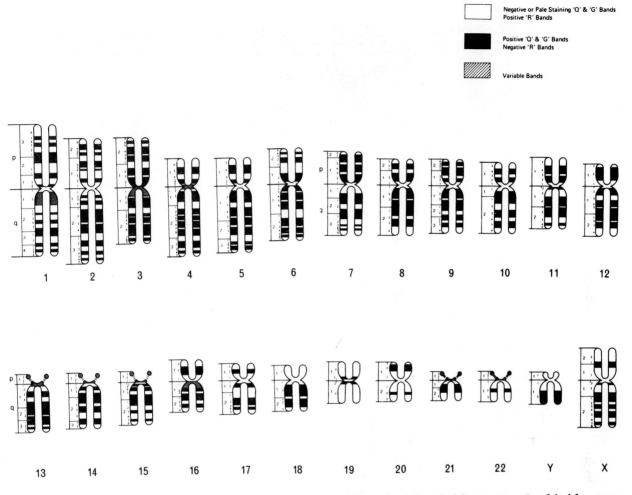

☐		Negative or Pale Staining 'Q' & 'G' Bands Positive 'R' Bands
■		Positive 'Q' & 'G' Bands Negative 'R' Bands
▨		Variable Bands

Figure 6-3 ■ A schematic representation of the banding pattern of a G-banded karyotype. In this ideogram 300 bands are represented. The short and long arms of the chromosomes are designated, and the segments are numbered according to the standard nomenclature adopted at the Paris conference, 1971. In this illustration, both sister chromatids are shown for each chromosome.

bridized with metaphase, prophase, or interphase chromosomes and then visualized under a fluorescence microscope. A common use of FISH is to determine whether a portion of a chromosome is deleted in a patient. In a normal individual, a probe will hybridize in two places, reflecting the presence of two homologous chromosomes in a somatic cell nucleus. If a probe from the chromosome segment in question hybridizes to only one of the patient's chromosomes, then the patient is likely to have the deletion on one chromosome. Excess chromosome material can also be detected using FISH. In this case the probe will hybridize in three places instead of two. Figure 6-4,*A*, illustrates a FISH result for a normal male and for his infant daughter who is missing a small distal piece of the short arm of chromosome 4 (Fig. 6-4,*B*). Only one fluorescent spot is seen in the daughter, indicating that the child has the deletion 4p syndrome or Wolf-Hirschhorn syndrome.

Fluorescence in situ hybridization (FISH) is a technique in which a labelled probe is hybridized to metaphase, prophase, or interphase chromosomes. FISH can be used to test for missing or additional chromosomal material.

■ ABNORMALITIES OF CHROMOSOME NUMBER

Polyploidy

A cell that contains a multiple of 23 chromosomes in its nucleus is said to be **euploid** (Greek, eu = "good," ploid = "set"). Thus haploid gametes and diploid somatic cells are euploid. **Polyploidy**, the presence of a complete set of extra chromosomes in a cell, is seen commonly in plants and often improves their agricultural value. Polyploidy also occurs in humans, although much less frequently. The polyploid conditions observed in humans are **triploidy** (69 chromosomes in the

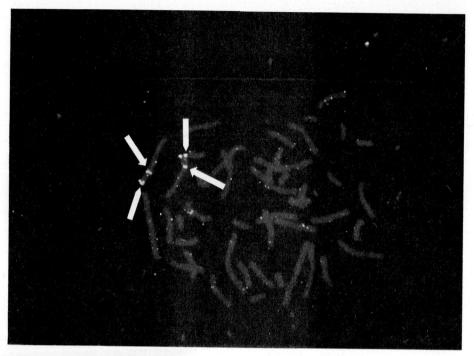

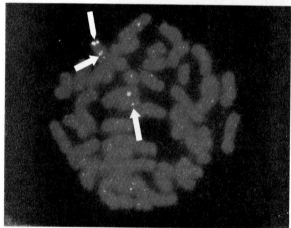

Figure 6-4 ■ A fluorescence in situ hybridization (FISH) result. The larger arrows point to a centromere-hybridizing probe for chromosome 4, and the smaller arrows point to a probe that hybridizes to 4p. A, In a normal male two fluorescent spots are seen for the probe that hybridizes to chromosome 4p. B, This probe reveals only one spot in his daughter, who has a deletion of chromosome 4p producing the Wolf-Hirschhorn syndrome. (Courtesy of Dr. Arthur Brothman, University of Utah Health Sciences Center) See color plates 4 and 5.

nucleus of each cell) and **tetraploidy** (92 chromosomes in each cell nucleus). The karyotypes for these two conditions would be designated 69,XXX and 92,XXXX, respectively (assuming that all of the sex chromosomes were X; other combinations of the X and Y chromosomes may be seen). Because the number of chromosomes present in each of these conditions is a multiple of 23, the cells are euploid in each case. However, the additional chromosomes encode a large amount of surplus gene product, causing multiple anomalies, such as defects of the heart and central nervous system. Triploidy and tetraploidy are both lethal.

Triploidy is seen among only 1 in 10,000 live births, but it accounts for an estimated 15% of the chromosome abnormalities occurring at conception. Thus the vast majority of triploid conceptions

are spontaneously aborted. The most common cause of triploidy is the fertilization of an egg by two sperm (**dispermy**). The resulting zygote then receives 23 chromosomes from the egg and 23 chromosomes from each of the two sperm cells. Triploidy can also be caused by the fusion of an ovum and a polar body, each containing 23 chromosomes, and subsequent fertilization by a sperm cell. **Meiotic failure**, in which a diploid sperm or egg cell is produced, can also produce a triploid zygote.

Tetraploidy is much rarer than triploidy, both at conception and among live births. It has been recorded among only a few live births, and these have survived only for short periods. Tetraploidy can be caused by a mitotic failure in the early embryo, in which all of the duplicated chromosomes migrate to one of the two daughter cells. It can also result from the fusion of two diploid zygotes.

Cells that have a multiple of 23 chromosomes are said to be euploid. Triploidy (69 chromosomes) and tetraploidy (92 chromosomes) are polyploid conditions found in the human. Most polyploid conceptions are spontaneously aborted, and all are incompatible with long-term survival.

Autosomal Aneuploidy

Cells that do not contain a multiple of 23 chromosomes are termed **aneuploid**. These cells are missing or contain additional chromosomes. Usually only one chromosome is affected, but it is possible for more than one chromosome to be missing or duplicated. Aneuploidies (or **aneusomies**) of the autosomes are among the most clinically important of the chromosome abnormalities. They consist primarily of **monosomy** (the presence of only one copy of a chromosome in an otherwise diploid cell) and **trisomy** (three copies

of a chromosome). Autosomal monosomies are nearly always incompatible with survival to term, so only a small number of them have been observed among liveborn individuals. In contrast, some trisomies are seen with appreciable frequencies among live births. The fact that trisomies produce less severe consequences than monosomies illustrates an important principle: *the body can tolerate excess genetic material more readily than it can tolerate a deficit of genetic material.*

The most common cause of aneuploidy is **nondisjunction**, the failure of chromosomes to disjoin normally during meiosis (Fig. 6-5). Nondisjunction can occur during meiosis I or meiosis II. The resulting gamete either lacks a chromosome or has two copies of it, producing a monosomic or trisomic zygote, respectively.

Aneuploid conditions consist primarily of monosomies and trisomies. They are usually caused by nondisjunction. Autosomal monosomies are virtually always lethal, whereas some autosomal trisomies are compatible with survival.

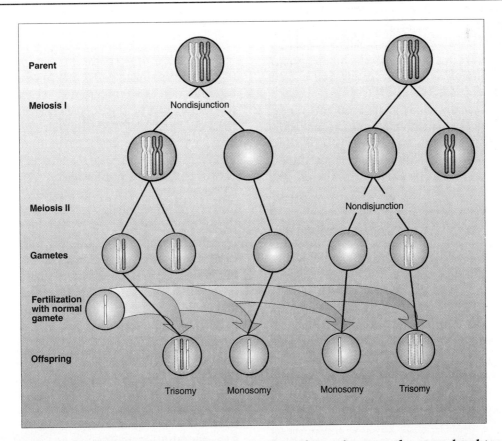

Figure 6-5 ■ In meiotic nondisjunction two chromosome homologs migrate to the same daughter cell instead of disjoining normally and migrating to different daughter cells. This produces monosomic and trisomic offspring.

Trisomy 21

Trisomy 21 (47,XY,+21 or 47,XX,+21)* is seen in approximately 1 in 800 live births, making it the most common aneuploid condition compatible with survival to term. This trisomy produces Down syndrome, a phenotype originally described by John Langdon Down in 1866 (SOL 34–40). Nearly 100 years elapsed between Down's description of this syndrome and the discovery (in 1959) that it is caused by the presence of an extra 21st chromosome.

Although there is considerable variation in the appearance of individuals with Down syndrome, they present a constellation of features that help the clinician to make a diagnosis. The facial features include a low nasal root, upslanting palpebral fissures, measurably small and sometimes overfolded ears, and a flattened maxillary and malar region, giving the face a characteristic appearance (Fig. 6-6). Some of these features led to the use of the term "mongolism" in earlier literature, but this term is inappropriate. The cheeks are round, and the corners of the mouth are sometimes downturned. The neck is short, and the skin is redundant at the nape of the neck, especially in newborns. The occiput is flat, and the hands and feet tend to be rather broad and short. Approximately 50% of individuals with Down syndrome have a deep, single flexion crease across their palms (termed a **simian crease**). Decreased muscle tone (hypotonia) is also a highly consistent feature and helpful in diagnosis.

Several medically significant problems occur with increased frequency among infants and children with Down syndrome. About 3% of these infants will develop an obstruction of the duodenum or atresia (closure or absence) of the esophagus, duodenum, or anus. Respiratory infections are common, and the risk of developing leukemia is 15 to 20 times higher among Down syndrome patients than among the general population. The most significant medical problem is that approximately 40% are born with structural heart defects. The most common of these is an **AV (atrioventricular) canal**, a defect in which the interatrial and interventricular septa fail to fuse normally during fetal development. The result is blood flow from the left heart to the right heart and then to the pulmonary vasculature, producing pulmonary hypertension. **Ventricular septal defects** (VSD) are also common

among babies with Down syndrome. Moderate to severe mental retardation (IQs ranging from 25 to 60) is seen in most individuals with Down syndrome. Down syndrome alone accounts for 10% of all cases of mental retardation in the United States.

Several other medical problems occur in infants and young children with this syndrome. Conductive and sometimes neural hearing loss, hypothyroidism, and various eye abnormalities are the most important and frequent. Clinical Commentary 6-1 (page 110) outlines a plan for routine medical care in infants and children with Down syndrome.

Because of the medical problems seen in children with Down syndrome, their survival rates are significantly decreased. Congenital heart defects are the most important single cause of decreased survival. In the early 1960s, only about half of children with this disorder survived until age 5. As a result of improvements in corrective surgery, antibiotic treatment, and management of leukemia, the survival rates have increased considerably in the past 30 years. Currently it is estimated that approximately 75% to 80% of children with Down syndrome survive to age 10. There is strong evidence that enriched environments can produce significant improvements in intellectual function.

Males with Down syndrome are nearly always sterile; only one case has been reported in which a male with Down syndrome has reproduced. Some females with this condition can reproduce, although approximately 40% fail to ovulate. Because reproduction is so uncommon, nearly all cases of trisomy 21 can be regarded as new mutations. The risk for a female with Down syndrome to produce a gamete with two copies of chromosome 21 (which would then produce a trisomic zygote) is 50%. However, because approximately 75% of trisomy 21 conceptions are spontaneously aborted, the Down syndrome female's risk of producing affected liveborn offspring is considerably lower than 50%.

Approximately 95% of Down syndrome cases are caused by nondisjunction, with most of the remainder being caused by chromosome translocations (page 109). Based on comparisons of chromosome morphology in the affected offspring and their parents, it was long thought that about 80% of chromosome 21 nondisjunctions occur in the mother. A more accurate assessment is now made possible by comparing RFLPs and other chromosome 21 polymorphisms in parents and offspring. This approach shows that the extra chromosome is contributed by the mother in about 95% of trisomy 21 cases. About 75% of these maternal nondisjunctions occur during meiosis I, with the remainder

---

*For brevity, the remainder of the karyotype designations for abnormalities not involving the sex chromosomes will indicate an affected male.

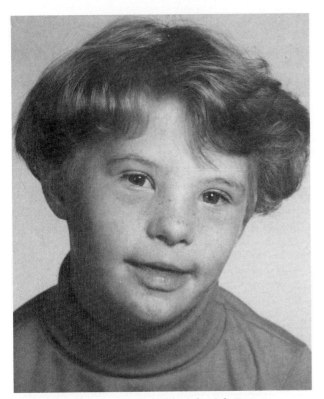

Figure 6-6 ■ *top,* **A 7-year-old girl with Down syndrome, illustrating upslanting palpebral fissures, redundant skin of the inner eyelid (epicanthic fold), and low nasal bridge.**
bottom, **A karyotype of a male with trisomy 21.**

occurring during meiosis II. As discussed in greater detail below, there is a strong correlation between maternal age and the risk of producing a child with Down syndrome.

Mosaicism is seen in approximately 1% to 3% of trisomy 21 live births. These individuals have some normal somatic cells and some cells with trisomy 21. This type of mosaicism in a male would be designated 47,XY, + 21/46,XY. Generally, mosaicism results in a milder clinical expression of Down syndrome. The most common cause of mosaicism for a trisomy is a trisomic conception followed by loss of the extra chromosome in some cells during mitosis in the embryo.

Depending on the timing and manner in which the mosaicism originated, some individuals may be **tissue-specific mosaics**. As the term suggests, this type of mosaicism is confined only to certain tissues. This can complicate diagnosis because karyotypes are usually made from a limited number of tissue types (usually circulating lymphocytes derived from a blood sample or, less commonly, fibroblasts derived from a skin clip).

Because of the prevalence and clinical importance of Down syndrome, considerable effort has been devoted to defining the critical portion of chromosome 21 responsible for this disorder. This region has been narrowed to 21q22, a portion of the distal long arm. Persons with a trisomy of only this part of the chromosome will develop Down syndrome. Molecular approaches, such as cloning

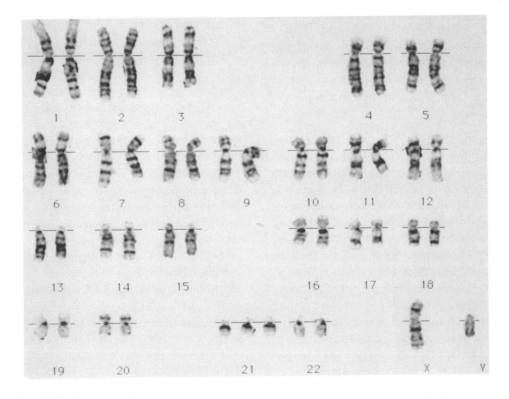

In recent years an approach termed "anticipatory guidance" has evolved in the care and treatment of individuals with genetic syndromes and chronic diseases. After a thorough study of the disease in question (including an extensive literature review), basic guidelines are established for the screening, evaluation, and care of patients. If followed by the primary care practitioner or the specialist, these guidelines should help to prevent further disability or illness. We will illustrate the anticipatory guidance approach with current guidelines for the care of children with Down syndrome.

• Evaluation of heart defects. As mentioned in the text, AV canals are the most common congenital heart defect seen in newborns with Down syndrome. Surgical correction for this condition is appropriate if it is detected before 1 year of age (after this time pulmonary hypertension has been present too long for surgery to be successful). Accordingly, it is now recommended that an *echocardiogram* be performed on children with Down syndrome before the age of 6 months.

• Because Down syndrome patients often have strabismus (deviation of the eye from its normal visual axis) and other eye problems, an *ophthalmologic examination* before the age of 4 is recommended.
• Hypothyroidism is common, especially during adolescence. Thus *thyroid hormone levels* should be measured annually.
• Sensorineural and conductive hearing loss is seen in children with Down syndrome. The routine follow-up should include a *hearing test* at 6 to 8 months of age and as needed afterward.
• Instability of the first and second vertebrae has led to spinal cord injuries in some older Down syndrome patients. It is thus suggested that *cervical spine x-rays* be obtained in children older than age 2.
• It is appropriate to refer children with Down syndrome to preschool programs to provide intervention for developmental disabilities.

Similar series of guidelines have been developed for children with trisomy 18 and Turner syndrome. In principle the anticipatory guidance approach can be applied to any genetic disease for which there is sufficient knowledge.

and sequencing, are being used to identify specific genes in this region that are responsible for the Down syndrome phenotype.

Trisomy 21, which causes Down syndrome, is the most common autosomal aneuploidy seen among live births. The most significant problems include mental retardation, GI tract obstruction, congenital heart defects, respiratory infections, and leukemia. The extra 21st chromosome is contributed by the mother in approximately 95% of cases. Mosaicism is seen in 1% to 3% of Down syndrome cases, and it usually accompanies a milder phenotype.

Trisomy 18 (47,XY, + 18)

This trisomy, also known as Edwards syndrome, is the second most common autosomal trisomy, with a prevalence of about 1 in 6000 live births. It is, however, much more common at conception and is the most common chromosome abnormality among stillborns with congenital malformations. The Edwards syndrome phenotype is as discernable as Down syndrome, but because it is less common, it is less likely to be recognized clinically. Trisomy 18 patients have prenatal growth deficiency (weight that is small for the gestational age), characteristic facial features, and a distinctive hand abnormality that often allows the clinician to make the initial diagnosis (Fig. 6-7). Minor anomalies of

diagnostic importance include small ears with unraveled helices, a small mouth that is often hard to open, short sternum, and rather short big toes. Most babies with trisomy 18 have structural defects. Congenital heart defects, particularly VSDs, are the most common. Other medically significant congenital malformations include omphalocele (protrusion of the bowel into the umbilical cord), diaphragmatic hernia, and, occasionally, spina bifida.

Recent studies have indicated that about 50% of children with trisomy 18 die in the first month, and only about 10% are still alive at 12 months of age. A combination of factors, including aspiration pneumonia, predisposition to infections and central apnea, and (most importantly) congenital heart defects, accounts for the high mortality rate.

Those with trisomy 18 who have survived infancy have a marked developmental disability. The degree of delay is much more significant than in Down syndrome, and most children are not able to walk. However, children with trisomy 18 do progress somewhat in their milestones, and older infants learn some communication skills.

More than 95% of individuals with Edwards syndrome have complete trisomy 18. A small percentage have mosaicism. As in trisomy 21, there is a significant maternal age effect. A recent molecular analysis evaluated 50 trisomy 18 cases and showed that 48 were the result of a maternally contributed extra chromosome.

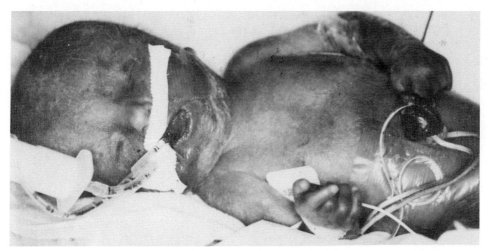

Figure 6-7 ▪ An infant with trisomy 18 (Edwards syndrome). Note the characteristic overlapping of the fingers. This infant also has an omphalocele (*SOL* 41-44). (Courtesy of Dr. Jan Byrne)

Trisomy 13 (47,XY,+13)

This condition, also termed Patau syndrome, is seen in about 1 in 10,000 births. The malformation pattern is distinctive and usually permits clinical recognition. It consists primarily of oral-facial clefts, microphthalmia (small, abnormally formed eyes) and postaxial polydactyly (Fig. 6-8). Malformations of the central nervous system are seen frequently, and cutis aplasia (a scalp defect on the posterior occiput) may also be seen (*SOL* 45-47).

The survival rate is similar to that of trisomy 18, with 90% of liveborn cases dying during the first year of life. As in trisomy 18, the children who survive infancy have significant developmental retardation, with skills seldom progressing beyond those of a child of 2 years. However, as in trisomy 18, children with trisomy 13 do progress somewhat in their development and are often able to communicate with their families.

About 80% of cases of Patau syndrome have full trisomy 13. Most of the remaining cases have trisomy of the long arm of chromosome 13 due to a translocation. As in trisomies 18 and 21, the risk of bearing a child with this condition increases with advanced maternal age. It is estimated that 95% or more of trisomy 13 and 18 conceptions are spontaneously lost during pregnancy.

Trisomies of the 13th and 18th chromosomes are sometimes compatible with survival to term, although 95% or more are spontaneously aborted. These trisomies are much less common at birth than trisomy 21, and they produce a much more seriously affected phenotype with 90% mortality during the first year of life.

Trisomies, Nondisjunction, and Maternal Age

The prevalence of Down syndrome among mothers of different ages is shown in Figure 6-9. Among mothers younger than the age of 30, the risk is less than 1 in 1,000. It increases to approximately 1 in 400 among women at age 35, to approximately 1% at age 40, and to 2% or more after age 45. Most other trisomies, including those that do not survive to term, also increase in prevalence as maternal age increases. This risk is one of the primary indications for prenatal diagnosis among women older than age 35 (see Chapter 11).

Several hypotheses have been advanced to account for this increase, including the idea that older women are less likely to spontaneously abort a trisomic pregnancy. It is most likely that the pattern is due to an increase in nondisjunction among older mothers. Recall that all of a female's oocytes are formed during her embryonic development. They remain suspended in prophase I until they are shed during ovulation. Thus an ovum produced by a 45-year-old woman is itself about 45 years old. This long period of suspension in prophase I may impair normal disjunction. However, the precise nature of this mechanism is not understood.

Many factors have been examined to determine whether they may affect the frequency of nondisjunction in women. These include hormone levels, cigarette smoking, autoimmune thyroid disease, alcohol consumption, and radiation (the latter does increase nondisjunction when administered in

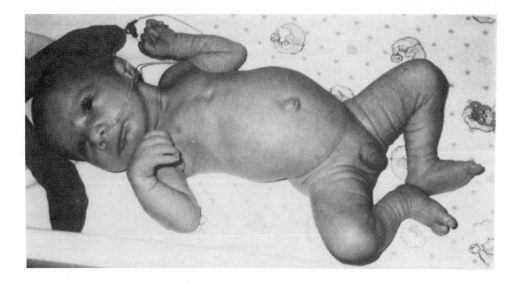

A

Figure 6-8 ■ A, A newborn male with full trisomy 13 (Patau syndrome). This baby has a cleft palate, atrial septal defect, inguinal hernia, and postaxial polydactyly of the left hand. He is deaf and legally blind. B, The same individual at age three (survival beyond the first year is uncommon). (Courtesy of Susan Barg.)

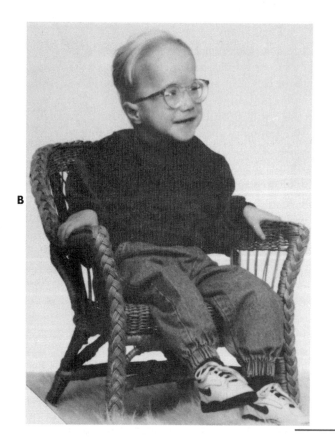

B

Number of Down syndrome cases per 1,000 births

Figure 6-9 ■ The prevalence of Down syndrome among live births in relation to age of the mother. The prevalence increases with maternal age and becomes especially notable after the age of 35. (Data from Hook EB, Chambers GM: Birth Defects: Original Articles Series, vol. 23, No. 3A, 123-141, 1977.)

large doses to experimental animals). None of these has shown consistent correlations with non-disjunction in humans, however, and maternal age remains the only known correlated factor.

Numerous studies have tested the hypothesis of a paternal age effect for trisomies, and the consensus is that such an effect, if it exists at all, is relatively minor. This may reflect the fact that spermatocytes, unlike oocytes, are generated throughout the life of the male.

Nearly all autosomal trisomies increase with maternal age. This is most likely due to an increased rate of nondisjunction among

older mothers. There is little evidence for a paternal age effect on nondisjunction.

Sex Chromosome Aneuploidy

Among live births, about 1 in 400 males and 1 in 650 females have some form of sex chromosome aneuploidy. Primarily because of X inactivation, the consequences of this class of aneuploidy are less severe than those of autosomal aneuploidy. With the possible exception of a complete absence of the X chromosome, all of the sex chromosome aneuploidies are compatible with survival in at least some cases.

Monosomy of the X Chromosome (Turner Syndrome)

The phenotype associated with a single X chromosome (45,X) was originally recognized by Henry Turner in 1939. Individuals with Turner syndrome are female and usually have a characteristic phenotype. The findings include the variable presence of (1) proportionate short stature, (2) sexual infantilism and ovarian dysgenesis, and (3) a pattern of major and minor malformations. The physical features may include a triangle-shaped face; posteriorly rotated, external ears; and a broad, "webbed" neck (Fig. 6-10). In addition, the chest is broad and shieldlike in shape. Lymphedema of the hands and feet is observable at birth. About 20% of patients with Turner syndrome have congenital heart defects, most commonly obstructive lesions of the left side of heart, including **coarctation** (narrowing) of the aorta. In a small percentage of cases, the coarctation can lead to necrosis and rupture of the aorta. About 50% of individuals with Turner syndrome have structural kidney defects, but these are usually unnoticed and do not cause medical problems. There is typically some diminution in spatial perceptual ability, but Turner females are not mentally retarded.

Girls with Turner syndrome do not undergo an adolescent growth spurt and thus have proportionate short stature. In recent years, evidence has accumulated that growth hormone administration may bring about increased height gain in these girls. **Gonadal dysgenesis** (lack of ovaries) is commonly seen in Turner syndrome. Instead of ovaries, most Turner females have streaks of connective tissue. Lacking normal ovaries, Turner females do not usually develop secondary sexual characteristics, and most women with this condition are infertile (about 5% to 10% have sufficient ovarian development to undergo menarche, and a small number have borne children). Girls with Turner syndrome are sometimes treated with estro-

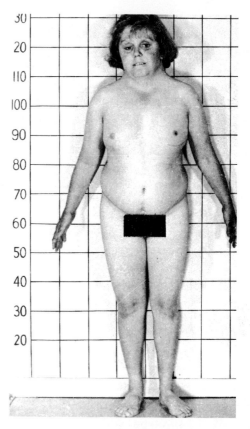

Figure 6-10 ▪ A female with Turner syndrome (45,X). Note the characteristically broad "webbed" neck. Stature is reduced, and sexual secondary characteristics are poorly developed. (SOL 48) (From K.L. McCance and S.E. Huether, Pathophysiology: The Biologic Basis for Disease in Adults and Children, p. 139, Mosby, 1994, St. Louis.)

gen to promote the development of secondary sexual characteristics. The dose is then continued at a minimal level to maintain these characteristics.

Frequently the diagnosis is made in the newborn infant, especially if there is a striking neck webbing coupled with a heart defect. The facial features are more subtle than the autosomal abnormalities described above, but the experienced clinician will often diagnose Turner syndrome because of one or more of the listed clues. If Turner syndrome is not diagnosed in infancy or childhood, it will often be diagnosed later because of short stature and/or amenorrhea.

The chromosome abnormalities in females with Turner syndrome are variable. About 50% of these patients have a 45,X karyotype in all of their peripheral lymphocytes. About 30% to 40% are mosaics, most commonly 45,X/46,XX and less commonly 45,X/46,XY. Mosaics who have Y chromosomes in some cells are predisposed to developing malignancies (gonadoblastomas) in their gonadal streaks. About 10% to 20% of patients with

Turner syndrome have structural X chromosome abnormalities involving a deletion of some or all of the short arm. This variation in chromosome abnormality helps to explain the considerable phenotypic variation seen in this syndrome.

Molecular studies have shown that approximately 80% of monosomy X cases are caused by meiotic error in the father (i.e., the offspring receives an X chromosome from the mother but no sex chromosome from the father). The prevalence of the 45,X karyotype is low compared with those of other sex chromosome abnormalities, with only about 1 in 2500 to 5000 liveborn females having the disorder. The 45,X karyotype is common among conceptions, however, and it accounts for 15% to 20% of the chromosome abnormalities seen among spontaneous abortions. Thus the great majority (>99%) of 45,X conceptions are lost prenatally. Among those that do survive to term, many are chromosomal mosaics, with mosaicism of the placenta alone (**confined placental mosaicism**) being especially common.

> **Turner syndrome is most commonly caused by a 45,X karyotype. Although common at conception, this disorder is relatively rare among live births, reflecting a high rate of spontaneous abortion. Mosaicism, including confined placental mosaicism, appears to increase the probability of survival to term.**

Klinefelter Syndrome

Like the Down and Turner syndromes, the syndrome associated with a 47,XXY karyotype was described long before the underlying chromosomal abnormality was understood. This disorder is a common cause of primary hypogonadism in the male and is seen in approximately 1 in 1000 male births. The phenotype is less striking than those of the syndromes described thus far. Males with Klinefelter syndrome tend to be taller than average, with disproportionately long arms and legs (Fig. 6-11). Clinical examination of postpubertal patients reveals small testes (<10 ml), and most Klinefelter males are sterile as a result of atrophy of the seminiferous tubules. Gynecomastia (breast development) is seen in approximately one third of Klinefelter males and leads to an increased risk of breast cancer. This risk can be reduced with mastectomy (breast removal). In addition, there is a predisposition for learning disabilities and subaverage intelligence. Although males with Klinefelter syndrome are not usually mentally retarded, the IQ is on average 10 to 15 points below that of the

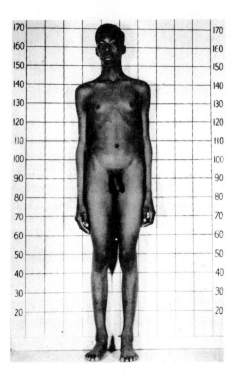

Figure 6-11 ■ A male with Klinefelter syndrome (47,XXY). Stature is increased, gynecomastia may be present, and body shape may be somewhat feminine. (From K.L. McCance and S.E. Huether, Pathophysiology: The Biologic Basis for Disease in Adults and Children, Mosby, 1994, St. Louis.)

affected individual's siblings. Because of the subtlety of this disorder, many Klinefelter patients are not diagnosed until after puberty and are sometimes first ascertained in fertility clinics.

The extra X chromosome is derived maternally in about 60% of Klinefelter cases, and the syndrome increases in incidence with advanced maternal age. Mosaicism is seen in about 15% of patients. Despite the relatively mild phenotypic features of this disorder, it is estimated that at least half of 47,XXY conceptions are spontaneously aborted.

Patients with the 48,XXXY and 49,XXXXY karyotypes have also been reported. Because they have a Y chromosome, they still have a male phenotype, but the degree of mental deficiency and physical abnormality increases with each additional X chromosome.

Testosterone therapy may enhance secondary sex characteristics in postpubertal Klinefelter males. There is some evidence that this treatment also improves general well-being, but this has not been clearly substantiated.

> **Klinefelter syndrome (47,XXY) males are taller than average, may have a reduction**

in IQ, and are usually sterile. Testosterone therapy and mastectomy for gynecomastia are sometimes recommended.

Trisomy X

The 47,XXX karyotype occurs in approximately 1 in 1000 females and usually has benign consequences. Overt physical abnormalities are rarely seen, but these females sometimes suffer from sterility, menstrual irregularity, or mild mental retardation. As in Klinefelter syndrome, 47,XXX females are often first ascertained in fertility clinics. The great majority of cases are the result of nondisjunction in the mother, and, as in other trisomies, the incidence increases among older mothers.

Females have also been seen with four, five, or even more X chromosomes. Each additional X chromosome is accompanied by increased mental retardation and physical abnormality.

47,XYY Syndrome

The final sex chromosome aneuploidy to be discussed is the 47,XYY karyotype. Males with this karyotype tend to be taller than average, and they have a 10- to 15-point reduction in average IQ. This condition, which causes few physical problems, achieved great notoriety when its incidence in male prison populations was discovered to be about 1 in 30, compared with 1/1000 in the general male population. This led to the suggestion that this karyotype might confer a predisposition to violent, criminal behavior. Several dozen studies have addressed this issue, and they have shown that XYY males are not inclined to commit violent crimes. There is, however, evidence of minor behavioral disorders, such as hyperactivity, attention deficit disorder, and learning disabilities.

The 47,XXX and 47,XYY karyotypes are seen in about 1 in 1000 females and males, respectively. Each involves a slight degree of reduction in IQ but few physical problems.

■ CHROMOSOME ABNORMALITIES AND PREGNANCY LOSS

For a long time it was difficult to detect the early stages of pregnancy with certainty. Thus it was possible for a woman to become pregnant but lose the embryo before knowing of the pregnancy. Sensitive urinary assays of chorionic gonadotropin levels, which show an increase when the embryo implants in the uterine wall, have allowed researchers to pinpoint accurately the occurrence of pregnancy at this early stage. Follow-up of women in whom implantation was verified in this way has shown that about one-third of pregnancies are lost after implantation (the number lost prior to implantation is unknown). Thus spontaneous pregnancy loss is common in the human.

As mentioned earlier, chromosome abnormalities are the leading known cause of pregnancy loss. It is estimated that a minimum of 10% to 15% of conceptions have a chromosome abnormality. At least 95% of these chromosomally abnormal conceptions are lost before term. Karyotype studies of miscarriages indicate that about half of the chromosome abnormalities are trisomies, 20% are monosomies, and 15% are triploids. The remainder consist of tetraploids and structural abnormalities. Some chromosome abnormalities that are common at conception seldom or never survive to term. For example, trisomy 16 is thought to be the most common trisomy at conception, but it is never seen in live births.

It is possible to study chromosome abnormalities directly in sperm and egg cells. Oocytes are typically obtained from unused material in in vitro fertilization studies. Karyotypes obtained from these cells indicate that 20% to 25% of oocytes have missing or extra chromosomes (this may be an underestimate because the oocyte's chromosomes are difficult to visualize and count). Human sperm cells can be studied after fusing them with hamster oocytes so that their DNA begins mitosis and condenses, allowing easier visualization. The frequency of aneuploidy in these sperm cells is about 3% to 4%. Structural abnormalities are seen in about 5% of sperm cells and about 1% of oocytes. Undoubtedly this high rate of chromosome abnormality contributes importantly to later pregnancy loss.

These approaches, although informative, may involve some biases. For example, mothers in whom in vitro fertilization is performed are not a representative sample of the population. In addition, their oocytes have been stimulated artificially, and only those oocytes that could not be fertilized by sperm cells are studied. Thus the oocytes themselves may not be a representative sample. The sperm cells studied in human–hamster hybrids represent only those that are capable of penetrating the hamster oocyte and again may not be a representative sample.

Recently, FISH has been used to detect missing or extra chromosomes in human sperm cells. This approach can evaluate thousands of cells fairly rapidly, giving it an important advantage over the human–hamster technique.

Clinical Commentary 6-2. XX Males, XY Females, and the Genetic Basis of Sex Determination

During normal meiosis in the male, crossover occurs between the tip of the short arm of the Y chromosome and the tip of the short arm of the X chromosome. These regions of the X and Y chromosomes contain highly similar DNA sequences. Because this crossover resembles the behavior of autosomes during meiosis, the distal portion of the Y chromosome is known as the **pseudoautosomal** region (Fig. 6-12). It spans approximately 2.5 MB. Just centromeric of the pseudoautosomal region lies a gene known as *SRY* (sex-determining region on the Y). This gene, which is expressed in embryonic development, encodes a product that interacts with other genes to initiate the development of the undifferentiated embryo into a male (e.g., Sertoli cell differentiation, secretion of mullerian inhibiting substance). The *SRY* gene product has DNA-binding characteristics, as expected of a protein that interacts with other genes in a developmental cascade. When the *SRY* gene is inserted experimentally into a female mouse embryo, a male mouse is produced. Mutations of *SRY* can produce individuals with an XY karyotype but a female phenotype. Thus there is good evidence that the *SRY* gene is the initiator of male sexual differentiation in the embryo.

Approximately 1 in 20,000 males presents with a condition similar to Klinefelter syndrome, but chromosome evaluation shows such males have a normal *female* karyotype (46, XX). It was demonstrated that these XX males have an X chromosome that includes the *SRY* gene. This is explained as a result of a faulty crossover between the X and Y chromosomes during male meiosis, such that the *SRY* gene, instead of remaining on the Y chromosome, is transferred to the X chromosome (Fig. 6-12). The offspring inheriting this X chromosome from the father consequently has a male phenotype. Conversely, it should be apparent that an offspring inheriting a Y chromosome that lacks the *SRY* gene would be an XY *female*. These females have gonadal streaks rather than ovaries and have poorly developed secondary sexual characteristics.

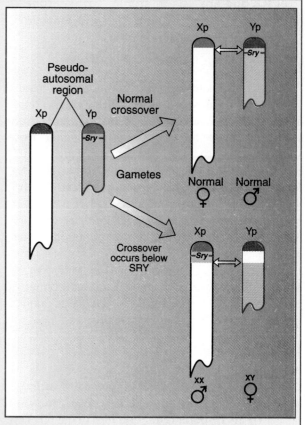

Figure 6-12 ■ The distal short arms of the X and Y chromosomes exchange material during meiosis in the male. The region of the Y chromosome in which this crossover occurs is called the pseudoautosomal region. The *SRY* gene, which triggers the process leading to male gonadal differentiation, is located just outside the pseudoautosomal region. Occasionally, the crossover occurs on the centromeric side of the *SRY* gene, causing it to lie on an X chromosome instead of a Y chromosome. An offspring receiving this X chromosome will be an XX male, and an offspring receiving the Y chromosome will be an XY female.

Pregnancy loss is common in the human, with approximately one-third of pregnancies lost spontaneously after implantation. Chromosome abnormalities, which have been studied in sperm cells, egg cells, and in miscarriages and stillbirths, are an important cause of pregnancy loss.

■ ABNORMALITIES OF CHROMOSOME STRUCTURE

In addition to the loss or gain of whole chromosomes, parts of chromosomes can be lost or duplicated as gametes are formed, and the arrangement of portions of chromosomes can be altered. Structural chromosome abnormalities may be unbalanced (the rearrangement causes a gain or loss of chromosomal material) or balanced (the rearrangement does not produce a loss or gain of chromosome material). Unlike aneuploidy and polyploidy, balanced structural abnormalities often do not produce serious health consequences. Nevertheless, abnormalities of chromosome structure, especially those that are unbalanced, can produce serious disease in individuals or their offspring.

Alterations of chromosome structure can occur when homologous chromosomes line up improperly during meiosis (e.g., unequal crossover, as described in Chapter 5). In addition, chromosome breakage during meiosis or mitosis can occur. Mechanisms exist to repair these breaks, and generally the break is repaired perfectly with no damage to the daughter cell. Sometimes, however, the breaks remain, or they heal in a fashion that alters the structure of the chromosome. The likelihood of chromosome breakage may be increased in the presence of certain harmful agents, called clastogens. Clastogens identified in experimental systems include ionizing radiation, some viral infections, and some chemicals. However, none of these agents has conclusively been shown to cause chromosome breakage in humans.

Translocations

A translocation is the interchange of genetic material between nonhomologous chromosomes. Balanced translocations represent one of the most common chromosomal aberrations in humans, with a prevalence of at least 1 in 500 individuals (Table 6-2). There are two basic types of translocations, termed reciprocal and Robertsonian.

Reciprocal Translocations

These translocations occur when breaks occur in two different chromosomes and the material is mutually exchanged. The resulting chromosomes are called derivative chromosomes. The carrier of a reciprocal translocation is usually normal because he or she has a normal complement of genetic material. However, the carrier's offspring can be normal, can carry the translocation, or can have duplications or deletions of genetic material.

An example of a reciprocal translocation between chromosomes 3 and 6 is shown in Figure 6-13. The distal half of the short arm of chromosome 6 is translocated to the short arm of chromosome 3, and a small piece of chromosome 3 is translocated to the short arm of chromosome 6. This karyotype is 46,XX,t(3p;6p). The offspring of this woman

Table 6-2 ■ Prevalence of chromosomal abnormalities among newborns

Abnormality	Prevalence at birth
Autosomal syndromes	
Trisomy 21	1/800
Trisomy 18	1/6000
Trisomy 13	1/10,000
Unbalanced rerrangements	1/17,000
Balanced rearrangements	
Robertsonian translocations	1/1000
Reciprocal translocations	1/11,000
Sex chromosome abnormalities	
47,XXY	1/1000 male births
47,XYY	1/1000 male births
45,X*	1/5000 female births
47,XXX	1/1000 female births
All chromosomal abnormalities	
Autosomal disorders and unbalanced rearrangements	1/230
Balanced rearrangements	1/500†

*Note that the 45,X karyotype accounts for about one half of the cases of Turner syndrome.
†This figure is based primarily on older studies of unbanded chromosomes. More recent studies using banded preparations (Jacobs et al, 1992) show that the prevalence of balanced structural abnormalities is approximately 1 in 200.

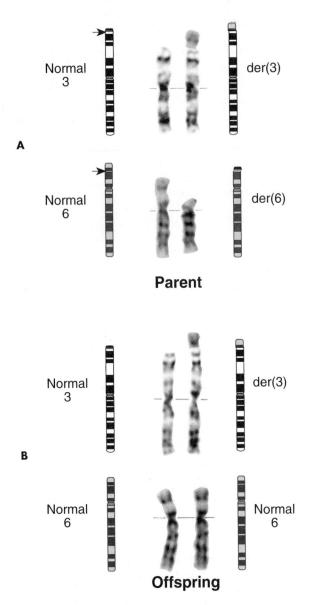

Figure 6-13 ■ A, The parent has a reciprocal balanced translocation involving the short arms of the 3 and 6 chromosomes. The distal short arm of the 6 has been translocated to the very distal tip of the 3 chromosome. A small piece of chromosome 3 is attached to the derivative 6. This individual had a child whose chromosomes are depicted in (B). The child received the derivative 3 chromosome (with part of the 6 short arm attached) and the normal 6. The child received a normal 3 and a normal 6 from the other parent. Thus, the child had a partial trisomy of the 6 short arm and presumably a small deletion of the 3 short arm (see text).

received the derivative chromosome 3 [der(3)] and the normal 6; thus the child has a **partial trisomy** of the distal portion of chromosome 6 (i.e., 6p trisomy). This is a well-established but rather uncommon chromosomal syndrome.

Reciprocal translocations are caused by two breaks on different chromosomes, with a subsequent exchange of material. While carriers of balanced reciprocal translocations usually have normal phenotypes, their offspring may have a partial trisomy or a partial monosomy and an abnormal phenotype.

Robertsonian Translocations

In this type of translocation, the short arms of two nonhomologous chromosomes are lost and the long arms fuse at the centromere, forming a single chromosome (Fig. 6-14). This type of translocation is confined to chromosomes 13–15, 21, and 22 because the short arms of these acrocentric chromosomes are small and contain no essential genetic material. When a Robertsonian translocation takes place, the short arms are usually lost during subsequent cell divisions. Because the carriers of

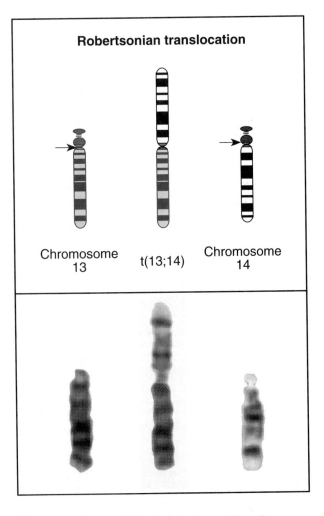

Figure 6-14 ■ In a Robertsonian translocation, shown here, the long arms of two acrocentric chromosomes (13 and 14) fuse, forming a single chromosome.

Robertsonian translocations lose no essential genetic material, they are phenotypically normal but have only 45 chromosomes in each cell. Their offspring, however, may inherit a missing or extra long arm of an acrocentric chromosome.

A common Robertsonian translocation involves the fusion of the long arms of chromosomes 21 and 14. The karyotype of a male carrier of this translocation would be $45,XY,-14,-21,+t(14q21q)$, with -14 and -21 showing that the carrier lacks one normal 14 and one normal 21. During meiosis, the translocation chromosome must still pair with its homologs (Figure 6-15). The figure illustrates the ways in which these chromosomes may segregate in the gametes formed by the translocation carrier. If **alternate segregation** occurs, then the offspring are either chromosomally normal or have a balanced translocation with a normal phenotype. If either of the **adjacent segregation** patterns occur, then the gametes are unbalanced and the

offspring may have trisomy 14, monosomy 14, monosomy 21, or trisomy 21 (note that these trisomies and monosomies are genetically the same as trisomies and monosomies produced by nondisjunction because only the long arms of these chromosomes contain genetically significant material). The former three possibilities do not survive to term, whereas the last results in an offspring with three copies of the long arm of chromosome 21 and a Down syndrome phenotype. Robertsonian translocations are responsible for approximately 5% of Down syndrome cases.

It is expected that the three types of conceptions compatible with survival would occur in equal frequencies. Thus one third would be completely normal, one third would carry the translocation but be phenotypically normal, and one third would have Down syndrome. In part because of prenatal loss, the actual proportion of liveborn offspring with Down syndrome is less than one third (about

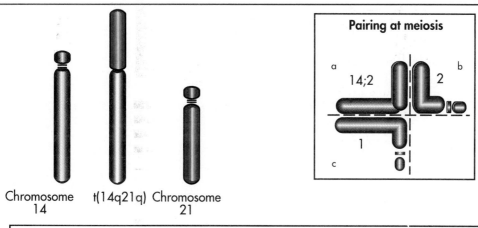

Chromosome
14

t(14q21q)

Chromosome
21

Pairing at meiosis

a   14;2   2   b

1

c

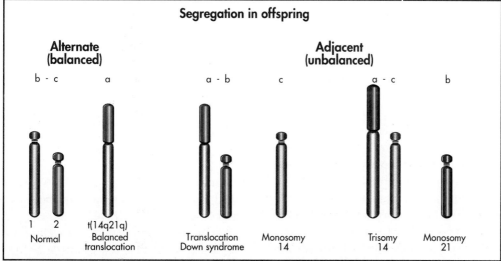

Segregation in offspring

**Alternate
(balanced)**

b - c   a

**Adjacent
(unbalanced)**

a - b   c   a - c   b

1   2
Normal

t(14q21q)
Balanced
translocation

Translocation
Down syndrome

Monosomy
14

Trisomy
14

Monosomy
21

Figure 6-15 ■ The possible segregation patterns for the gametes formed by a carrier of a Robertsonian translocation. Alternate segregation (quadrant A alone or quadrant B with quadrant C) produces either a normal chromosome constitution or a translocation carrier with a normal phenotype. Adjacent segregation (quadrant A with C or quadrant A with B) produces unbalanced gametes and will result in conceptions with trisomy 14, trisomy 21, monosomy 14, or monosomy 21.

10% to 15% for mothers carrying the translocation, and only 1% to 2% for fathers that carry it). This recurrence risk, however, is greater than the risk for parents of a child who has the nondisjunction type of Down syndrome, which is 1% for mothers younger than age 30. This difference in recurrence risks demonstrates why it is critical to order a chromosome study whenever a trisomy such as Down syndrome is suspected.

> **Robertsonian translocations occur when the long arms of two acrocentric chromosomes fuse at the centromere. The carrier of a Robertsonian translocation can produce conceptions with monosomy or trisomy.**

Deletions

A **deletion** is caused by a chromosome break and subsequent loss of genetic material. A single break leading to a loss that includes the chromosome's tip is called a **terminal deletion**. When two breaks occur and the material between the breaks is lost, an **interstitial deletion** has occurred. For example, a chromosome segment with normal DNA might be symbolized ABCDEFG. An interstitial deletion could produce the sequence ABEFG, and a terminal deletion could produce ABCDE.

Usually a gamete containing a chromosome with a deletion unites with a normal gamete to form a zygote. The zygote then has one normal chromosome and a homolog with the deletion. Microscopically visible deletions generally involve multiple genes, and the consequences of losing this much genetic material on even one member of the chromosome pair can be severe.

After the three autosomal aneuploidies described earlier, the autosomal deletion syndromes are the most common group of clinically significant chromosome abnormalities. A well-known example of a chromosome deletion syndrome is the *cri-du-chat* syndrome. This term (French for "cry of the cat") describes the distinctive cry of the child. This cry usually becomes less obvious as the child ages, making a clinical diagnosis more difficult after 2 years of age. *Cri-du-chat* syndrome is caused by a deletion of the short arm of chromosome 5- [karyotype 46,XY,del(5p)]. Seen in approximately 1 in 50,000 live births, it is also characterized by mental retardation (average IQ about 35), microcephaly (small head), and a characteristic but not distinctive facial appearance. Survival to adulthood has been observed but is not common.

Wolf-Hirschhorn syndrome (Fig. 6-16) is another well-characterized deletion syndrome, caused by a deletion of the short arm of chromosome 4 (4p-).

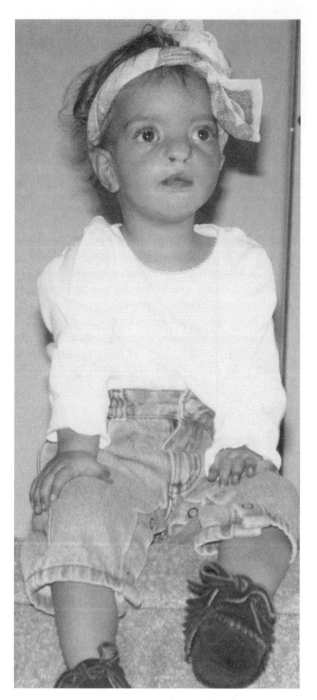

Figure 6-16 ■ A child with Wolf-Hirschhorn syndrome [46,XX,del(4p)]. Note the wide-spaced eyes and repaired cleft lip.

In addition to the 4p- and 5p- syndromes, other well-known deletions include those of 18p, 18q, and 13q. With the exception of the 18p- syndrome, each of these disorders is relatively distinctive, and the diagnosis can often be made before obtaining the karyotype. The features of the 18p- syndrome are much more subtle, and usually children with this condition are recognized when chromosome analysis is performed for evaluation of developmental disability.

Microscopically observable chromosome deletions, which may be either terminal or interstitial, usually affect a fairly large number of genes and produce recognizable syndromes.

Microdeletion Syndromes

The deletions described thus far all involve relatively large segments of chromosomes. Each of these was described before chromosome-banding techniques were developed. With the advent of banding, and especially high-resolution banding, it has become possible to identify microscopically a large number of deletions that were previously too small for detection. In addition, advances in molecular genetics, particularly the development of large numbers of easily identified polymorphisms, have permitted the detection of deletions too small to be observed microscopically. Such deletions are detected by showing that a series of RFLPs in a defined chromosome region all produce single, relatively faint bands, indicating that one copy of this region of the chromosome is missing (Figure 6-17).

Prader-Willi syndrome, a disorder discussed in Chapter 4, is a good example of a **microdeletion syndrome**. Although this condition was described in the 1950s, it was not until 1981 that advanced banding techniques detected a small deletion of

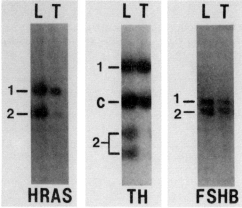

Figure 6-17 ■ RFLP loss of heterozygosity demonstrates a microdeletion in tumor cells. Autoadiograms for three RFLPs on the tip of the short arm of chromosome 11 are shown. In each autoradiogram, the lane labeled "L" contains DNA taken from a patient's lymphocytes, while the lane labeled "T" contains DNA taken from the patient's malignant astrocytoma. Because a tiny part of 11 p was deleted in the tumor cells, the tumor DNA is homozygous for the HRAS and TH RFLPs, whereas the lymphocyte DNA is heterozygous for these markers. The FSHB marker lies outside the region of the deletion and is thus heterozygous in both the tumor and the lymphocyte DNA. (Courtesy of Dr. Dan Fults, University of Utah Health Sciences Center.)

chromosome bands 15q11-q13 in about 50% of these patients. By using molecular techniques, deletions that were too small to be detected cytogenetically were also discovered. In total, about 70% of Prader-Willi cases are due to microdeletions of 15q. Because of imprinting, the inheritance of a microdeletion of the paternal chromosome 15 material produces Prader-Willi syndrome, whereas a microdeletion of the maternally derived chromosome 15 produces the phenotypically distinct Angelman syndrome (see Chapter 4).

High-resolution banding and molecular genetic techniques have often led to a more precise specification of the critical chromosome region that must be deleted to cause a given syndrome. Wolf-Hirschhorn syndrome, for instance, can be produced by the deletion of only a small telomeric segment of 4p. In some instances, specific genes responsible for chromosome abnormality syndromes can be pinpointed. For example, individuals with a deletion of 11p may present with a series of features including Wilms tumor (a kidney tumor), aniridia (absence of the iris), genitourinary abnormalities,* and mental retardation (sometimes termed the WAGR syndrome). The genes responsible for the kidney tumor and for aniridia have now each been identified and cloned. Because the WAGR syndrome involves the deletion of a series of adjacent genes, it is sometimes referred to as an example of a **contiguous gene syndrome**. In addition to microdeletions, microduplications can also produce contiguous gene syndromes.

Several examples of microdeletion syndromes are given in Table 6-3. Some of these conditions, including the Prader-Willi, Miller-Dieker, and velo-cardio-facial syndromes (Clinical Commentary 6-3), are now diagnosed using the FISH technique.

Microdeletions are a subtype of chromosome deletion that can only be observed using banded chromosomes or, in some cases, using molecular genetic approaches. Because these abnormalities generally involve the deletion of a series of adjacent genes, they are also sometimes called contiguous gene syndromes.

Uniparental Isodisomy

As just mentioned, about 70% of Prader-Willi cases are caused by microdeletions. The remainder have **uniparental disomy** (di = "two"), a

*Because individuals with the WAGR syndrome also have gonadoblastomas (gonadal tumors), some authorities believe that the "G" should stand for gonadoblastoma rather than genitourinary abnormality.

Clinical Commentary 6-3. The DiGeorge Anomaly, the Velo-Cardio-Facial Syndrome, and Microdeletions of Chromosome 22

The DiGeorge anomaly consists of a pattern of structural or functional defects of the thymus, hypoparathyroidism (reduced parathyroid function), secondary hypocalcemia (decreased serum calcium), and congenital heart defects. This pattern is a malformation complex probably caused by an alteration of the embryonic migration of neural crest cells to the developing structures of the neck. In the 1980s it was learned that some children with the DiGeorge anomaly had a deletion of the long arm of chromosome 22, often related to an unbalanced translocation between this and another chromosome. This led to the hypothesis that genes on chromosome 22 were responsible for the DiGeorge anomaly.

Independently, a condition called the velo-cardio-facial (VCF) or Shprintzen syndrome was described in the late 1970s. This autosomal dominant syndrome involves palate (velum) abnormalities (including clefts), a characteristic facial appearance, and, in some cases, heart disease. In addition, these patients have learning disabilities and developmental delay. Later it was discovered that some individuals with VCF

have dysfunctional T-cells (these cells mature in the thymus), and some have all features of the DiGeorge anomaly. This suggested that the DiGeorge anomaly was somehow related to VCF.

The resemblance between the DiGeorge anomaly and VCF led to the hypothesis that both conditions were caused by abnormalities on chromosome 22. High-resolution chromosome studies in patients with DiGeorge anomaly and in patients with VCF revealed small deletions of chromosome 22 in both sets of patients. This analysis also helped to narrow the critical region that causes both conditions. Approximately 80% of infants with DiGeorge anomaly have a microdeletion of the 22q11 region, and about 70% of VCF patients have the same microdeletion. It is now postulated that alterations of a gene(s) in this region can produce a variable phenotype ranging from the DiGeorge anomaly to the full VCF syndrome. It is possible that the VCF syndrome is a contiguous gene syndrome, and the gene(s) causing DiGeorge anomaly is a subset of those that cause VCF.

This example illustrates how cytogenetic studies can demonstrate potential biologic relationships between genetic syndromes. Further studies are under way to identify the individual genes that cause DiGeorge anomaly and VCF.

condition in which one parent has contributed two copies of a chromosome and the other parent has contributed no copies. If the parent has contributed two copies of one homolog, the condition is termed **isodisomy**. If the parent has contributed one copy of each homolog, it is termed **heterodis-**

omy. This phenomenon, only recently discovered in humans, can arise in a number of ways. For example, a trisomic conception can lose one of the extra chromosomes, resulting in an embryo that has two copies of the chromosome contributed by one parent. Disomy can also arise from a monosomic

Table 6-3 ■ Microdeletion syndromes

Syndrome	Clinical features	Chromosomal deletions	FISH available
Prader-Willi	Mental retardation, short stature, obesity, hypotonia, characteristic facies, small feet	15q11–13	Yes
Angelman	Mental retardation, microcephaly, seizures, characteristic gait	15q11	Yes
Langer-Giedion	Characteristic facies, sparse hair, exostosis, variable mental retardation	8q24	Possible
Miller-Dieker	Lissencephaly, characteristic facies	17p13.3	Yes
DiGeorge anomaly/ velo-cardio-facial syndrome	DiGeorge anomaly/characteristic facies, cleft palate, heart defect	22q11	Yes
Rubinstein Taybi syndrome	Developmental disability, characteristic face, broad thumbs	16p13	Possible
Williams syndrome	Developmental disability, characteristic facies, supravalvular aortic stenosis	7q1	Yes
Retinoblastoma	Eye tumor presenting in infancy	13q14	Yes
Aniridia/Wilms tumor	Mental retardation, aniridia, predisposition to Wilms tumor, genital defects	11p13	Yes

conception followed by mitotic nondisjunction, producing cells with two copies of the monosomic chromosome. Uniparental disomy, although fairly rare, has been observed in several conditions besides Prader-Willi and Angelman syndromes. These include cystic fibrosis (see Chapter 4) and the Beckwith-Wiedemann syndrome (see Chapter 12).

Duplications

A partial trisomy, or a **duplication**, of genetic material may be seen in the offspring of individuals who carry a reciprocal translocation. Duplications can also be caused by unequal crossover during meiosis, as described for the X-linked color vision loci (see Chapter 5). Duplications tend to produce less serious consequences than deletions, again illustrating the principle that a loss of genetic material is more serious than is an excess of genetic material.

> **Duplications can arise from unequal crossover or can occur among the offspring of reciprocal translocation carriers. Duplications generally have less serious consequences than deletions.**

Ring Chromosomes

Sometimes deletions occur at both tips of a chromosome. The remaining chromosome ends can then fuse, forming a **ring chromosome** (Fig. 6-18). The karyotype of a female with a ring X chromosome would be 46,X,r(X). If the ring chromosome includes a centromere, it can often proceed through cell division, but its structure can create difficulties. Ring chromosomes are often lost, resulting in monosomy for the chromosome in at least some cells (i.e., mosaicism for the ring chromosome may be seen). Ring chromosomes have been described in at least one case in each of the human autosomes.

Inversions

An **inversion** is the result of two breaks on a chromosome followed by the reinsertion of the missing fragment at its original site but in inverted order. Thus a chromosome symbolized as ABCDEFG might become ABEDCFG after an inversion. When the inversion includes the centromere, it is called a **pericentric inversion**. Inversions not involving the centromere are termed **paracentric inversions**.

Like reciprocal translocations, inversions are a balanced structural rearrangement. Thus they usually have no apparent physical effect (recall from Chapter 5, however, that an inversion that inter-

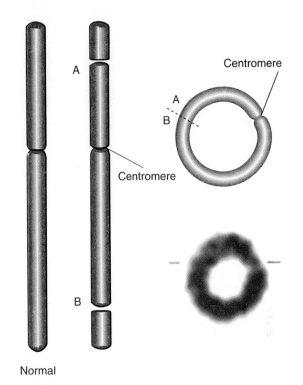

Normal

Figure 6-18 ■ Both tips of a chromosome can be lost, leaving sticky ends that attach to each other, forming a ring chromosome. A chromosome 12 ring is show here.

rupts the factor VIII gene produces severe hemophilia A). Inversions can interfere with meiosis, however, producing chromosome abnormalities in the offspring of inversion carriers. Because chromosomes must line up in perfect order during prophase I, a chromosome with an inversion must form a loop to line up with its normal homolog (Fig. 6-19). Crossing over within this loop can result in duplications or deletions in the chromosomes of daughter cells. Thus the offspring of individuals who carry inversions often have chromosome deletions or duplications. It is estimated that about 1 in 1000 people carries an inversion and is therefore at risk for producing gametes with duplications or deletions.

Figure 6-19 gives an example of a pericentric inversion that has occurred on chromosome 8 [46,XX,inv(8)]. About 5% of the offspring of those who carry this inversion will receive a duplication or deletion of the distal portion of 8q. This combination results in the relatively well-described recombinant 8 syndrome.

> **Chromosome inversions are a relatively common structural abnormality and may be either pericentric (including the centromere) or paracentric (not including the centromere). Parents with inversions are usually**

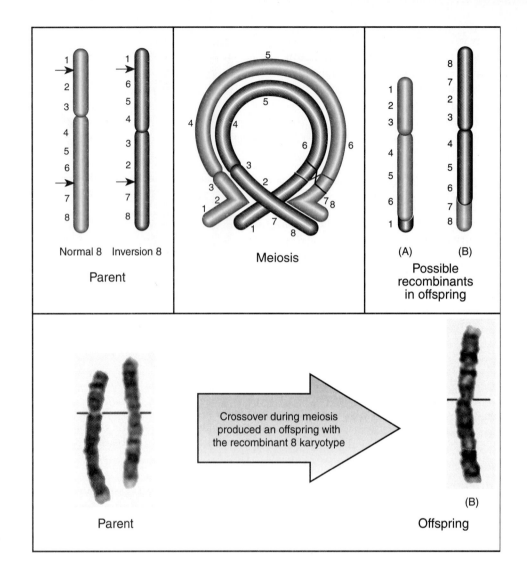

Figure 6-19 ■ A pericentric inversion in chromosome 8 causes the formation of a loop during the alignment of homologous chromosomes in meiosis. Crossing over in this loop can produce duplications or deletions of chromosome material in the resulting gamete. The offspring in the lower panel received one of the recombinant 8 chromosomes from this parent.

normal in phenotype but can produce off-spring with deletions or duplications.

Isochromosomes

Sometimes a chromosome divides along the axis perpendicular to its usual axis of division (Fig. 6-20). The result is an **isochromosome**, a chromosome that has two copies of one arm and no copies of the other. Because the genetic material is substantially altered, isochromosomes of most autosomes are lethal. Most isochromosomes observed in live births involve the X chromosome, and babies with isochromosome Xq [46,X,i(Xq)] usually have features of Turner syndrome. Isochromosome 18q, producing an extra copy of the long arm of chromosome 18, has been observed in infants

with Edwards syndrome. Although most isochromosomes appear to be formed by faulty division, they can also be created by Robertsonian translocations of homologous acrocentric chromosomes.

■ CHROMOSOME ABNORMALITIES AND CLINICAL PHENOTYPES

As we have seen, most autosomal aberrations induce consistent patterns of multiple malformations, minor anomalies, and phenotypic variations with variable degrees of developmental retardation. Although the individual features are usually nonspecific (e.g., simian creases can be seen both in Down syndrome and trisomy 18), the general pattern of features is usually distinctive enough to

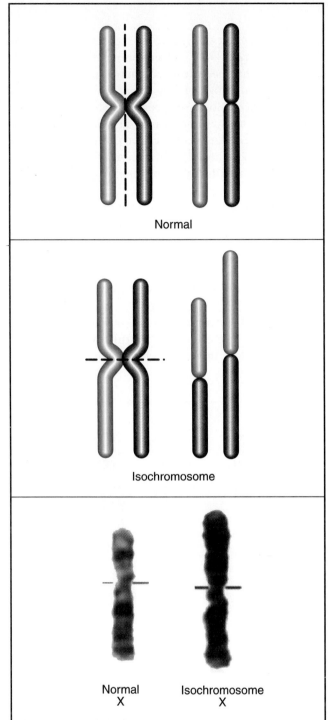

Figure 6-20 An isochromosome is formed when a chromosome divides along an axis perpendicular to its usual axis of division. This produces one chromosome with only the short arms and another with only the long arms. A normal X chromosome is compared with an isochromosome of Xq.

permit a clinical diagnosis. This is especially true of the well-known chromosome syndromes: Down syndrome, Edwards syndrome, Patau syndrome, and Turner syndrome. However, there is considerable phenotypic variability even within these syn-

dromes. No one patient has every feature; most congenital malformations (e.g., heart defects) are seen in only some affected individuals. This phenotypic variability (and the attendant potential for misdiagnosis) underscores the need to order a karyotype whenever clinical features suggest a chromosome abnormality.

Usually the biologic basis for this phenotypic variability is unknown, although mechanisms such as mosaicism, which leads to milder expression, are being uncovered. The basis of variable expression of chromosome syndromes will be better understood as the individual genes involved in these abnormalities are identified and characterized.

Despite the variability of chromosome syndromes, it is possible to make several generalizations:

1. Most chromosome abnormalities (especially those involving autosomes) are associated with developmental delay in children and mental retardation in older individuals. This reflects the fact that a large number of our genes, perhaps 30,000, are involved in the development of the central nervous system. Thus a chromosome abnormality, which typically may affect hundreds or thousands of genes, is likely to involve genes affecting nervous system development.

2. Most chromosome syndromes involve alterations of facial morphogenesis that produce characteristic facial features. For this reason the patient often resembles other individuals with the same disorder more than members of his or her own family. Usually the facial features and minor anomalies of the head and neck are the best aids to diagnosis (see Chapter 12).

3. Growth delay (short stature and/or poor weight gain in infancy) is commonly seen in autosomal syndromes.

4. Congenital malformations, especially congenital heart defects, occur with increased frequency in most autosomal chromosome disorders. These defects occur in specific patterns. For example, although AV canals and ventricular septal defects are common in children with Down syndrome, other congenital heart defects, such as aortic coarctation or hypoplastic (underdeveloped) left ventricle, are seldom seen in these children.

The most common clinical indications for a chromosome analysis are the newborn with multiple congenital malformations or a child with developmental retardation. A summary of clinical situations in which a chromosome evaluation should be considered is given in Box 6-1.

Chromosome abnormalities typically result in developmental delay, mental retardation, characteristic facial appearances, and various types of congenital malformations. Despite some overlap of phenotypic features, many chromosome abnormalities can be recognized by clinical examination.

■ CANCER CYTOGENETICS

Most chromosome abnormality syndromes are caused by errors that occur in the meiotic process leading to gamete formation. However, chromosome rearrangements in somatic cells are responsible for a number of important cancers in humans. The first of these to be recognized was a chromosome alteration seen consistently in patients with chronic myelogenous leukemia (CML). Initially it was suggested that the chromosome alteration was a deletion of the long arm of either chromosome 21 or 22. With the subsequent development of chromosome-banding techniques, the abnormality was identified as a reciprocal translocation between chromosomes 9 and 22. The **Philadelphia chromosome**, as this translocation is commonly known, consists of a translocation of most of chromosome 22 onto the long arm of chromosome 9. A small distal portion of 9q in turn is translocated to chromosome 22. The net effect is a smaller chromosome 22, which explains why the Philadelphia chromo-

some was first thought to be a deletion. This translocation (Fig. 6-21) is seen in most cases of CML.

Much has been learned about the effects of this translocation by isolating the genes that are located near the translocation **breakpoints** (i.e., the locations on the chromosomes at which the breaks occur preceding translocation). A proto-oncogene called *abl* is moved from its normal position on 9q to 22q. This alters the *abl* gene product, causing it to exhibit increased tyrosine kinase activity. This appears to bring about malignancy in hematopoietic cells (i.e., cells that form blood cells such as lymphocytes). In fact, the introduction of this altered gene into the bone marrow of normal mice causes them to develop malignancies, including CML.

A second example of a translocation that produces cancer is given by Burkitt lymphoma, a childhood jaw tumor that is common in equatorial Africa but rare elsewhere. In this case a reciprocal translocation involving chromosomes 8 and 14

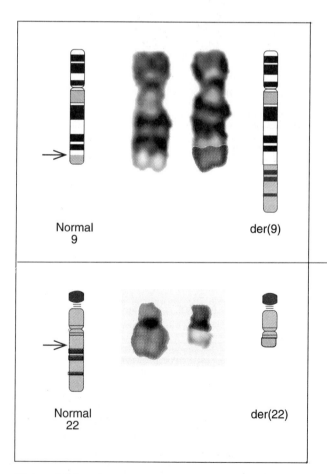

Normal
9   der(9)

Normal
22   der(22)

Figure 6-21 ■ **A reciprocal translocation between chromosome 22 and the long arm of chromosome 9 (the Philadelphia chromosome). The occurrence of this translocation in hematopoietic cells can produce chronic myelogenous leukemia.**

moves the *myc* proto-oncogene from 8q24 to 14q32, near the immunoglobulin heavy chain loci (see Chapter 8). There is good evidence that transcription regulation sequences near the immunoglobulin genes then activate *myc,* causing malignancies to form.

More than 100 different rearrangements involving nearly every chromosome have been observed in over 40 different types of cancer. Some of these are summarized in Table 6-4. In some cases identification of the chromosome rearrangement leads to more accurate prognosis and therapy. Hence the cytogenetic evaluation of bone marrow cells from leukemia patients is a routine part of diagnosis. Furthermore, identification and characterization of the genes that are altered in translocation syndromes are leading to a better understanding of carcinogenesis in general.

Balanced translocations in somatic cells can sometimes cause malignancies by interrupting or altering genes or their regulatory sequences.

■ CHROMOSOME INSTABILITY SYNDROMES

Several autosomal recessive disease conditions exhibit an increased incidence of chromosome breaks under specific laboratory conditions. These conditions, which are termed **chromosome instability syndromes**, include ataxia-telangiectasia, Bloom syndrome, Fanconi anemia, and xeroderma pigmentosum (the latter was discussed in Chapter 2). Among Fanconi anemia patients, the frequency of breaks can be increased further when the chromosomes are exposed to certain alkylating agents. Patients with Bloom syndrome also have a high incidence of somatic cell **sister chromatid exchange** (exchange of chromosome material between sister chromatids, see Chapter 2). Each of these syndromes is associated with a significant increase in cancer risk. All are thought to be the result of faulty DNA replication or repair. DNA repair defects were discussed at length for xeroderma pigmentosum. In Bloom syndrome, normal DNA replication is impaired by a reduction in the activity of DNA ligase I. The protein product of the recently cloned Bloom syndrome gene is similar to the RecQ helicases, which are involved in maintaining accurate DNA replication.

The chromosome instability syndromes all involve increased frequencies of chromo-

Table 6-4 ■ Specific cytogentic changes observed in selected leukemias and solid tumors

	Most common Chromosome aberration
Leukemias	
Chronic myelogenous leukemia	t(9;22)(q34;q11)
Acute myeloblastic leukemia	t(8;21)(q22;q22)
Acute promyelocytic leukemia	t(15;17)(q22;q11.2−12)
Acute nonlymphocytic leukemia	+8,−7,−5,del(5q),del(20q)
Selected solid tumors	
Burkitt lymphoma	t(8;14)(q24;q32)
Ewing sarcoma	t(11;22)(q24;q12)
Meningioma	Monosomy 22
Retinoblastoma	del(13)(q14)
Wilms tumor	del(11)(p13)

some breakage and an increased risk of malignancy. All are associated with defects in DNA replication or repair.

■ STUDY QUESTIONS

1. Distinguish among haploidy, diploidy, polyploidy, euploidy, and aneuploidy.
2. Describe three ways in which triploidy could arise.
3. Studies of karyotypes obtained by prenatal diagnosis at 10 weeks gestation (chorionic villus sampling, see Chapter 11) reveal prevalence rates of chromosome abnormalities that differ from those obtained in karyotypes at 16 weeks gestation (amniocentesis, Chapter 11). Explain this.
4. Even though conditions such as Down syndrome and Edwards syndrome can usually be diagnosed accurately by clinical examination alone, a karyotype is always recommended. Why?
5. Females with the 49,XXXXX karyotype have been reported. Explain how this karyotype could occur.
6. A male with hemophilia A and a normal female produce a child with Turner syndrome (45,X). The child has normal factor VIII activity. In which parent did the meiotic error occur?
7. A cytogenetics laboratory reports a karyotype of 46,XY,del(8p) for one patient and a karyotype of 46,XY,dup(8p) for another patient. Based on this information alone, which patient is expected to be more severely affected?

■ ADDITIONAL READING

Antonarakis SE: Parental origin of the extra chromosome in trisomy 21 as indicated by analysis of DNA polymorphisms, N Engl J Med 324:872–876, 1991.

Baty BJ, Blackburn BL, and Carey JC: Natural history of trisomy 18 and trisomy 13. I. Growth, physical assessment, medical histories, survival, and recurrence risk, Am J Med Genet 49:175–188, 1994.

Baty BJ, Jorde LB, Blackburn BL, and Carey JC: Natural history of trisomy 18 and trisomy 13. II. Psychomotor development, Am J Med Genet 49:189–194, 1994.

Carey JC: Health supervision and anticipatory guidance for children with genetic disorders (including specific recommendations for trisomy 21, trisomy 18, and neurofibromatosis I), Pediatr Clin North Am 39:25–53, 1992.

Cohen MM, Rosenblum-Vos LS, Prabhakar G: Human cytogenetics: a current overview, Arch Disease Child 147:1159–1166, 1993.

Cooper CS: Translocations in solid tumors, Curr Opin Genet Dev 6:71–75, 1996.

Epstein CJ: Down syndrome (trisomy 21). In Scriver CR, Beaudet AL, Sly WS, and Valle D, editors: The metabolic basis of inherited disease, ed. 7 vol 1, New York, 1995, McGraw-Hill.

Fisher JM, Harvey JF, Lindenbaum RH, Boyd PA, and Jacobs PA: Molecular studies of trisomy 18, Am J Hum Genet 52:1139–1144, 1993.

Greenberg F: Contiguous gene syndromes, Growth, Genetics Hormones 9:5–10, 1993.

Hall JG: Turner syndrome. In King RA, Rotter JI, and Motulsky AG, editors: The genetic basis of common disease, pp. 895-914, Oxford, 1992, Oxford University Press.

Hassold T, Hunt PA, and Sherman S: Trisomy in humans: incidence, origin and etiology, Curr Opin Genet Dev 3:398–403, 1993.

Hawkins JR: Sex determination, Hum Molec Genet 3:1463–1467, 1994.

Jacobs PA, Betts P, Cockwell AE, Cholla JA, MacKenzie MJ, Robinson DO, Youings, SA: A cytogenetic and molecular reappraisal of a series of patients with Turner's syndrome, Ann Hum Genet 54:209–223, 1990.

Jacobs PA, Browne C, Gregson N, Joyce C, and White H: Estimates of the frequency of chromosome abnormalities detectable in unselected newborns using moderate levels of banding, J Med Genet 29:103–108, 1992.

Ledbetter DH, Engel E: Uniparental disomy in humans: development of an imprinting map and its implications for prenatal diagnosis, Hum Molec Genet 4:1757–1764, 1995.

Lindsay EA, Greenberg F, Shaffer LG, Shapira SK, Scambler PJ, Baldini A: Submicroscopic deletions at 22q11.2: variability of the clinical picture and delineation of a commonly deleted region, Am J Hum Genet 56:191–197, 1995.

Lott IT, McCoy EE, editors: Down syndrome: advances in medical care, New York, 1992, Wiley-Liss.

Martin RH, Ko E, and Rademaker A: Distribution of aneuploidy in human gametes: comparison between human sperm and oocytes, Am J Med Genet 39:321–331, 1991.

Mitelman F: Catalog of chromosome aberrations in cancer, ed 5, New York, 1994, Wiley-Liss.

Paulsen CA and Plymate SR: Klinefelter's syndrome. In King RA, Rotter JI, and Motulsky AG, editors: The genetic basis of common disease, pp. 876-894, Oxford, 1992, Oxford University Press.

Rabbitts TH: Chromosomal translocations in human cancer, Nature 372:143–149, 1994.

Sandberg A: Cancer cytogenetics for clinicians, CA Cancer J. Clin. 44:136-159, 1994.

Therman E: Human chromosomes: structure, behavior, effects, ed 3, New York, 1993, Springer-Verlag.

van Ommen GB, Breuning MH, Raap AK: FISH in genome research and molecular diagnostics, Curr Opin Genet Dev 5:304–308, 1995.

Williams BJ, Ballenger CA, Malter HE, Bishop F, Tucker M, Zwingman TA, Hassold TJ: Non-disjunction in human sperm: results of fluorescence in situ hybridization studies using two and three probes, Hum Mol Genet 2:1929–1936, 1993.

Witkin HA, Mednick SA, Schulsinger F, Bakkeström E, Christiansen KO, Goodenough DR, Hirschhorn K, Lundsteen C, Owen DR, Philip J, Rubin DB, Stocking M: Criminality in XYY and XXY men, Science 193:547–555, 1976.

Yoon PW, Freeman SB, Sherman SL, Taft LF, Gu Y, Pettay D, Flanders WD, et al.: Advanced maternal age and the risk of Down syndrome characterized by the meiotic stage of the chromosomal error: a population-based study, Am J Hum Genet 58:628–633, 1996.

7 Gene Mapping

The mapping of genes to specific locations on chromosomes is a central focus of medical genetics. Dramatic advances in molecular genetic technology, coupled with important developments in the statistical analysis of genetic data, have greatly increased the rate at which genes are being mapped (Fig. 7-1). Currently, protein-coding genes are being mapped at the rate of about one per day, and over 4000 such genes have been assigned to chromosome locations. Although this is an admirable rate of progress, this number represents only a small fraction of the estimated 50,000 to 100,000 genes that compose the human genome. Clearly a great deal of work remains to be done. One goal of the Human Genome Project, discussed below, is to map all of our genes to specific chromosome locations. As this work progresses, our understanding of the biologic basis of genetic disease will surely progress as well.

Gene mapping is a critical step in the understanding, diagnosis, and eventual treatment of a genetic disease. When a disease gene's location is pinpointed, it is often possible to provide a more accurate prognosis for individuals at risk for a genetic disease. Locating a disease gene is also often necessary to clone the gene. Once a gene is cloned, its DNA sequence and protein product can be studied. This can contribute to our understanding of the actual cause of the disease. Furthermore it opens the way to the manufacture of a normal gene product through recombinant DNA techniques, permitting more effective treatment of many genetic diseases. Gene therapy, the insertion of normal genes into the bodies of individuals affected with a genetic disease, also becomes a possibility. Thus gene mapping contributes directly to many of the primary goals of medical genetics.

In this chapter we discuss the approaches commonly used in gene mapping. Two major types of gene mapping can be distinguished. In **genetic mapping,** the frequency of meiotic crossovers between loci is used to determine interlocus distances. **Physical mapping** involves the use of cytogenetic and molecular techniques to determine the actual physical location of genes on chromosomes. In addition to discussing mapping procedures, we see how these techniques lead to more accurate prediction of disease risk in families and how they lead to the isolation and cloning of disease genes.

■ GENETIC MAPPING
Linkage Analysis

One of Gregor Mendel's laws, the principle of independent assortment, states that an individual's genes will be transmitted to the next generation independently of one another (Chapter 4). Mendel was not aware that genes are located on chromosomes and that genes located near one another on the same chromosome are transmitted together, not independently. Thus Mendel's principle of independent assortment holds true for most pairs

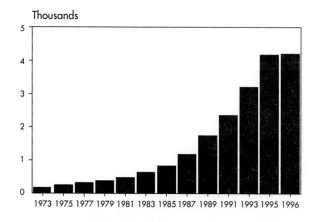

Figure 7-1 ■ **The number of coding genes mapped to specific chromosome locations.** (From Guyer and Collins, 1995; and the online Genome Data Base, March 1996)

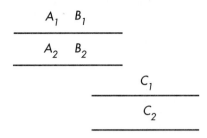

Figure 7-2 ■ Loci A and B are linked on the same chromosome, so alleles A₁ and B₁ are usually inherited together. Locus C is on a different chromosome, so it is not linked to A and B, and its alleles are transmitted independently of the alleles of A and B.

of loci, but not those that occupy the same region of a chromosome. Such loci are said to be **linked**.

Figure 7-2 depicts two loci, *A* and *B,* that are located close together on the same chromosome. A third locus, *C,* is located on another chromosome. In the individual in our example, each of these loci has two alleles, designated 1 and 2. *A* and *B* are linked, so A_1 and B_1 are inherited together. Because *A* and *C* are on different chromosomes and thus unlinked, their alleles do follow the principle of independent assortment. Hence, if the process of meiosis places A_1 in a gamete, the probability that

C_1 will be found in the same gamete is 50%.

Recall from Chapter 2 that homologous chromosomes sometimes exchange portions of their DNA during prophase I (crossing over, or crossover). The average chromosome will experience one to three crossover events during meiosis. As a result of crossover, new combinations of alleles can be formed on a chromosome. Consider the linked loci, *A* and *B,* discussed above. Alleles A_1 and B_1 are located together on one chromosome, and alleles A_2 and B_2 are located on the homologous chromosome. The combination of allelles on each chromosome is termed a **haplotype** (from ''haploid genotype''). The two haplotypes of this individual are denoted as A_1B_1/A_2B_2. As Figure 7-3, *A* shows, A_1B_1 is found in one gamete and A_2B_2 is found in the other gamete in the absence of crossover. When there is a crossover, new allele combinations, A_1B_2 and A_2B_1, are found in each gamete (Fig. 7-3, *B*). The process of forming such new arrangements of alleles is called **recombination**. Crossover does not necessarily lead to recombination, however, because a **double crossover** can occur between two loci, resulting in no recombination (Fig. 7-3, *C*).

As Figure 7-4 shows, crossovers are more likely to occur between loci that are situated far apart on a

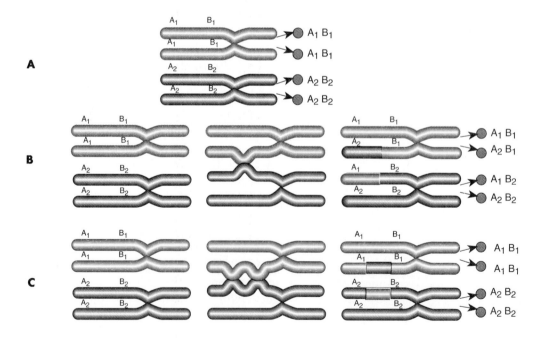

Figure 7-3 ■ The genetic results of crossover. A, No crossover: A₁ and B₁ remain together after meiosis; B, A crossover between A and B results in a recombination: A₁ and B₂ are inherited together on a chromosome, and A₂ and B₁ are inherited together on another chromosome; C, A double crossover between A and B results in no recombination of alleles. (Modified from McCance KL and Huether SE: Pathophysiology, ed 2, St Louis, 1994, Mosby.)

chromosome than between loci that are situated close together. Thus the distance between two loci can be inferred by estimating how frequently recombinations occur in families (this is called the **recombination frequency**). If, in a large series of meioses studied in families, the alleles of *A* and *B* undergo recombination 5% of the time, then the recombination frequency for *A* and *B* would be 5%.

The genetic distance between two loci is measured in **centiMorgans (cM),** in honor of T.H. Morgan, who discovered the process of crossing over in 1910. 1 cM is approximately equal to a recombination frequency of 1%. The relationship between recombination frequency and centiMorgans is approximate because double crossovers produce no recombination. The recombination frequency thus underestimates map distance, especially as the recombination frequency increases above 5% to 10%. Mapping functions have been devised to correct for this underestimate.

Loci that are on the same chromosome are said to be **syntenic** ("same thread"). If two syntenic loci are 50 cM apart, they are considered to be unlinked. This is because their recombination frequency is just as large as if they were on different chromosomes.

> Crossovers between loci on the same chromosome can produce recombination. Loci on the same chromosome that experience recombination less than 50% of the time are said to be linked. The distance between loci can be expressed in centiMorgans; 1 cM represents a recombination frequency of approximately 1%.

Recombination frequencies can be estimated by observing the transmission of genes in pedigrees. Figure 7-5, *A* is an example of a pedigree in which neurofibromatosis type 1 (*NF1*) is being transmitted. The members of this pedigree have also been typed for a two-allele RFLP termed *1F10,* which, like the *NF1* gene, is located on chromosome 17. The *1F10* genotypes are shown below each individual in the pedigree. Examination of generations 1 and 2 allows us to determine that the *NF1* gene must be on the same chromosome as allele 1 of the *1F10* system in this family because individual I-2, who is homozygous for allele 2, is unaffected with the disease. The arrangement of these alleles on each chromosome is referred to as **linkage phase**. Knowing the linkage phase, individual II-2's haplotypes would then be *N1/n2*, where *N* indicates the allele causing *NF1*, *n* indicates the normal allele, and 1 and 2 are the two *1F10* alleles. This woman's

husband (individual II-1) is unaffected with the disease and is a homozygote for allele 2 at *1F10*. He must have the haplotypes *n2/n2*. Because the *NF1* and *1F10* loci are linked, the children of this union who are affected with NF1 should usually have *IF10* allele *1,* whereas those who are unaffected should have allele *2.* In seven of eight children in genera-

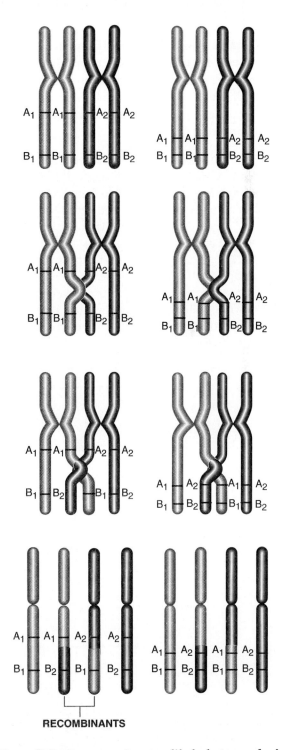

RECOMBINANTS

Figure 7-4 ■ Crossover is more likely between loci that are far apart on chromosomes *(left)* than when they are close together *(right).*

tion 3, we find this to be true. In one case a recombination occurred (individual III-6). This gives a recombination frequency of 1/8 = 12.5%.

In actual practice a much larger sample of families would be used to ensure statistical accuracy of this result (if this were done, it would show that *1F10* and *NF1* are in fact much more closely linked than indicated by this example, with a recombination frequency less than 1%).

> **Estimates of recombination frequencies are obtained by observing the transmission of alleles in families. Determination of the linkage phase (i.e., the chromosome on which each allele is located) is an important part of this procedure.**

Polymorphisms such as *1F10,* which can be used to follow a disease gene through a family, are termed **markers**. Because linked markers can be typed in an individual of any age (even in a fetus), they are useful for the early diagnosis of genetic disease (see Chapter 11).

In general, 1 cM corresponds to approximately 1 million bp (1 Mb) of DNA. However, this is only an approximate relationship because several factors are known to influence crossover rates. First, crossovers are roughly 1.5 times more common in female meiosis (oogenesis) than in male meiosis

(spermatogenesis). Also, crossovers tend to be more common near the telomeres of chromosomes than near the centromeres. Finally, some chromosome regions exhibit much higher crossover rates than most others. These regions are termed **recombination hot spots**. It is not yet known what causes recombination hot spots in humans, although specific DNA sequences, possibly including *Alu* sequences (see Chapter 2), are thought to be especially prone to crossover.

> **Although there is a correlation between centiMorgans and the actual physical distances between loci, this relationship is complicated by gender differences in recombination, higher recombination frequencies near telomeres, and the existence of recombination hot spots.**

LOD Scores: Determining the Significance of Linkage Results

As in any statistical study, we must be careful to ensure that the results obtained in a linkage study are not due simply to chance. For example, consider a two-allele marker locus that has been typed in a pedigree. It is possible *by chance* for all affected offspring to inherit one allele and for all unaffected offspring to inherit the other allele even if the marker is not linked to the disease gene. This

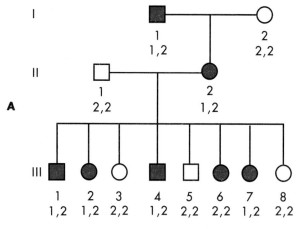

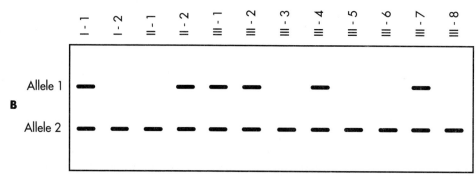

Figure 7-5 ■ An NF1 pedigree in which each member has been typed for the 1F10 polymorphism (A). Genotypes for this two-allele marker locus are shown below each individual in the pedigree. Affected pedigree members are indicated by a shaded symbol. An autoradiogram for the 1F10 polymorphism in this family (B).

misleading result becomes less likely as we increase the number of subjects in our linkage study (just as the chance of a strong deviation from a 50–50 heads–tails ratio becomes smaller as we toss a coin many times).

How do we determine whether a linkage result is likely to be due to chance alone? In linkage analysis a standard method is used. We begin by comparing the **likelihood** (a likelihood is similar in concept to a probability) that two loci are linked at a given recombination frequency (denoted θ) versus the likelihood that the two loci are not linked (recombination frequency = 50%, or $\theta = 0.5$). Suppose we wish to test the hypothesis that two loci are linked at a recombination frequency of $\theta = 0.1$ versus the hypothesis that they are not linked. We use our pedigree data to form a **likelihood ratio**:

$$\frac{\text{likelihood of observing pedigree data if } \theta = 0.1}{\text{likelihood of observing pedigree data if } \theta = 0.5}$$

If our pedigree data indicate that θ is more likely to be 0.1 than 0.5, then the likelihood ratio (or "odds") will be greater than 1. If, however, the pedigree data argue against linkage of the two loci, then the denominator will be greater than the numerator, and the ratio will be less than 1.0. For convenience the common logarithm* of the ratio is usually taken; this "logarithm of the odds" is termed a **LOD score**. Conventionally, a LOD score of 3.0 is accepted as evidence of linkage; a score of 3.0 indicates that the likelihood in favor of linkage is 1000 times greater than the likelihood against linkage. Conversely, a LOD score less than -2 (odds of 100 to 1 *against linkage*) is considered to be evidence that two loci are not linked.

A simple example will help to illustrate the concepts of likelihood ratios and LOD scores. Consider the pedigree in Figure 7-6, which illustrates another family in which *NF1* is being transmitted. The family has been typed for the *1F10* marker, as in Figure 7-5. The male in generation 2 had to receive the *1F10-1* allele from his mother because she can transmit only this marker allele. Thus his *1F10-2* allele had to come from his father, on the same chromosome as the *NF1* disease gene. This allows us to establish linkage phase in this pedigree: the affected male in generation 2 must have

the haplotypes *N2/n1*. He marries an unaffected woman who is a homozygote for the *1F10-2* allele. Thus the hypothesis of close linkage ($\theta = 0.0$) predicts that each child in generation 3 who receives allele 2 from his or her father must also receive the *NF1* disease allele. Under the hypothesis of linkage, the father can transmit only two possible combinations: either the chromosome having the disease gene and *1F10-2* (*N2*) or the other chromosome, which has the normal gene and *1F10-1* (*n1*). The probability of each of these events is 1/2. Thus if $\theta = 0.0$, the probability of observing four children with the genotypes shown in Figure 7-6 is $(1/2)^4$, or 1/16. This is the numerator of the likelihood ratio.

Now consider the likelihood of observing these genotypes if *1F10* and *NF1* were *not* linked ($\theta = 0.5$). Under this hypothesis, there is *independent assortment* of alleles at *1F10* and *NF1*. Thus the father can transmit any of four combinations, *N1*, *N2*, *n1*, and *n2*, with equal probability (1/4). The probability of observing four children with the observed genotypes is then $(1/4)^4 = 1/256$. This likelihood is the denominator of the likelihood ratio. The likelihood ratio is then $1/16 : 1/256 = 16$. Thus the data in this pedigree tell us that *linkage*, at $\theta = 0.0$, is 16 times more likely than *nonlinkage*. If we take the common logarithm of 16, we find that the LOD score is 1.2, which is still far short of the value of 3.0 usually accepted as evidence of linkage. To prove linkage, then, we would need to examine data from additional families. LOD scores obtained from individual families can be added together to obtain an overall score.

Suppose that a recombination had occurred in the meiosis producing one of the children in

---

*Recall that the common logarithm of a number is the power to which 10 is raised to obtain the number. Thus the common logarithm of 100 is 2, the common logarithm of 1000 is 3, and so on.

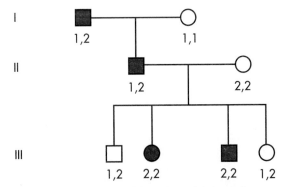

Figure 7-6 ■ An NF1 pedigree in which each member has been typed for the 1F10 polymorphism. Again the marker genotypes are shown below each individual in the pedigree.

generation 3. This event is impossible under the hypothesis that $\theta = 0.0$, so the numerator of the likelihood ratio becomes 0, and the LOD score is $-\infty$.

When doing linkage analysis, a series of θ values is usually tested, comparing the likelihood of each value of θ with the likelihood that $\theta = 0.5$. This produces a LOD score for each value of θ that is tested. These LOD scores are then graphed against the θ values, as shown in Figure 7-7. The highest LOD score on the graph is the **maximum likelihood estimate** of θ. That is, it is the *most likely* distance between the two loci being analyzed.

In practice, the analysis of human linkage data is not as simple as in the previous example. Linkage phase is often unknown, penetrance of the disease gene may be incomplete, and the mode of inheritance of the disease may be unclear. Thus linkage data are analyzed using one of several available computer software packages. These packages also allow one to carry out **multipoint mapping**, an approach in which the map locations of several markers are estimated simultaneously.

> **The statistical odds that two loci are a given number of centiMorgans apart can be calculated by measuring the ratio of two likelihoods: the likelihood of linkage at a given distance divided by the likelihood of no link-**

> **age. The logarithm of this odds ratio is a LOD score. LOD scores >3.0 are taken as evidence of linkage, and LOD scores <-2.0 are taken as evidence that two loci are not linked.**

Linkage Analysis and the Human Gene Map

Suppose that we are studying a disease gene in a series of pedigrees, and we wish to map it to a specific chromosome location. Typically we would type the members of our pedigree for marker loci distributed along each chromosome, testing for linkage between the disease gene and each marker. Most of these tests would yield negative LOD scores, indicating no linkage between the marker and the disease gene. Eventually this exercise will reveal linkage between a marker and the disease gene. Because of the large size of the human genome, one may have to type dozens, or even hundreds, of markers before finding linkage. Many important diseases have been localized using this approach, including cystic fibrosis, Huntington disease, Marfan syndrome, and NF1.

A little over a decade ago, linkage analyses had little chance of success because there were only a few dozen useful polymorphic markers in the entire human genome. Thus it was unlikely that a disease gene would be located near enough to a marker to yield a significant linkage result. This situation has changed dramatically over the past few years, as thousands of new polymorphic markers (RFLPs, VNTRs, and microsatellite polymorphisms; see Chapter 3) have been generated (Fig. 7-8). It is now commonplace to map a disease gene

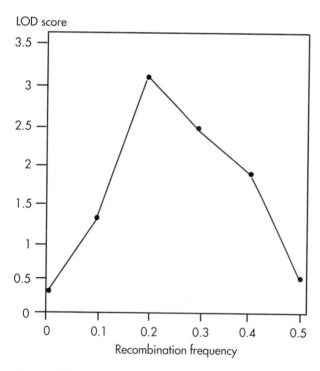

Figure 7-7 ■ The LOD score (logarithm of the odds, y-axis) is plotted against the recombination frequency (x-axis) to determine the most likely recombination frequency for a pair of loci.

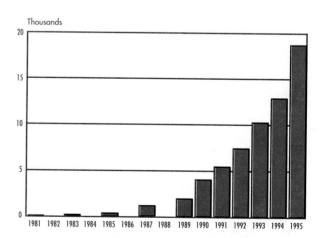

Figure 7-8 ■ The number of known polymorphic marker loci, showing a rapid rate of increase during the past decade. (From Guyer and Collins, 1995; online Genome Data Base, March 1996)

with only a few months of laboratory and statistical analysis.

To be useful for gene mapping, marker loci should have several properties. First, they should be codominant (i.e., homozygotes should be distinguishable from heterozygotes). This makes it easier to determine linkage phase. RFLPs, VNTRs, and microsatellite polymorphisms fulfill this criterion, whereas some of the older types of markers, such as the ABO and Rh blood groups, do not. Second, marker loci should be numerous, so that close linkage to the disease gene is likely. As Figure 7-8 shows, this requirement has largely been fulfilled. Our chromosomes are rapidly becoming saturated with markers (Fig. 7-9). Finally, the marker loci are most useful when they are highly polymorphic (i.e., when the locus has many different alleles in the population). A high degree of polymorphism ensures that most parents will be heterozygous for the marker locus, making it easier to establish linkage phase in families. VNTRs and microsatellite repeat polymorphisms typically have many alleles

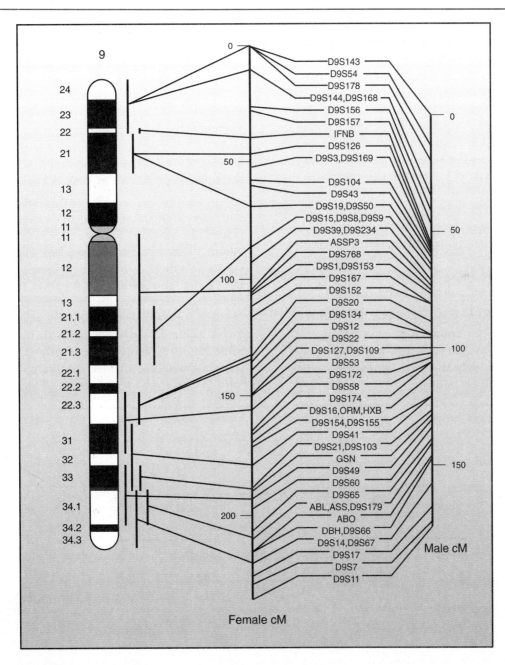

Figure 7-9 ■ A genetic map of chromosome 9, showing the locations of a large number of polymorphic markers. Because recombination rates are usually higher in female meiosis, the distances between markers (in cM) are larger for females than for males. (From Atwood, Atwood J, Chiano M, Collins A, et al. Genomics 19:203–214, 1994.)

and are thus especially well suited to gene mapping.

An example will illustrate this last point. Consider the pedigree in Figure 7-10, *A*. The affected man is a homozygote for an RFLP that is closely linked to the disease locus and has two alleles (recall that most RFLPs are caused by the presence or absence of a restriction site and thus have only two alleles in a population). His wife is a heterozygote. Their affected daughter is homozygous for the marker allele. Based on these genotypes, it is impossible to determine linkage phase in this generation, so we cannot predict which children will be affected with the disorder and which will not. The mating in generation 1 is called an **uninformative mating**. In contrast, a microsatellite repeat polymorphism with six alleles has been typed in the same family in Figure 7-10, *B*. Because the mother in generation 1 has two alleles that differ from those of the affected father, it is now possible to determine that the affected daughter in generation 2 has inherited the disease gene on the single chromosome that contains marker allele 1. Because she married a man who has alleles 4 and 5, we can predict that each offspring who receives allele 1 from her will be affected, while each one who receives allele 2 will be normal. Exceptions will be due to recombination. This example demonstrates the value of highly polymorphic markers both for linkage analysis and diagnosing genetic disease (see Chapter 11).

> To be useful in gene mapping, linked markers should be codominant, numerous, and highly polymorphic. A high degree of polymorphism increases the probability that matings will be informative.

Sometimes, linkage analysis will show that a disease gene is linked to a specific marker in some families but not in others. If LOD scores near 0 are obtained for a subset of families, this could mean simply that these families are uninformative (a LOD score of 0 indicates that the likelihoods of linkage and nonlinkage are approximately equal). However, highly negative LOD scores obtained for a subset of families provide evidence of locus heterogeneity. For example, osteogenesis imperfecta type I can be caused either by mutations on chromosome 7 or chromosome 17 (see Chapter 4). A study of families with this disease could show linkage to markers on chromosome 17 in some families and linkage to chromosome 7 in others. Linkage analysis has helped define locus heterogeneity in a large number of diseases, including retinitis pigmentosa, a major cause of blindness (Clinical Commentary 7-1).

Linkage Disequilibrium, the Nonrandom Association of Alleles at Linked Loci

Within families, one allele of a marker locus will be transmitted along with the disease allele if the marker and disease loci are linked. For example, allele 1 of a linked two-allele marker could co-occur with the Huntington disease (HD) allele in a family. This association is part of the definition of linkage. However, if one examines a series of families for linkage between HD and the marker locus, allele 1 will co-occur with the disease in some families, while allele 2 of the marker will co-occur with the disease in others. This reflects the fact that, even for closely linked loci, crossovers

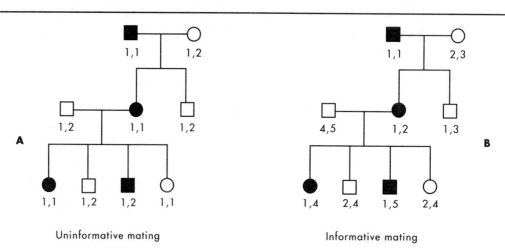

Uninformative mating   Informative mating

Figure 7-10 ■ An autosomal dominant disease gene is segregating in this family. A, A closely linked two-allele RFLP has been typed for each member of the family, but linkage phase cannot be determined (uninformative mating). B, A closely linked six-allele microsatellite polymorphism has been typed for each family member, and linkage phase can now be determined (informative mating).

Clinical Commentary 7-1. Retinitis Pigmentosa, a Genetic Disorder Characterized by Locus Heterogeneity

Retinitis pigmentosa (RP) describes a collection of inherited retinal defects that together are the most common inherited cause of human blindness, affecting 1 in 3000 to 4000 individuals. The first clinical signs of RP are seen as the rod photoreceptor cells begin to die, causing night blindness. With the death of rod cells, other tissue begins to degenerate as well. Cone cells die, and the vessels that supply blood to the retinal membranes begin to attenuate. This leads to a reduction in daytime vision. Patients develop tunnel vision and may eventually lose all sight. The name "retinitis pigmentosa" comes from the pigments that are deposited on the retinal surface as pathologic changes accumulate (Fig. 7-11; *SOL* 61). RP is neither preventable nor curable.

RP is known to be inherited in different families in autosomal dominant, autosomal recessive, and X-linked recessive fashion. Linkage analysis of the X-linked form produced conflicting results at first, but extensive analysis of a large series of families resolved the conflict by demonstrating that there are two RP genes on the X chromosome. Both are located on the short arm, with one fairly close to the centromere and the other roughly 10 million bp away.

Further locus heterogeneity is indicated by the autosomal modes of inheritance seen in many families. Linkage analysis mapped an autosomal dominant form of RP to the long arm of chromosome 3. This was a significant finding because the gene for rhodopsin (a retinal visual pigment) had also been mapped to this region. Because of its role in vision, rhodopsin was a reasonable "candidate gene" for RP. Linkage analysis was performed using a polymorphism located within the rhodopsin gene, and a LOD score of 20 was obtained for zero recombination in a large Irish pedigree. Subsequently, various mutations in the rhodopsin gene were shown to cause RP, confirming the role of this locus in causing the disease.

Additional studies showed that autosomal dominant RP in other families was not always caused by mutations at the rhodopsin locus. Linkage analyses in these families localized another RP gene to the short arm of chromosome 6. Again, a candidate gene, peripherin, was located in the region indicated by linkage analysis. Peripherin is a structural component of rod cells that had been studied extensively in mice suffering from retinal degeneration. Peripherin mutations were identified in human patients with RP, verifying the pathogenic role of this locus.

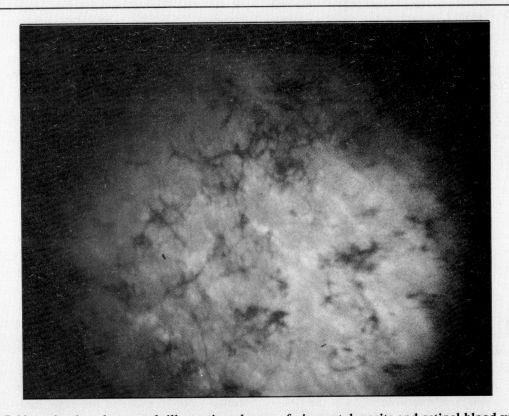

Figure 7-11 ■ A fundus photograph illustrating clumps of pigment deposits and retinal blood vessel attenuation in retinitis pigmentosa (Courtesy of Dr. Don Creel, University of Utah Health Sciences Center).

Continued.

occurring through time will eventually result in recombination of the marker and disease alleles. A specific marker allele and the disease allele will thus be associated *within* families but not necessarily *between* families. If we study a large collection of families and find that there is no preferential association between the disease gene and a specific allele at a linked marker locus, the two loci are said to be in **linkage equilibrium**.

Sometimes, however, we do observe the preferential association of a specific marker allele and the disease allele in a population (i.e., the chromosome haplotype consisting of one marker allele and the disease allele is found more often than we would expect based on the frequencies of the two alleles in the population). This nonrandom association of alleles at linked loci is termed **linkage disequilibrium**. Figure 7-12 illustrates how linkage disequilibrium can come about. Imagine two RFLPs linked to the myotonic dystrophy locus on chromosome 19. Marker B is closely linked, at less than 1 cM away. Marker A is less closely linked, at about 5 cM away. Because each of these marker loci has two alleles (denoted 1 and 2), there are four possible combinations of marker alleles at the two loci, as shown in Figure 7-12. When a myotonic dystrophy mutation first occurs in a population, it can be found only on one chromosome, in this case the one with the A_1B_2 marker combination. As the disease mutation is passed through multiple generations, crossovers will occur between it and the two markers. Because the disease locus is more closely linked to marker B than marker A, fewer crossovers will occur between the disease mutation and marker B. As a result, the disease mutation is found on a B_2 chromosome 90% of the time, while it is found on an A_1 chromosome 72% of the time. The degree of linkage disequilibrium is stronger between marker B and the disease allele than between marker A and the disease allele. Notice also that *both* the A_1 and B_2 alleles are still positive-

ly associated with the disease allele, because each allele has a much lower frequency (50%) in the population of individuals lacking the disease allele (Fig. 7-12). If enough generations elapse, recombination would eventually eliminate the allelic associations completely, and the loci would be in linkage equilibrium.

Because linkage disequilibrium is a function of the distance between loci, it can be used to help infer the order of genes on chromosomes. However, linkage disequilibrium can be influenced by evolutionary forces, such as natural selection, that have acted during the history of a population. For example, some loci in the major histocompatibility complex on chromosome 6 (see Chapter 8) are in disequilibrium, presumably because certain allelic combinations confer a selective advantage for immunity to some diseases.

> Linkage disequilibrium is the nonrandom association of alleles at linked loci. Linkage disequilibrium between loci diminishes through time as a result of recombination.

Linkage versus Association in Populations

The phenomena of linkage and association are sometimes confused. Linkage refers to the positions of loci on chromosomes. When two loci are linked, specific combinations of alleles at these loci will be transmitted together (on the same chromosome) *within families*. But as the HD example cited above showed, the specific combinations of alleles transmitted together can vary from one family to another. **Association**, however, refers to a statistical relationship between two traits (which may or may not be genetic) *in the general population*. The two traits occur together in the same individual more often than expected by chance.

If two associated traits happen to be encoded by two linked loci, then the association would reflect linkage disequilibrium. In this case a population

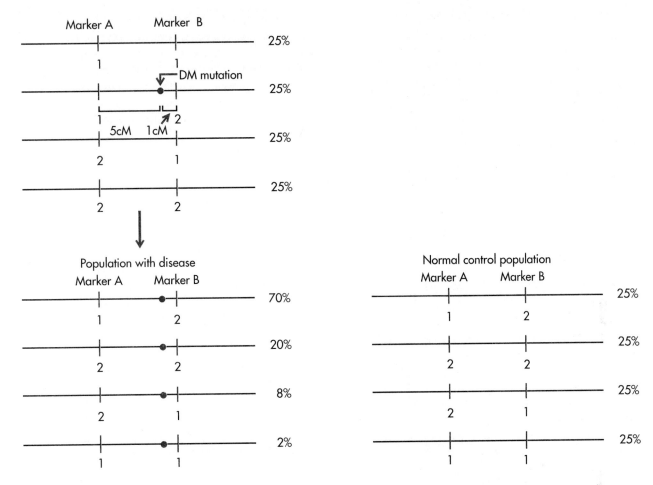

Figure 7-12 ■ Linkage disequilibrium between the myotonic dystrophy (DM) locus and two linked loci, A and B. The DM mutation first arises on the chromosome with the A_1B_2 haplotype. After a number of generations have passed, most chromosomes carrying the DM mutation still have the A_1B_2 haplotype, but as a result of recombination the DM mutation is also found on other haplotypes. Because the A_1B_2 haplotype is seen in 70% of DM chromosomes but only 25% of normal chromosomes, there is linkage disequilibrium between DM and loci A and B. Because locus B is closer to DM, it has greater linkage disequilibrium with DM than does locus A.

association can lead to mapping of a disease gene. An example is given by idiopathic hemochromatosis, an autosomal recessive disorder in which the body accumulates iron, which is then deposited in vital organs, such as the heart, pancreas, and liver. One association study showed that 78% of hemochromatosis patients had the A3 allele of the HLA-A locus on chromosome 6 (see Chapter 8 for further discussion of the HLA system), whereas only 27% of unaffected subjects (controls) had this allele. This strong statistical association prompted linkage analyses using HLA polymorphisms and led to the mapping of the hemochromatosis gene to chromosome 6.

Population associations can also be due to a causal relationship between an allele and a disease condition. An example of such an association involves ankylosing spondylitis, a joint disease that primarily affects the sacroiliac area (Fig. 7-13). Inflammation of the ligaments leads to their ossification and eventually to fusion of the joints (ankylosis). The HLA-B27 allele is found in about 90% of individuals who have ankylosing spondylitis, but only 5% to 10% of the U.S. white population has this allele. Because the population incidence of ankylosing spondylitis is low (<1%), most people who have the HLA-B27 allele do not develop ankylosing spondylitis. However, those who have the HLA-B27 allele are about 90 times more likely to develop the disease than are those who do not have the B27 allele (i.e., 9% of the HLA-B27 individuals shown in Table 7-1 have ankylosing spondylitis, whereas only about 0.1% of those without HLA-B27 have the disease). Because of this strong

Ossification of discs,
joints, and ligaments
of spinal column

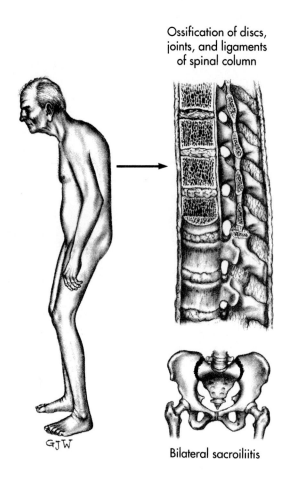

GJW

Bilateral sacroiliitis

Figure 7-13 ▪ Ankylosing spondylitis, caused by ossification of discs, joints, and ligaments in the spinal column. Note the characteristic posture.
(From K.L. McCance and S.E. Huether, Pathophysiology: The Biologic Basis for Disease in Adults and Children, St. Louis 1994, Mosby.)

association, a test for HLA-B27 is sometimes included as part of the diagnosis of ankylosing spondylitis. It is important to emphasize that the genetic and environmental factors causing ankylosing spondylitis remain unclear and that the observed *population association* between HLA-B27 and this disorder does not necessarily imply genetic *linkage*. Because ankylosing spondylitis is thought to be an autoimmune disorder, the association may reflect the fact that the HLA system is a key element in the body's immune response (see Chapter 8).

A population association is also seen between the HLA-DR3 and HLA-DR4 alleles and type I diabetes (see Chapter 10). Because autoimmunity appears to be a factor in the etiology of type I diabetes, there may well be a causative relationship between the HLA-DR3/DR4 alleles and increased susceptibility to this form of diabetes.

Association studies should be interpreted cautiously, because many things can produce spurious associations between a disease and a potential risk factor. An example is ethnic stratification in a population: certain diseases are more frequent in certain ethnic groups, and allele frequencies may also differ among these groups because of their evolutionary histories. Thus, if one compares disease cases and controls without proper matching for ethnicity, a false association, due simply to ethnic differences in the two groups, could be found. For example, type II diabetes (see Chapter 10) has been studied extensively among the Pima and Papago Native American population, where the disease is much more common than among whites. It was observed that the absence of haplotype Gm3;5,13,14 of human immunoglobulin G (abbreviated here as Gm3) was strongly associated with type II diabetes among the Pima and Papago. This suggested initially that the absence of Gm3 might be involved in the causation of type II diabetes. However, further analysis revealed that the proportion of white ancestry varied substantially among members of the Pima/Papago population and that the Gm3 frequency *also* varied with the degree of white ancestry: Gm3 is absent in Pima and Papago individuals with no white ancestry but increases to 65% among whites. Because type II diabetes is much less common among whites, the apparent association between type II diabetes and the absence of Gm3 was most likely a consequence of the level of white mixture. Once the degree of white ancestry in the study subjects was taken into account, there was no evidence of an association.

Other factors that may produce false associations include imprecise definition of the disease state, inadequate sample sizes, and improper matching of cases and controls on variables such as age and gender. The inability to replicate an association in multiple study populations is a good indication that the association may be invalid. An example is given by an association reported, but not replicated,

Table 7-1 ▪ Association of ankylosing spondylitis and the HLA-B27 allele in a hypothetical population†

HLA-B27	Ankylosing spondylitis*	
	+	−
+	90	1000
−	10	9000

†This table shows that individuals with ankylosing spondylitis are much more likely to have the HLA-B27 allele than are normal controls.
*+, present; −, absent.

between alcoholism and a polymorphism near the dopamine D2 receptor locus (discussed further in Chapter 10).

> **Population associations refer to the nonrandom co-occurrence of factors at the population level. Associations are distinguished from linkage, which refers to the positions of loci on chromosomes.**

■ PHYSICAL MAPPING

Linkage analysis allows us to determine the relative distances between loci, but it does not assign specific locations to markers or disease genes. Physical mapping, which involves a variety of methods, accomplishes this goal, and considerable progress has been made in developing high-resolution physical mapping approaches.

Chromosome Morphology

A simple and direct way of mapping disease genes is to show that the disease is consistently associated with a cytogenetic abnormality, such as a duplication, deletion, or other variation in the appearance of a chromosome. Such abnormalities may have no clinical consequences themselves (thus serving as a marker), or they may cause the disease. Because these approaches are historically the oldest of the physical mapping approaches, we will discuss them first.

Heteromorphisms

A **heteromorphism** is a variation in the appearance of a chromosome. Conceptually, heteromorphisms are similar to polymorphisms: they are natural variations that occur among individuals in populations. The difference is that polymorphisms are not detectable microscopically, whereas heteromorphisms are.

A well-known example of a heteromorphism is an "uncoiled" (and thus elongated) region of chromosome 1, a rare feature that is transmitted regularly in families. In the 1960s researcher R.P. Donahue was practicing cytogenetic analysis on his own chromosomes and found that he had this heteromorphism. He studied other members of his family and found that the heteromorphism was transmitted through his family as a mendelian trait. He then typed his family members for several blood groups. He found that the heteromorphism was perfectly associated in his family with allele *A* of the Duffy blood group. Linkage analysis of the "uncoiler" locus and the Duffy locus showed that they were

closely linked, leading to the first assignment of a gene to a specific autosome.

It should be emphasized that heteromorphisms, like marker loci, do not *cause* a genetic variant or disease, but they may be associated with it within a family, thus indicating the gene's location. Although such heteromorphisms can be useful in mapping genes, they are not common and thus have been useful in only a few instances.

Deletions

Karyotypes of patients with a genetic disease will occasionally reveal deletions of a specific region of a chromosome. This provides a strong hint that the locus causing the disease may lie within the deleted region. The extent of the deletion may vary from patient to patient. Deletions are compared in many patients to define the region that is deleted in all patients, thus narrowing the location of the disease gene (Fig. 7-14). Deletion mapping has been used,

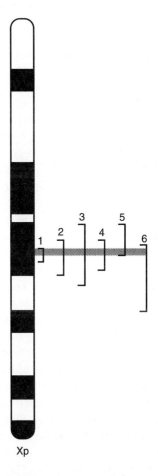

Xp

Figure 7-14 ■ Localization of a disease gene through deletion mapping. A series of overlapping deletions is studied in which each deletion produces the disease phenotype. The region of overlap of all deletions defines the location of the disease gene.

for example, in locating the genes responsible for retinoblastoma (see Chapters 4 and 9), Prader-Willi and Angelman syndromes (see Chapter 4), and Wilms tumor, a childhood kidney tumor that can be caused by mutations on chromosome 11 (*SOL* 62). As opposed to the heteromorphisms just discussed, deletions of genetic material are the direct cause of the genetic disease.

Note that these deletions affect only one member of the homologous pair of chromosomes, making the patient heterozygous for the deletion. If a region large enough to be microscopically observable were missing in both chromosomes, it would usually produce a lethal condition.

Translocations

As discussed in Chapter 6, balanced chromosome translocations often have no effect on a translocation carrier because the individual still has a complete copy of his or her genetic material. However, when a translocation happens to interrupt a gene, it can produce genetic disease. For example, linkage analysis had mapped the NF1 gene approximately to the long arm of chromosome 17. A more refined location was obtained when two patients were identified, one with a balanced translocation between chromosomes 17 and 22 and another with a balanced translocation between chromosomes 17 and 1. The breakpoints of these translocations on chromosome 17 were located close to one another in the same region implicated by linkage analysis. They provided a physical starting point for experiments that subsequently led to cloning of the NF1 gene.

A similar example is provided by translocations observed between the X chromosome and autosomes in females affected with Duchenne muscular dystrophy (DMD). Because this is a lethal X-linked recessive disorder, fully affected homozygous females are rare. The translocation breakpoint on the X chromosome was in the same location (Xp21) in several affected females, suggesting that the translocation interrupted the DMD gene. This proved to be the case, and these translocations aided considerably in mapping and cloning the DMD gene. (Although these females also carried a normal X chromosome, the normal X was preferentially inactivated, leaving only the interrupted X as the active chromosome.)

Dosage Mapping Using Deletions and Duplications

When a deletion occurs on a chromosome, it stands to reason that the protein products encoded by genes in the deleted region would be present in only half the normal quantity. This is the basis of a simple approach known as **dosage mapping**. For example, it was observed that a 50% reduction in the level of the enzyme adenylate kinase was consistently associated with a deletion on chromosome 9, mapping the adenylate kinase gene to this chromosome region. Dosage mapping was also used to map the gene for red cell acid phosphatase to chromosome 2.

Similarly, a duplication of chromosome material should be associated with an increase in gene product levels. Because three genes are present instead of two, the increase should be approximately 50% above normal. This form of dosage mapping was used to assign the gene encoding superoxide dismutase-1 (SOD-1) to the long arm of chromosome 21.

A gene can be physically mapped to a chromosome region by associating cytogenetically observable variations (heteromorphisms, translocations, deletions, duplications) with gene expression (including the presence of a genetic disease).

In Situ Hybridization

In situ hybridization, illustrated in Figure 7-15, is a direct and intuitively simple approach to mapping DNA segments. Suppose that we have a segment of DNA, taken from a polymorphic marker or disease gene, whose location we wish to determine. This DNA can be cloned into a probe using the recombinant DNA methods outlined in Chapter 2. The probe is labeled with a radioactive substance, such as tritium. The probe is then exposed to a slide containing metaphase chromosomes whose DNA has been denatured in place (in situ). The labeled probe undergoes complementary base pairing with the denatured DNA of a specific chromosome segment. Because the probe emits radiation, its position on a chromosome can be pinpointed by placing x-ray film over the slide (autoradiography, see Chapter 3). The probe DNA often hybridizes nonspecifically with random chromosomal segments, so it is usually necessary to repeat the experiment many times to pinpoint the most likely chromosomal location of the probe DNA.

In situ hybridization using radioactive probes is usually a slow process, and the degree of resolution (2 to 5 million bases) is rather low. In recent years nonradioactive fluorescent probes, which can be visualized under a fluorescence microscope, have become popular. Fluorescence in situ hybridi-

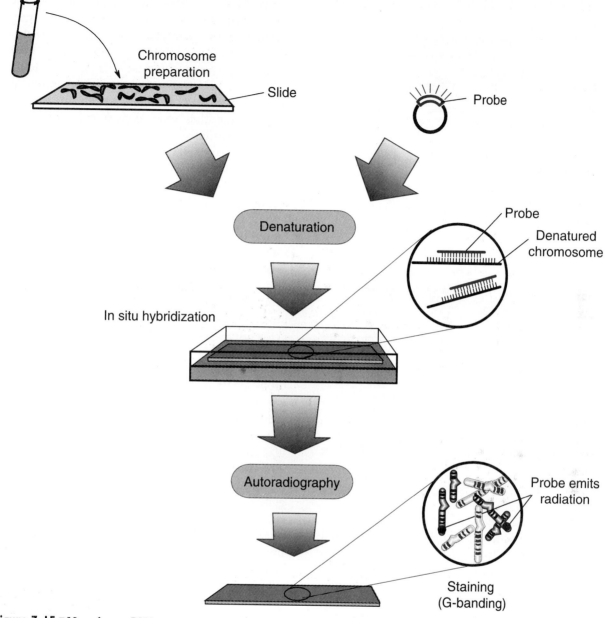

Figure 7-15 ▪ Mapping a DNA segment to a chromosome location through in situ hybridization.

zation (FISH), discussed and illustrated in Chapter 6, is faster than radioactive hybridization, largely because there is little nonspecific hybridization. It also offers better resolution of a probe's location, often within 1 million bp. For these reasons FISH is rapidly supplanting in situ hybridization as a physical mapping technique.

In situ hybridization is a physical mapping technique in which a labeled probe is hybridized to fixed metaphase chromosomes to determine the chromosomal location of the DNA in the probe.

Somatic Cell Hybridization

Another common method of gene localization exploits the somewhat surprising fact that somatic cells from different species, when grown in the same culture in the presence of agents such as polyethylene glycol or Sendai virus, will sometimes fuse together to form hybrid cells (**somatic cell hybridization**, shown in Fig. 7-16). When mouse and human cells are grown together in this way, the resulting hybrid cells contain 86 chromosomes: the 46 human chromosomes together with the 40 mouse chromosomes. The cells are exposed to selective media such as a combination of hypoxan-

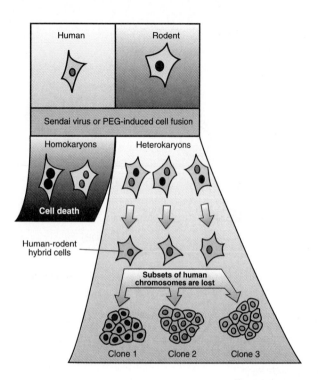

Figure 7-16 ■ Gene mapping by somatic cell hybridization. The human and rodent cells that fused are selected using a medium such as HAT. The hybrid cells preferentially lose human chromosomes, resulting in clones that each have only a few human chromosomes. Each clone is examined to determine whether the gene is present, thus assigning the gene to a specific chromosome.

sions. Eventually cells remain that have a full set of mouse chromosomes but only one or a few human chromosomes. The cells are karyotyped to determine which human chromosomes remain (human and mouse chromosomes are distinguishable from each other on the basis of size and banding patterns). These sets of cells can then be studied to determine which ones consistently contain the gene in question (Table 7-2). For example, if the gene is always found in cells that contain human chromosome 1 but never found in those that do not, we would conclude that the gene must be located on this chromosome.

Presence of the gene in the hybrid cell can be detected in several ways. If the gene encodes an enzyme that is produced by the cell, then an enzyme assay can be used. Protein electrophoresis (see Chapter 3) may be used to detect a human protein product and to distinguish it from the equivalent mouse protein product. These approaches, however, require that a known protein product can be detected. More often, investigators now test for hybridization of the fused cell lines with a labeled probe containing the DNA of interest using Southern blotting or PCR techniques (Fig. 7-17).

Sometimes a gene can be assigned to a specific *segment* of a chromosome using somatic cell hybridization. Translocations infrequently occur in which only part of a single human chromosome is attached to one of the mouse chromosomes. If the gene or DNA segment of interest is detectable in a cell containing such a translocation, then the gene must be located on the translocated segment of the human chromosome. Similarly, if a gene is consistently absent in cell lines containing a known deletion, then the gene can be localized to the region that is deleted.

thine, aminopterin, and thymidine (HAT) to eliminate those that did not fuse. The hybrid cells are then cloned. For reasons that are not well understood, these cells will begin to lose some of their human chromosomes as they undergo cell divi-

Table 7-2 ■ Somatic cell hybridization panel*

Clone	DNA segment	1	2	3	4	5	6	7	8	9	10	11	12	13	14	15	16	17	18	19	20	21	22	X	Y
1	+	−	−	−	+	−	+	+	+	+	−	+	+	−	−	+	−	+	−	+	−	−	−	+	−
2	−	+	+	+	−	+	−	+	−	−	+	−	−	−	+	+	+	−	−	+	+	+	+	−	−
3	+	−	−	−	−	+	+	+	+	+	−	−	−	+	−	+	−	+	−	+	+	−	+	−	−
4	+	+	−	+	−	−	−	+	−	+	−	+	+	−	−	−	+	−	+	−	−	+	−	−	−
5	−	−	+	+	+	+	+	−	−	−	+	−	+	−	+	−	+	−	−	+	+	−	+	+	+
6	−	+	−	+	−	−	+	−	−	−	+	+	−	+	+	−	+	−	+	−	−	−	+	+	−
7	+	−	+	−	+	−	+	+	+	+	−	+	−	−	−	+	+	−	+	−	+	+	−	+	−
8	−	−	+	+	+	+	−	−	+	−	+	+	+	−	+	−	+	+	−	+	+	−	−	−	−

*Note that the DNA segment being tested shows a positive hybridization signal to clones 1, 3, 4, and 7. Each of these clones contains chromosome 9, whereas clones 2, 5, 6, and 8 do not contain this chromosome. This pattern localizes the DNA segment to chromosome 9.

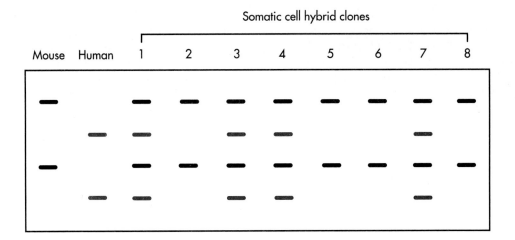

Figure 7-17 ■ A Southern blot used in a somatic cell hybridization gene mapping experiment (compare with panel shown in Table 7-2). Human and mouse bands differ in size because the two species have different recognition sequences. The human gene probe hybridizes only to the hybrid cells 1, 3, 4, and 7, showing that the probe hybridizes only when chromosome 9 is present.

Somatic cell hybridization is a physical mapping technique in which human and rodent cells are hybridized, resulting in cells that have a reduced number of human chromosomes. Panels of such cells are used to correlate the presence of a gene with the consistent presence of one chromosome (or when translocations are available, a specific segment of a chromosome).

Closing in on the Gene: Positional Cloning

Sometimes, the gene product responsible for a genetic disease is known before the gene itself is identified. This was the case with the β-globin polypeptide and sickle cell disease, for example. Then one can deduce the DNA sequence from the amino acid sequence of the polypeptide; this DNA sequence can be used to make a probe in order to locate the disease gene using the techniques just described.

In other cases, however, we have only a linkage result, localizing the disease gene to a region that may be as much as 1 Mb in size. Such a region can contain as many as several dozen genes, interspersed with noncoding DNA. Because cloning the disease gene is an important goal of any gene mapping study, we now turn our attention to ways in which specific disease genes are identified and cloned. One may begin with a DNA segment (e.g., a linked marker) and then canvas the region around the marker to locate and clone the disease gene itself. This process, previously known as "reverse genetics," is now usually referred to as **positional cloning**.

Suppose that we know the approximate location of a polymorphic marker that is tightly linked (less than 1 cM, or approximately 1 Mb) to the disease gene we wish to isolate. A technique commonly used to proceed toward the gene is called **chromosome walking**. DNA from the marker is used as a probe to pick out partially overlapping segments of DNA from a genomic library (Box 7-1). The overlap can be determined by testing for hybridization between the probe and each DNA segment taken from the library (Fig. 7-18, page 148). Once identified, the overlapping DNA segment itself is used as a probe to pick out another DNA segment from the genomic library with which it partially overlaps. In this way one uses partially overlapping DNA segments to "walk" along the chromosome until the disease gene itself is reached. Because we usually cannot be certain whether the disease gene is on one side of the marker or the other, chromosome walking typically proceeds in both directions away from the marker (a "bidirectional" walk).

The DNA segments may be cloned into vectors, such as plasmids, cosmids, or yeast artificial chromosomes (YACs), as discussed in Chapter 3. Plasmids accommodate the smallest DNA inserts, whereas YACs accommodate the largest ones, about 1000 kb. Figure 7-20 (page 148) depicts a map of overlapping YACs and cosmids in the adenomatous polyposis coli region (a form of colon cancer; see Chapter 9). These maps of contiguous DNA segments are often termed "contig" maps.

The process of chromosome walking can be further illustrated with an analogy. Suppose that we have been placed somewhere in the state of

Box 7-1. Probes and Libraries: Their Construction and Use in Gene Mapping

Probes and libraries play central roles in gene mapping. A DNA **library** is much like an ordinary library, except that the library is composed of pieces of DNA rather than books. There are several types of DNA libraries. The most general is termed a **genomic library** and consists of fragments of DNA that are the result of a restriction digest of whole genomic DNA. The DNA is partially digested, so that some recognition sites are cleaved while others are not. This produces fragments that will overlap with one another. These fragments are then cloned into phage, cosmids, or YACs using the recombinant DNA techniques discussed in Chapter 3. A genomic library contains all of the human genome: introns, exons, promoters, and the vast stretches of noncoding DNA that separate genes.

A **cDNA library** is much more limited (and thus often easier to search), containing only the DNA corresponding to exons. It is obtained by purifying mRNA from a specific tissue, such as liver or skeletal muscle, and then exposing the mRNA to an enzyme called **reverse transcriptase**. This enzyme copies the mRNA into the appropriate complementary DNA (hence cDNA) sequence. DNA polymerase can then be used to convert this single-stranded DNA to double-stranded DNA, after which it is cloned into phage or other vectors, as in the genomic library. The steps involved in making genomic and cDNA libraries are summarized in Figure 7-19.

Yet another type of DNA library is the **chromosome-specific library**. Chromosomes are sorted using a method called **flow cytometry**, which separates chromosomes according to the proportion of AT base pairs in each one. The result is a library consisting mostly of DNA from only one chromosome. For example, after the gene for Huntington disease was mapped to a region on the short arm of chromosome 4, a library specific for this chromosome was used to refine the location of the gene.

DNA libraries are often used in making new polymorphic markers. For example, phage probes from a genomic library can be radioactively labeled and then hybridized to a Southern blot (recall from Chapter 3 that a Southern blot consists of DNA fragments that have been cleaved with a restriction enzyme such as *Eco*RI, sorted according to length by electrophoresis, and then fixed on a membrane). If the genomic DNA inserted in the phage contains an *Eco*RI restriction site that is present in some individuals and absent in others, then the Southern blot will reveal bands of different lengths in different individuals (i.e., a poly-

morphism). A number of different phage probes can be extracted from the genomic library and tested against various restriction enzymes to define new polymorphisms in this way. The polymorphism can then be mapped to a specific location by using the probe in conjunction with physical mapping techniques, such as somatic cell hybridization and in situ hybridization.

Microsatellite polymorphisms can be obtained from DNA libraries by constructing a probe that contains multiple repeated DNA sequences (e.g., multiple CA repeats). Then the DNA library is "screened" with this probe to find fragments in the library that hybridize with the probe. These fragments can be tested in a series of individuals to determine whether they are polymorphic.

Probes are also highly useful in isolating specific disease genes. In this context they can be made in several different ways. If the defective protein (or part of it) has been identified, the protein's amino acid sequence can be used to deduce part of the DNA sequence of the gene. Generally a short DNA sequence, only 20 to 30 bp in length, is sufficiently unique so that it will hybridize only to the complementary DNA in the disease gene. These sequences can be synthesized in a laboratory instrument to make oligonucleotide probes (Chapter 3). Because of the degeneracy of the DNA code, more than one triplet codon may specify an amino acid. For this reason, different possible combinations of base pairs must be tried. These combinations of oligonucleotide probes are mixed together, and the mixture is then used to probe a DNA library (e.g., a cDNA library). When one of the oligonucleotide probes in the mixture hybridizes with a fragment in the library, a portion of the desired gene has been identified. This fragment can be mapped using the physical techniques mentioned in the text.

Often the investigator has no knowledge of the sequence of the gene product. In this case it is sometimes possible to isolate the gene by purifying mRNA produced by specialized cell types. For example, reticulocytes (immature red blood cells) produce mostly globin polypeptides. mRNA taken from these cells can be converted to cDNA using reverse transcriptase, as discussed above, and then used as a probe to find larger fragments of the gene in a DNA library. It is sometimes easier to obtain mRNA from an experimental animal, such as a pig or rodent. Because of sequence similarity between these animals and humans, the animal-derived probe will usually hybridize appropriately with segments of a human DNA library.

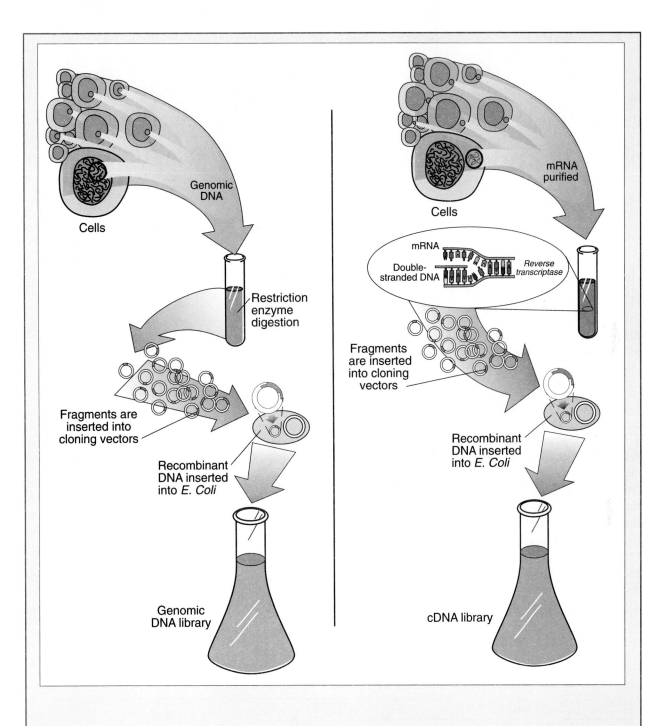

Figure 7-19 ■ **The creation of human DNA libraries.** *left,* A total genomic library is created using a partial restriction digest of human DNA and then cloning the fragments into vectors, such as phage, cosmids or YACs. *right,* A cDNA library is created by purifying mRNA from a tissue, exposing it to reverse transcriptase to create cDNA sequences. These are cloned into vectors.

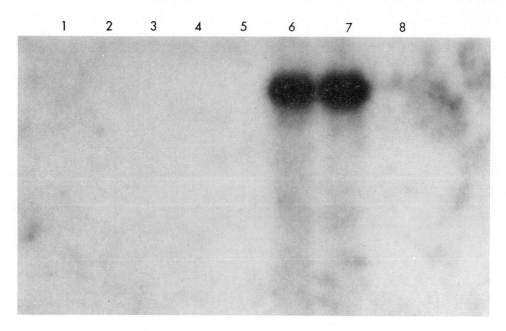

Figure 7-18 ■ A probe was tested against eight clones taken from a human YAC library. The probe hybridized with two of the clones (lanes 6 and 7), indicating overlap between the DNA in the probe and the DNA in each of the two YAC clones.

California and that our ultimate destination is Los Angeles. We do not know in which direction Los Angeles lies, nor do we know exactly how far away it is. We are given a map of the county in which we are currently located, and we have access to a library of highway maps of each county of California. These maps are not labeled, but, like most highway maps, there is a small region of overlap between maps of adjacent counties. We then use the first map we were given to search the library for maps that overlap in either direction. Finding such maps, we then use them to search the library again, ultimately progressing to Los Angeles.

Chromosome walking typically involves the isolation of partially overlapping DNA segments from genomic libraries in an attempt to progress along the chromosome toward a disease gene.

As chromosome walking proceeds, how do we know when we have reached the disease gene? Several approaches may be used.

Analysis of Cross-species Conservation

This approach helps to distinguish whether the DNA segment under consideration consists of coding DNA or noncoding DNA. This is important

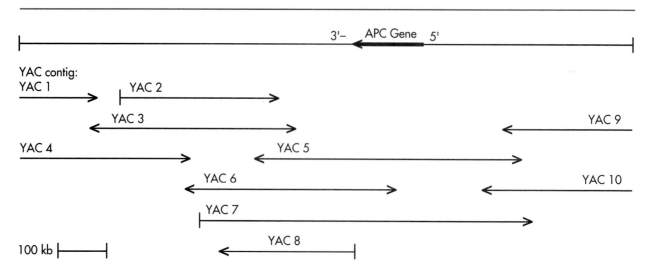

Figure 7-20 ■ An example of a YAC contig map used in "walking" along chromosome 5 in the region of the adenomatous polyposis coli (APC) gene.

because most of the region under consideration is likely to contain noncoding DNA, but a disease gene must contain coding DNA. Because it is likely to perform an important function, coding DNA generally cannot change much through evolution. This means that it will be **conserved**, or similar in DNA sequence, in a large number of different species. However, noncoding DNA is likely to change rapidly and differ substantially among species. Thus, if the sequence we are currently considering in our chromosome walk consists of coding DNA, it is more likely to hybridize (i.e., undergo complementary base pairing) with the DNA of many other species. A nonconserved sequence is less likely to show cross-species hybridization. To test whether a DNA segment is conserved across species, a probe containing the DNA segment is constructed and then exposed to denatured DNA from several species to determine whether it hybridizes (this is sometimes whimsically termed a "zoo blot"). Although this approach does not neccessarily identify the disease gene itself, it alerts us to the possibility that a DNA segment is part of a coding gene.

Identification of CG Islands

As discussed in Chapter 3, most CG dinucleotides are methylated. However, the 5′ regions of genes are often rich in *unmethylated* CG dinucleotides. Probable genes can thus be identified when such **CG islands** are encountered.

Further Linkage Analysis

As chromosome walking proceeds, polymorphisms within the overlapping segments can be analyzed as new markers for the disease gene. These markers are then used in new linkage analyses in families. If we find that the recombination frequency has increased between our new markers and the disease gene, then we are likely to be moving away from the disease gene rather than toward it. Because recombination in genomic regions smaller than 1 Mb is rare, additional linkage analysis is often of limited usefulness.

Screen for Mutations in the Sequence

Once a portion of coding DNA has been isolated, it can be examined for mutations using techniques such as SSCP, DGGE, and direct DNA sequencing (see Chapter 3). If a DNA sequence represents the disease gene, then mutations should be found in individuals with the disease, but they should not be found in normal individuals. To help distinguish disease-causing mutations from polymorphisms

that vary naturally among individuals, it is particularly useful to compare the DNA of patients whose disease is caused by a *new mutation* with the DNA of their unaffected parents. Although a harmless polymorphism will be seen in both the affected offspring and the unaffected parents, a mutation responsible for the disease in the offspring will not be seen in the parents. This approach was especially useful in identifying mutations that cause NF1.

Another type of mutation that can be tested is a submicroscopic deletion (i.e., a deletion too small to be observable under a microscope). Small deletions can be detected using Southern blotting techniques, described in Chapter 3. A deletion will produce a smaller-than-normal restriction fragment, which migrates more quickly through a gel. Somewhat larger deletions can be detected through **pulsed field gel electrophoresis**, a variation on the Southern blotting technique in which restriction digests are done with enzymes that, because their recognition sequences are rare, cleave the DNA infrequently. This produces restriction fragments that can be tens or hundreds of thousands of bp in length. These fragments are too large to be distinguished from one another using standard gel electrophoresis, but they will migrate differentially according to size when the electrical charge is turned off and on (pulsed) for a few seconds or minutes at a time.

Test for Gene Expression

To help verify that a gene is responsible for a given defect, one can test various tissues to determine the ones in which the gene is expressed (i.e., transcribed into mRNA). This is done by purifying mRNA from the tissue and hybridizing it with a probe made from the gene. This is done using a technique known as **Northern blotting** (Fig. 7-21), which is conceptually similar to Southern blotting except that mRNA, rather than DNA, is being probed. If the gene in question causes the disease, the mRNA should be expressed in tissues known to be affected by the disease. For example, one would expect the phenylalanine hydroxylase gene (in which mutations can cause PKU) to be expressed in the liver, where this enzyme is known to be synthesized.

A more direct gene expression test involves injecting the normal version of the DNA sequence into a defective cell from a diseased individual (or animal model), using recombinant DNA techniques. If the normal sequence corrects the defect, then it is likely to represent the disease gene of interest. This approach has been used, for example,

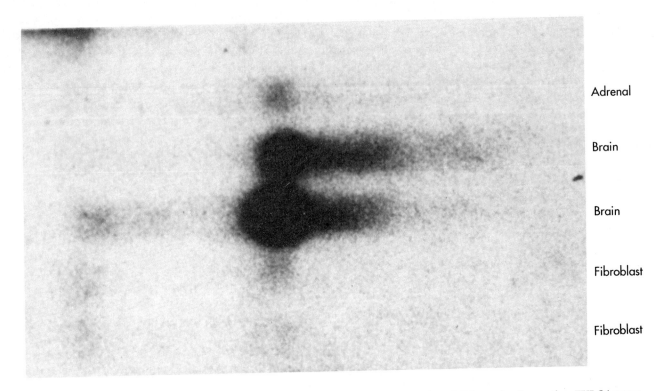

Adrenal

Brain

Brain

Fibroblast

Fibroblast

Figure 7-21 ▪ An example of a Northern blot, showing hybridization of a cDNA probe from the *EVI 2A* gene (a gene embedded within an intron of the *NF1* gene) with mRNA from the adrenal gland, brain, and fibroblasts. This result indicates that the *EVI 2A* gene is expressed in the brain at a much higher level than in the other two tissues. (Courtesy of Dr. Richard Cawthon, University of Utah Health Sciences Center.)

to prove that mutations in the CFTR gene can cause cystic fibrosis.

Many things can complicate the positional cloning procedure. For example, the isolation of overlapping DNA sequences can become difficult when long sequences of repetitive DNA are encountered. As a result, this process can be laborious and time-consuming. The Huntington disease gene, for example, was localized to chromosome 4p by linkage analysis in 1983, but 10 years of hard work by a large group of dedicated researchers elapsed before the disease gene itself was cloned. Four years of positional cloning were required to isolate the cystic fibrosis gene. The positional cloning process has been accelerated somewhat as better and faster cloning techniques and vectors have been devised (e.g., YACs, which can carry much larger inserts than cosmids). However, positional cloning may still require long and intense effort.

During the course of chromosome walking, one needs to determine whether the DNA segment currently under consideration is part of a disease gene. Tests that are used for this purpose include cross-species hybridization, identification of unmethylated CG islands, further linkage analysis using polymorphisms in the newly isolated DNA segment as markers, mutation screening in affected individuals, and tests of gene expression.

Candidate Genes

The gene hunting process can be expedited considerably when a **candidate gene** is available. As the name implies, these are genes whose known protein product makes them a likely candidate for the disease in question. For example, the various collagen genes were considered to be reasonable candidates for Marfan syndrome, because collagen is an important component of connective tissue. However, linkage analysis using collagen gene markers in Marfan syndrome families consistently yielded negative results. Another candidate gene emerged when the *fibrillin* gene was identified on chromosome 15. Fibrillin, as discussed in Chapter 4, is also a connective tissue component. Linkage analysis had localized the Marfan syndrome gene to chromosome 15, so the fibrillin gene became an even stronger candidate. Analysis of mutations in the *fibrillin* gene showed that they were consistently associated with Marfan syndrome, confirming *fibrillin* mutations as a cause of the disease.

A similar example is provided by hyperkalemic periodic paralysis, an autosomal dominant muscle disorder characterized by transient episodes of weakness or paralysis. The electrophysiologic abnormalities observed in this disorder suggested that a defect in a voltage-gated sodium channel could be involved. A sodium channel gene on chromosome 17 thus presented itself as a likely candidate, and a polymorphism in this gene showed perfect linkage with the disease phenotype in large families. Subsequent analyses verified the pathogenic role of the sodium channel gene by detecting mutations in affected individuals.

Candidate genes are those whose characteristics (such as protein product) suggest that they may be responsible for a genetic disease.

Table 7-3 ▪ Some important genetic diseases that have been mapped to specific chromosome locations

Disease	Chromosome location	Gene cloned*
Achondroplasia	4p	Yes
Huntington disease	4p	Yes
Cystic fibrosis	7q	Yes
Hemophilia A, Hemophilia B	Xq	Yes
von Willebrand disease	12q	Yes
Marfan syndrome	15q	Yes
Sickle cell anemia	11p	Yes
β-thalassemia	11p	Yes
α-thalassemia	16p	Yes
Familial breast cancer	13q, 17q	Yes
Fragile X syndrome	Xq	Yes
Phenylketonuria	12q	Yes
Duchenne/Becker muscular dystrophy	Xp	Yes
Retinoblastoma	13q	Yes
Hemochromatosis	6p	No
Familial hypercholesterolemia (LDL receptor defect)	19p	Yes
Adult polycystic kidney disease	4q, 16p	16p gene cloned
α-1-antitrypsin deficiency	14q	Yes
Familial Alzheimer disease	1q, 14q, 19q, 21q	Yes
Isolated cleft palate	Xq	No
Tay-Sachs disease	15q	Yes
Neurofibromatosis (classical)	17q	Yes
Neurofibromatosis (bilateral acoustic form)	22q	Yes
Familial polyposis coli	5q	Yes
Familial melanoma	1p, 9p	9p gene cloned
Hereditary nonpolyposis colorectal cancer	2p, 3p	Yes
Myotonic dystrophy	19q	Yes
Retinitis pigmentosa	1q, 3q, 4p, 5q, 6p, 7q, 7p, 8p, 11q, 11p, 14q, 15q, 16q, 17p, 19q, Xp	Some genes cloned
Long QT syndrome	3p, 4q, 7q, 11p	3p, 7q, and 11p genes cloned
Albinism, oculocutaneous type 1	11q	Yes
Albinism, oculocutaneous type 2	15q	Yes
Albinism, X-linked ocular	Xp	Yes
Charcot-Marie-Tooth disease	1q, 1p, 3q, 8q, 17p, Xq, Xp	Some genes cloned
Amyotrophic lateral sclerosis	21q	Yes
Bloom syndrome	15q	Yes
Ataxia telangiectasia	11q	Yes

*Cloning may be partial or complete.

Using the techniques described in this chapter, a large number of important disease genes have now been mapped, and many of them have also been cloned. Some examples are given in Table 7-3.

■ PROGRESS TOWARD A COMPLETE HUMAN GENE MAP

A coordinated effort is now under way to achieve a "complete" map of the human genome. The Human Genome Project, a 15-year endeavor initiated in 1991, has several goals. The first, scheduled for completion by 1995, is to create a genetic map in which highly informative markers are placed at least every 2 to 5 cM throughout the human genome. A second goal is to form a contiguous map (overlapping sets of DNA segments) for the entire genome, using small DNA sequences known as sequence-tagged sites (STS) to mark the map every 100 to 300 kb. This will provide a detailed physical map of the genome. The final goal of the project is to provide a complete sequence of the 3 billion bp of the human genome. Currently the sequencing portion of the project is directed at developing cheaper and more rapid sequencing methods so that sequencing can proceed at a cost of about $.50 per base.

The human gene map offers many important benefits:

1. Marker genes will be available to establish close linkage for virtually all single-gene disorders. Linkage studies are sometimes hampered by a lack of informative markers in the region of interest.

2. A complete map will help resolve issues of locus heterogeneity. The demonstration of linkage to different markers in different families is conclusive proof of heterogeneity (examples include retinitis pigmentosa and osteogenesis imperfecta).

3. Knowing the location of disease genes can help us understand the underlying pathology of a genetic disease. An example is the multiple X-linked genes that can undergo unequal crossover to produce various forms of color blindness.

4. The mapping of genes is an important step toward cloning them. Once a gene is cloned, the function of the gene product can be analyzed. A cloned gene can be placed in a nonhuman host (e.g., bacteria) using recombinant DNA techniques. This has enabled scientists to artificially produce large quantities of otherwise scarce proteins, such as insulin, interferon, clotting factor VIII, and human growth hormone. Cloning a gene may also lead to gene therapy, as discussed in Chapter 11.

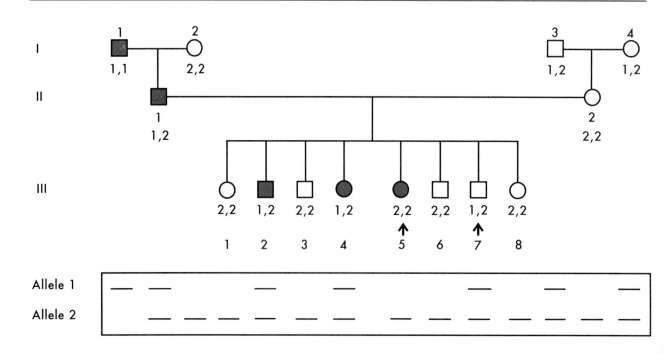

■ STUDY QUESTIONS

1. In the accompanying pedigree for an autosomal dominant disease, each family member has been typed for a two-allele RFLP marker, as shown in the Southern blot below the pedigree. Determine the linkage phase for the disease and marker locus in the affected male in generation 2. Based on the meioses that produced the offspring in generation 3, what is the recombination frequency for the marker and the disease locus?

2. In the accompanying Huntington disease pedigree, the family has been typed for two two-allele markers, A and B. The genotypes for each marker are shown below each family member; the genotype for marker A is shown above the genotype for marker B. Under the hypothesis that $\theta = 0.0$, what is the LOD score for linkage between each marker locus and the Huntington disease locus?

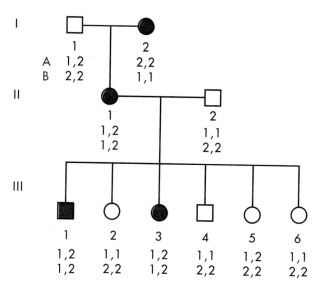

3. Interpret the following table of LOD scores and recombination frequencies (θ):

θ	0.0	0.05	0.1	0.2	0.3	0.4	0.5
LOD	$-\infty$	1.7	3.5	2.8	2.2	1.1	0.2

4. The family shown in the accompanying pedigree has been presented for genetic diagnosis. The disease in question is autosomal dominant. The family members have been typed for a closely linked two-allele marker locus. What can you tell the family about the risks for their offspring?

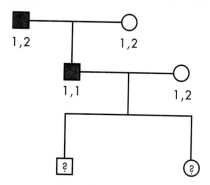

5. Distinguish the differences among the concepts of synteny, linkage, linkage disequilibrium, and association.

6. A recent study showed no linkage disequilibrium between neurofibromatosis type 1 and a closely linked marker locus. Explain this, keeping in mind that the neurofibromatosis type 1 has a high rate of new mutations.

7. The somatic cell hybridization panel below indicates the clones that yielded a positive hybridization signal for a cDNA segment. Based on this information, on which chromosome is the cDNA segment likely to reside?

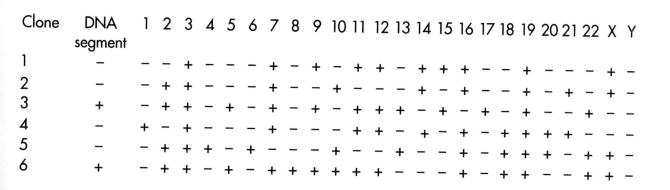

Clone	DNA segment	1	2	3	4	5	6	7	8	9	10	11	12	13	14	15	16	17	18	19	20	21	22	X	Y
1	−	−	−	+	−	−	−	−	+	−	+	−	+	+	−	+	+	+	−	−	+	−	−	−	+	−
2	−	−	+	+	−	−	−	+	−	−	+	−	−	−	+	−	+	−	−	+	−	+	−	+	−
3	+	−	+	+	−	+	−	+	−	+	−	+	+	+	−	+	−	+	−	+	−	−	+	−	−
4	−	+	−	+	−	−	−	+	−	−	−	+	+	−	+	−	+	−	+	−	+	+	+	−	−	−
5	−	−	+	+	+	−	+	−	−	−	+	−	−	+	−	−	+	−	+	+	+	−	+	+	−
6	+	−	+	+	−	+	−	+	+	+	+	+	+	−	−	−	+	−	+	+	−	−	+	+	−

■ ADDITIONAL READING

Bentley DR, Dunham I: Mapping human chromosomes, Curr Opin Genet Dev 5:328–334, 1995.

Collins FS: Positional cloning moves from perditional to traditional, Nature Genet 9:347–350, 1995.

Cross SH, Bird AP: CpG islands and genes, Curr Opin Genet Dev 5:309–314, 1995.

Davies KE, editor: Human genetic disease analysis: a practical approach, London, 1993, Oxford University Press.

de Belleroche J, Orrell R, King A: Familial amyotrophic lateral sclerosis/motor neurone disease (FASLS): a review of current developments, J Med Genet 32:841–847, 1995.

Dib C, Fauré S, Fizames C, Samson D, Droucot N, Vignal A, Millasseau P: A comprehensive genetic map of the human genome based on 5,624 microsatellites, Nature 380:152–154, 1996.

Dryja TP, Li T: Molecular genetics of retinitis pigmentosa, Hum Molec Genet 4:1739–1743, 1995.

Guyer MS, Collins FS: How is the Human Genome Project doing, and what have we learned so far? Proc Natl Acad Sci USA 92:10841–10848, 1995.

Hudson TJ, Stein LD, Gerety SS, Ma J, Castle AB, Silva J, Slonim DK, et al.: An STS-based map of the human genome, Science 270:1945–1954, 1995.

Jorde LB: Invited editorial: Linkage disequilibrium as a gene mapping tool, Am J Hum Genet 56:11–14, 1995.

Lander E, Kruglyak L: Genetic dissection of complex traits: guidelines for interpreting and reporting linkage results, Nature Genet 11:241–247, 1995.

Morton NE: LODs past and present, Genetics 140:7–12, 1995.

Murray JC, Buetow KH, Weber JL, Ludwigsen S, Scherpbier-Heddema T, Manion F, Quillen J, et al.: A comprehensive human linkage map with centimorgan density, Science 265:2049–2054, 1994.

Nelson DL: Positional cloning reaches maturity, Curr Opin Genet Devel 5:298–303, 1995.

Ott J: Analysis of human genetic linkage, rev ed, Baltimore, 1991, Johns Hopkins University Press.

Sheffield VC, Nishimura DY, Stone EM: Novel approaches to linkage mapping, Curr Opin Genet Dev 5:335–341, 1995.

Southern EM: Genome mapping: cDNA approaches, Curr Opin Genet Dev 2:412–416, 1992.

Weeks DE, Lathrop GM: Polygenic disease: methods for mapping complex disease traits, Trends Genet, 11:513–523, 1995.

8 Immunogenetics

Each day our bodies are confronted with a formidable series of invaders: viruses, bacteria, and many other disease organisms whose goal is to overcome our natural defenses. These defenses, known collectively as the immune system, consist of a complex collection of trillions of cells. The immune system must be able to cope with a multitude of invading microorganisms, and it must be able to distinguish "self" from "non-self" with a high degree of accuracy.

As one might expect, the genetic basis of the immune system is complex. The study of the genetics of the immune system, known as **immunogenetics**, has benefitted enormously from new developments in gene mapping and cloning. Most of the techniques discussed in earlier chapters (e.g., linkage analysis, chromosome walking, DNA sequencing) have been used to study the genes responsible for the immune response. Many new genes have been uncovered, and their functions and interactions have been studied intensely. This chapter provides a brief review of basic immunology, and it discusses the genes underlying our capacity to defend against a highly diverse array of disease pathogens. Aspects of autoimmune disease are examined, and some of the major immunodeficiency disorders are discussed.

■ THE IMMUNE RESPONSE: BASIC CONCEPTS

Innate Immune System

When a foreign microorganism is encountered, the body's first line of defense includes **phagocytes** (a type of cell that engulfs and destroys the microorganism) and the **complement system**. The complement proteins can destroy microbes directly by perforating their cell membranes, and they can also attract phagocytes and other immune system agents to microbes by coating the microbial surface (it is because of this assisting role that the term "complement" originated). These components of the immune system can distinguish foreign bodies in a variety of ways. For example, bacteria are often identified because they produce distinctive peptides beginning with formyl methionine. Viruses are often recognized because they produce double-stranded RNA, which is relatively rare in mammals. These components of the early phase of the immune response, termed the **innate immune system**, recognize only general features of foreign microbes.

> The innate immune system, which includes some phagocytes and the complement system, is an early part of the immune response and recognizes general features of invading microorganisms.

Adaptive Immune System

Although the innate immune system may help hold an infection in check in its early phases, it is often incapable of overcoming the infection. This is the task of a more specialized component of the immune system, the **adaptive immune system**. As its name suggests, this part of the immune system is capable of "adapting" to features of the invading microorganism to mount a more specific and more effective immune response.

Key components of the adaptive immune response include **T lymphocytes** (or **T cells**) and **B lymphocytes** (or **B cells**). These cells are created in the body's primary lymphoid organs (bone marrow for B cells and the thymus for T cells). In the thymus, T cells that can tolerate the body's own peptides are selected, and those that would attack the body's peptides are eliminated. The B and T cells then progress to secondary lymphoid tissues, such as the lymph nodes, spleen, and tonsils, where they encounter foreign microorganisms. Mature B lymphocytes produce circulating **antibodies**, which combat infections. Because it involves agents that circulate in the bloodstream, this portion of the immune system is sometimes called the **humoral immune system**. T lymphocytes help B lymphocytes respond to infections more effectively, and they can directly kill infected cells. This part of the immune system is sometimes called the **cellular immune system**. It is estimated that the body contains several trillion B and T cells.

> B lymphocytes are a component of the adaptive immune system; they produce circulating antibodies in response to infection. T lymphocytes, another component of the adaptive immune system, interact directly with infected cells to kill these cells, and they aid in the B cell response.

B Cell Response: Humoral Immune System

A major element of the adaptive immune response begins when specialized types of phagocytes engulf invading microbes and then present peptides derived from these microbes on their cell surfaces. These cells, which include **macrophages** and **dendritic cells**, are termed **antigen presenting cells (APCs)**. B cells are also capable of presenting foreign peptides on their cell surfaces. The foreign peptide is transported to the surface of the APC by a **class II major histocompatibility complex (MHC)** molecule, which carries the foreign peptide in a specialized groove (Fig. 8-1). This complex, which projects into the extracellular environment, is recognized by another cell, the **helper T lymphocyte**. This cell has a **receptor** on its surface capable of binding (i.e., forming noncovalent bonds) to the MHC–peptide complex. As shown in Figure 8-2 (page 158), other cell-surface proteins, such as the various **cell adhesion molecules** and **costimulatory molecules**, also participate in the binding process. Binding the MHC–peptide complex stimulates the helper T lymphocyte to secrete **cytokines**, which are substances that cause other cells to proliferate. In particular, these cytokines help stimulate the subset of B lymphocytes whose cell surface receptors, termed **immunoglobulins**, can bind to the invading microorganism's peptides. The immunoglobulin's capacity to bind a specific foreign peptide (i.e., its **affinity** for the peptide) is determined by its shape and other characteristics.

> In the humoral immune response, foreign particles are displayed in conjunction with class II MHC molecules by APCs. These are recognized by helper T cells, which then stimulate proliferation of B cells whose immunoglobulins can bind to the foreign pathogen.

It is estimated that, upon initial exposure to a foreign microbe, only about 1 in every million B lymphocytes happens to produce immunoglobulins capable of binding to the microbe. This number is too small to fight an infection effectively. Furthermore, the immunoglobulins' binding affinity is likely to be relatively poor. However, once this relatively small population of B lymphocytes is stimulated, they begin an adaptive process in which minor DNA sequence variations are introduced with each mitotic division (somatic hypermutation, see below). These DNA sequence variations in turn produce variations in the binding characteristics of immunoglobulins (e.g., the shape of the protein). Some of these variant immunoglobulins will possess a higher level of binding affinity for the microorganism. The B cells producing these immunoglobulins are favorably selected and proliferate rapidly. These B cells then become **plasma cells**, which secrete immunoglobulins into the bloodstream. The secreted immunoglobulins, which are structurally identical to the immunoglobulins that act as receptors on the B cell's surface, are antibodies. It can now be seen how the adaptive immune system gets its name: it involves the initial selection of B cells whose receptors can bind with the pathogen and subsequent fine-tuning of these B cells to achieve higher binding affinity.

> During the B-cell response to a foreign peptide, the binding affinity of immunoglobulins for the invading pathogen increases. When mature, the B cell becomes an antibody-secreting plasma cell.

After initial stimulation by the disease pathogen, the process of B-cell differentiation and maturation into antibody-producing plasma cells requires about 5 to 7 days for completion. Each plasma cell is capable of secreting approximately 10 million antibody molecules per hour. Antibodies bind to the pathogen's surface **antigens** (antigen = "*anti*body *gene*rating") and may destroy the microorganism directly. More often, the antibody "tags" the pathogen for destruction by other components of the immune system, such as complement proteins and phagocytes.

Another important activity of the humoral immune response is the creation of **memory cells**, a subset of high affinity–binding B cells that persist in the body after the infection has subsided. These cells, which have already been highly selected for

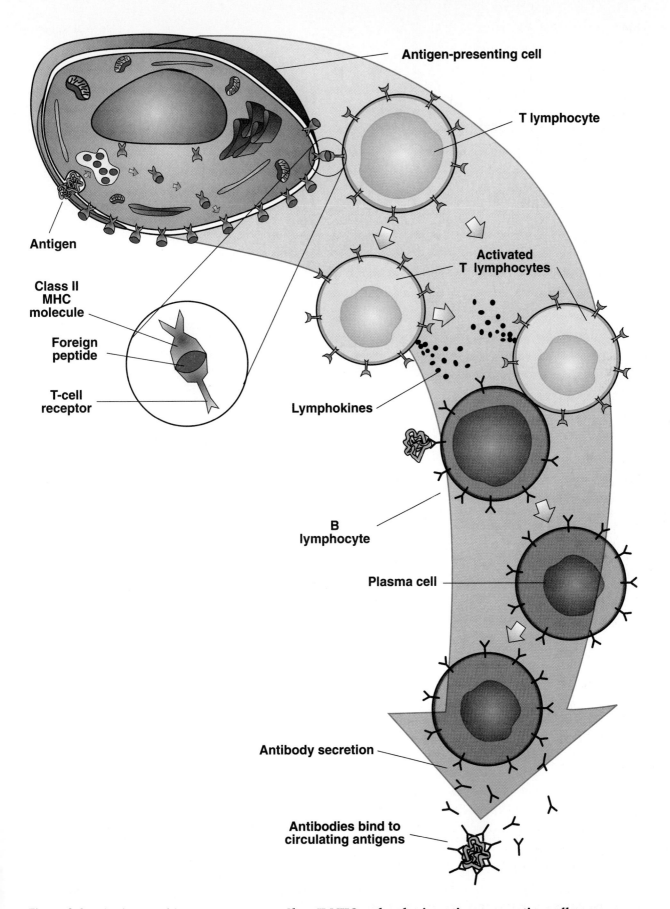

Antigen-presenting cell

T lymphocyte

Activated T lymphocytes

Antigen

Class II MHC molecule

Foreign peptide

T-cell receptor

Lymphokines

B lymphocyte

Plasma cell

Antibody secretion

Antibodies bind to circulating antigens

Figure 8-1 ■ The humoral immune response. Class II MHC molecules in antigen-presenting cells carry foreign peptides to the surface of the cell, where the foreign peptide is recognized by a helper T cell. The T cell secretes cytokines that stimulate B cells whose immunoglobulins will bind to the foreign peptide. These B cells become plasma cells, which secrete antibodies into the circulation to bind with the microbe, helping to combat the infection. (Modified from Nossal JVN: Sci Am 269:53–62, 1993.)

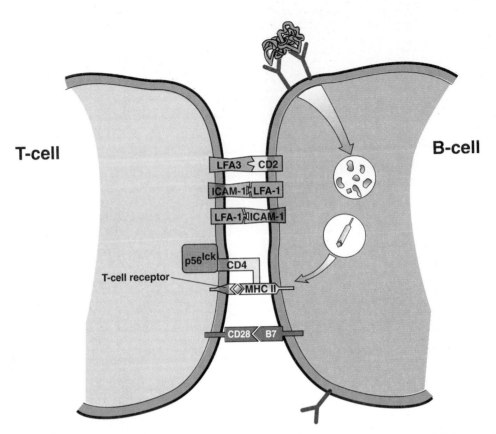

T-cell

LFA3 ⟨ CD2
ICAM-1 ⟩ LFA-1
LFA-1 ⟩ ICAM-1
p56^{lck} ⟩ CD4
T-cell receptor
⟨◇⟩ MHC II
CD28 ⟨ B7

B-cell

Figure 8-2 ■ **A detailed view of the binding between a helper T cell and a B cell. In addition to the binding of the T-cell receptor to the MHC–peptide complex, a number of other molecules interact with one another, such as the costimulatory B7-CD28 complex.** (Adapted from DeFranco, Nature 351:603, 1991.)

response to the pathogen, provide a more rapid response should the pathogen be encountered again later in the individual's life. Vaccinations are effective because they induce the formation of memory cells that can respond to a specific pathogen.

Cellular Immune System

Some microorganisms, such as viruses, are adept at quickly inserting themselves into the body's cells. Here they are inaccessible to antibodies, which are water-soluble proteins that cannot pass through the cell's lipid membrane. To combat such infections, a second component of the adaptive immune system, the cellular immune system, has evolved. A key member of the cellular immune system is the **class I MHC molecule**, which is found on the surfaces of nearly all of the body's cells. In a normal cell the class I MHC molecule binds with small peptides (8 to 10 amino acids in length) derived from the interior of the cell. It migrates to the cell's surface, carrying the peptide with it and displaying it outside the cell. Because this is one of the body's *own* peptides, no immune response is elicited. In an infected cell, however, the class I MHC molecule binds to small peptides that are derived from the infecting organism. Cell-surface presentation of the *foreign peptide* by the class I MHC molecule alerts the immune system, T cells in particular. Recall that T lymphocytes learn to tolerate "self" peptides while developing in the thymus, but they are highly intolerant of foreign peptides. The MHC–peptide complex binds to a receptor on the appropriate T cell's surface, which prompts the T cell to emit a chemical that destroys the infected cell (Fig. 8-3). Because of their ability to destroy cells in this way, these T lymphocytes are termed **cytotoxic T lymphocytes** (or **killer T lymphocytes**). They are also known as CD8 T cells because of the presence of CD8 molecules on their surfaces (helper T cells have a CD4 molecule on their cell surfaces and are thus a type of CD4 T lymphocyte). Each cytotoxic T lymphocyte can destroy one infected cell every 1 to 5 minutes.

The cellular immune system is capable of destroying the body's cells once they are infected. Peptides from the pathogen are

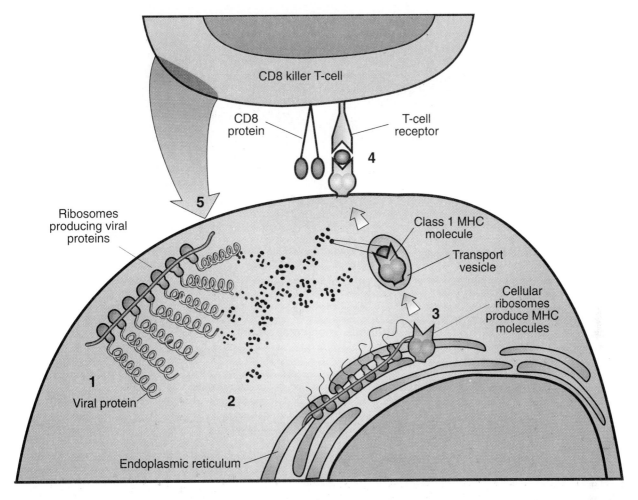

Figure 8-3 ■ In a cell infected by a virus, the viral peptides (1, 2) are carried to the cell surface by class I MHC molecules (3). The T-cell receptor of a CD8 cytotoxic T cell binds to the peptide–MHC complex (4). Recognizing the peptide as foreign, the cytotoxic T cell secretes chemicals that kill the infected cell (5). (Modified from Janeway CA: Sci Am 269:73–79, 1993.)

displayed on cell surfaces by class I MHC molecules. These are recognized by cytotoxic (killer) T lymphocytes, which destroy the infected cell.

As with B lymphocytes, only a small proportion of the body's T cells will have binding affinity for the infecting pathogen. By secreting cytokines, helper T cells stimulate the proliferation of the cytotoxic T lymphocytes that can bind to the infected cells. In addition, circulating dendritic cells present the foreign peptides on their cell surfaces and migrate to secondary lymphoid tissues, where most of the T cells reside, helping to alert the appropriate T cells to the infection.

The humoral immune system is specialized to combat extracellular infections, such as circulating bacteria. The cellular immune system combats intracellular infections, such as viruses and cellular parasites. However, this division of labor is not strict, and there is a great deal of interaction between the two components of the adaptive immune system.

■ IMMUNE RESPONSE PROTEINS: GENETIC BASIS OF STRUCTURE AND DIVERSITY

Immunoglobulin Genes and Structure

As illustrated in Figure 8-4, each antibody (or immunoglobulin) molecule is composed of four chains: an identical pair of longer **heavy chains** and an identical pair of shorter **light chains**. The chains are linked together by disulfide bonds. There are five different types of heavy chains (termed γ, μ, α, δ, and ϵ) and two types of light chains (κ and λ). The five types of heavy chains determine the major **class** (or **isotype**) to which an immunoglobulin (Ig) molecule belongs: γ, μ, α, δ, and ϵ correspond to the immunoglobulin iso-

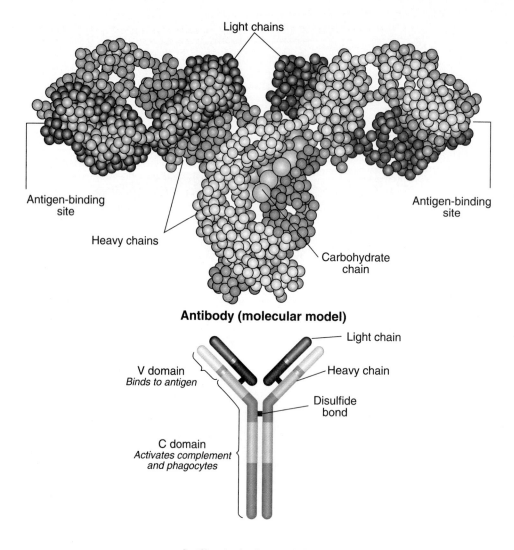

Light chains

Antigen-binding
site

Heavy chains

Antigen-binding
site

Carbohydrate
chain

Antibody (molecular model)

Light chain

Heavy chain

V domain
Binds to antigen

Disulfide
bond

C domain
*Activates complement
and phagocytes*

Antibody (schematic)

Figure 8-4 ■ An antibody molecule consists of two identical light chains and two identical heavy chains. The light chain includes variable, joining, and constant regions, and the heavy chain includes these regions as well as a diversity region located between its variable and joining regions. The upper portion of the figure depicts a molecular model of antibody structure.

types IgG, IgM, IgA, IgD, and IgE, respectively. Immature B lymphocytes produce only IgM, but as they mature, a rearrangement of heavy chain genes called **class switching** occurs. This produces the four other major classes of immunoglobulins, each of which differs in amino acid composition, charge, size, and carbohydrate content. Each class tends to be localized in certain parts of the body, and each tends to respond to a different type of infection. The two types of light chains can be found in association with any of the five types of heavy chains.

The heavy and light chains both contain a **constant** and a **variable** region, which are located at the C-terminal and N-terminal ends of the chains, respectively. The arrangement of genes encoding

the constant region determines the major class of the Ig molecule (e.g., IgA, IgE). The variable region is responsible for antigen recognition and binding and thus varies within immunoglobulin classes. Three distinct gene segments encode the light chains: C for the constant region, V for the variable region, and J for the region joining the constant and variable regions. Four gene segments encode the heavy chains, with C, V, and J coding again for the constant, variable, and joining regions, respectively, and a "diversity" (D) region located between the joining and variable regions. The genes encoding the κ light chain are located on chromosome 2, and those encoding the λ light chain are on chromosome 22. The genes that encode the heavy chains are on chromosome 14.

Immunoglobulin molecules consist of two identical heavy chains and two identical light chains. The heavy chain constant region determines the major class to which an immunoglobulin belongs. The variable regions of the light and heavy chains recognize and bind antigens.

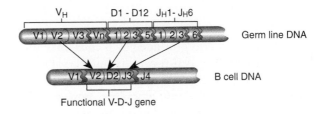

Figure 8-5 ■ **Somatic recombination in the formation of a heavy chain of an antibody molecule. The functional heavy chain is encoded by only one segment each from the multiple V, D, and J segments.** (Modified from Roitt I, Brostoff J, and Male D, editors: Immunology, ed 3, St Louis 1993, Mosby.)

Basis of Immunoglobulin Diversity

Our bodies face an enormous variety of infectious organisms. Because the immune system cannot "know" in advance what types of microbes it will encounter, the system must contain a huge reservoir of structurally diverse immune cells so that at least a few cells can respond (i.e., bind) to any invading microbe. Indeed, the humoral immune system is capable of generating at least 10 billion structurally distinct antibodies. At one time it was thought that, because each antibody has a unique amino acid sequence, each must be encoded by a different gene. However, this "one gene–one antibody" hypothesis could not possibly be correct because the human has only 50,000 to 100,000 genes. Further study has shown that several mechanisms are responsible for generating antibody diversity:

1. *Multiple germline immunoglobulin genes.* Molecular genetic studies (cloning and DNA sequencing) have shown that, for each heavy and light chain, an individual has 100 to 200 different V segments located contiguously in his/her germline and six different J segments. In the heavy chain region there are at least 30 D segments.
2. *Somatic recombination (VDJ recombination).* As immunoglobulin molecules are formed during B lymphocyte maturation, a specific combination of single V and J segments is selected for the light chain, and another combination of single V, J, and D segments is selected for the heavy chain. This is accomplished by specific deletion of the DNA sequences separating the single V, J, and D segments before they are transcribed into mRNA (Fig. 8-5). This process is carried out by enzymes called **recombinases**, which are encoded in part by the *RAG1* and *RAG2* genes. This "cutting and pasting" process is known as **somatic recombination**, as opposed to the germline recombination that takes place during meiosis. Somatic recombination produces a rather unique result: unlike most other cells of the body, whose DNA composition is identical, mature B lymphocytes *vary* in terms of their rearranged immunoglobulin

DNA sequences. Because there are many possible combinations of single V, J, and D segments, somatic recombination can generate a large number of different types of antibody molecules.

3. *Junctional diversity.* As the V, D, and J regions are assembled, slight variations occur in the position at which they are joined, and small numbers of nucleotides may be deleted or inserted at the junctions joining the regions. This creates even more variation in antibody amino acid sequence.
4. *Somatic hypermutation.* After stimulation by a foreign antigen, the B lymphocytes undergo a "secondary differentiation" process characterized by **somatic hypermutation**, as mentioned above. The mutation rate of the genes encoding the immunoglobulins increases to approximately 10^{-3} per base pair per cell division. This causes minor variation in the DNA sequences encoding immunoglobulins and thus in their peptide-binding characteristics. Somatic hypermutation of the V, D, and J genes produces considerable antibody diversity and may be caused by mutational hotspots in these genes.
5. *Multiple combinations of heavy and light chains.* Further diversity is created by the random combination of different heavy and light chains in assembling the immunoglobulin molecule.

Each of these mechanisms contributes to antibody diversity. Considering all of them together, it has been estimated that as many as 10^{10} to 10^{14} distinct antibodies can potentially be produced.

Mechanisms that produce antibody diversity include multiple germline gene segments, somatic recombination of the germline gene segments, junctional diversity, somatic hypermutation, and the potential for multiple combinations of heavy and light chains.

T-Cell Receptors

The T-cell receptors are similar in many ways to the immunoglobulins produced by B cells. Like the immunoglobulins, T-cell receptors must be able to bind to a large variety of peptides from invading organisms. Unlike immunoglobulins, however, T-cell receptors are never secreted from the cell, and T-cell activation requires the presentation of foreign peptide along with an MHC molecule. T-cell receptors are heterodimers composed of either an α and a β chain, or a γ and a δ chain (Fig. 8-6). The genes encoding the α and δ chains are both located on chromosome 14, and those encoding the β and γ chains are both located on chromosome 7. A given T cell will have either the α-β receptor or the γ-δ receptor. The γ-δ T-cell receptor was discovered more recently than the α-β receptor, and many of its properties are not yet well understood.

As in immunoglobulin formation, multiple germ-line gene segments, VDJ somatic recombination (mediated by recombinases), and junctional diversity are important in generating T-cell receptor diversity. However, somatic hypermutation does not occur in the genes that encode the T-cell receptors. This may be related to the requirements that T-cell receptors must be able to tolerate normal ''self'' peptides and also recognize MHC molecules.

> **T-cell receptors are similar in function to B-cell receptors (immunoglobulins). Their diversity is created by the same mechanisms that produce immunoglobulin diversity, with the exception of somatic hypermutation.**

■ THE MAJOR HISTOCOMPATIBILITY COMPLEX

Class I, II, and III Genes

The major histocompatibility complex (MHC) includes a series of at least 80 genes that lie in a 4-Mb region on the short arm of chromosome 6 (Fig. 8-7). The MHC is commonly classified into three groups: class I, class II, and class III. As previously mentioned, the class I MHC molecule forms a complex with foreign peptides that is recognized by receptors on the surfaces of cytotoxic T lymphocytes. Class I MHC molecules are composed of a single heavy glycoprotein chain (encoded by loci on chromosome 6) and a single light chain, called β_2-microglobulin, encoded by a gene on chromosome 15 (Fig. 8-8, *A*). The most

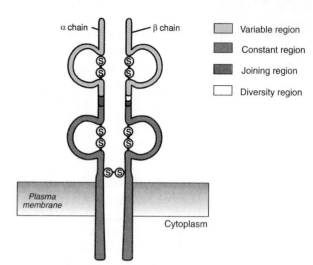

Figure 8-6 ■ The T-cell receptor, a heterodimer, which consists of either an α and a β chain, or a γ and a δ chain. (Modified from Raven PH, Johnson GB: Biology, ed 3, St. Louis, 1992, Mosby.)

important of the class I loci are labeled **HLA*** A, B, and C. Each of these loci has dozens of alleles, resulting in a high degree of class I MHC variability among different individuals. It is thought that this interindividual variation has evolved so that infections will spread less easily in populations.

The class I region spans 1.8 Mb and includes at least 20 genes, but the other genes in this region are less polymorphic than the HLA A, B, and C genes and play a lesser role in T-cell receptor recognition. The region also includes several **pseudogenes** (genes that are similar in DNA sequence to other genes but that have been altered so that they cannot be transcribed or translated).

The class I molecules were first discovered in the 1940s by scientists who were experimenting with tissue grafts in mice. When the class I alleles in donor and recipient mice differed, the grafts were rejected. This is the historical basis for the term *major histocompatibility complex.* In humans, matching of the donor and recipient's class I alleles increases the probability of graft or transplant tolerance. Because grafts and transplants are a relatively new phenomenon in human history, the MHC obviously did not evolve to effect transplant rejection. Instead, T cells, when confronted with foreign MHC molecules on donor cells, interpret these as foreign peptides and attack the cells.

---

* HLA stands for ''human leukocyte antigen,'' reflecting the fact that these molecules were seen in early studies of leukocyte (white cell) surfaces. However, as mentioned previously, they are found on the surfaces of nearly all cells.

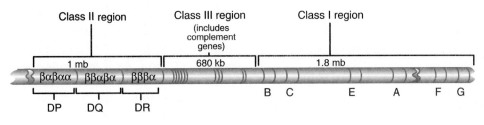

Chromosome 6p

Figure 8-7 ▪ A map of the human MHC. The 4-mb complex is divided into three regions: classes I, II, and III.

The class I MHC molecules are encoded by the highly polymorphic **HLA A, B, and C loci on chromosome 6.** In addition to presenting foreign peptides on the surfaces of infected cells, they can also bring about transplant rejection when foreign **MHC molecules** stimulate cytotoxic **T cells.**

While the class I MHC molecules are found on the surfaces of nearly all cells and can bind with cytotoxic T-cell receptors, the class II MHC molecules ordinarily are found only on the surfaces of the immune system's APCs (phagocytes and B lymphocytes). When associated with foreign peptides, they bind to receptors on the surfaces of helper T cells, as described above. The class II molecules are heterodimers consisting of an α and a β chain, each of which is encoded by a different gene located on chromosome 6 (Fig. 8-8, *B*). In addition to including the genes encoding major class II systems (such as HLA DP, DQ, and DR), the class II region includes genes that encode peptide transporter proteins (TAP1 and TAP2) that help to transport peptides into the endoplasmic reticulum, where they initially form complexes with class I molecules before migration to the cell surface.

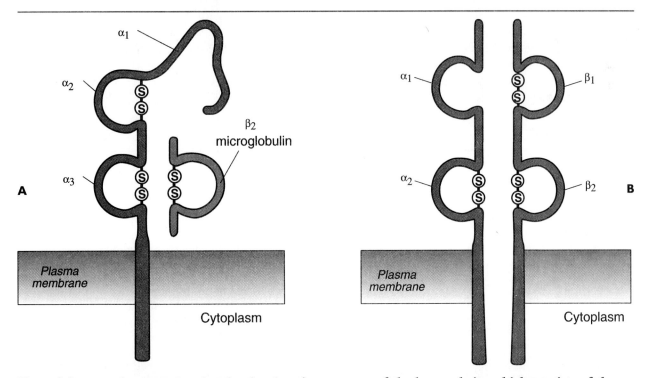

Figure 8-8 ▪ A, A class I MHC molecule, showing the structure of the heavy chain, which consists of three extracellular domains (α_1, α_2, and α_3), a membrane-spanning domain, and a cytoplasmic domain. A groove formed by the α_1 and α_2 domains carries peptide for presentation to T-cell receptors. The α_3 domain associates closely with the β_2-microglobulin chain. B, A class II MHC molecule, showing the structure of the α and β chains. Each has two globular extracellular domains, a membrane-spanning domain, and a cytoplasmic domain. The α_1 and β_1 domains apparently form a groove into which peptide nestles for presentation to T-cell receptors. (Modified from Raven PH, Johnson GB: Biology, ed 3, St. Louis, 1992, Mosby.)

Class II MHC molecules are heterodimers encoded by genes on chromosome 6. Like the class I MHC molecules, class II molecules are highly polymorphic.

It can be seen that both class I and class II MHC molecules guide T-cell receptors (cytotoxic and helper, respectively) to specific cells. This is called **MHC restriction**. Not all components of the immune system are MHC restricted. The complement system, for example, does not require direct interaction with MHC molecules. In addition, about 15% of lymphocytes belong to a group termed **natural killer cells**. These cells, which provide an early defense against some viral infections and some tumors, do not appear to recognize MHC surface molecules and are thus not MHC restricted.

The class III MHC region spans 680 kb and contains at least 36 genes, only some of which are involved in the immune response. Among the most important of these are the genes encoding the complement proteins.

The genes encoding the immunoglobulins, the T-cell receptors, and the class I and class II MHC proteins all share similar DNA sequences and structural features. Thus they are members of a gene family, like the globin genes, the color vision genes, and the collagen genes described in earlier chapters. Table 8-1 provides a summary of the major genes of the immune system and their chromosome locations.

It is important to emphasize that the class I and class II MHC molecules differ greatly *among* individuals, but each cell within an individual has the same class I and class II molecule (this uniformity is necessary for recognition by T cells). In contrast, after VDJ recombination the T-cell receptors and immunoglobulins differ from cell to cell *within* individuals, allowing the body to respond to a large variety of different infectious agents.

The immunoglobulin, T-cell receptor, and MHC genes are members of a gene family. Whereas immunoglobulins and T-cell receptors vary within individuals, MHC molecules vary between individuals.

MHC–Disease Associations

A number of diseases show significant associations with specific MHC alleles: those individuals who have the allele are much more likely to develop the disease than are those who lack it. Some examples, mentioned in earlier chapters, include the HLA-B27 (i.e., allele 27 of the HLA-B locus) association with ankylosing spondylitis and the HLA-DR3/HLA-DR4 association with type I diabetes. An especially strong association is seen between HLA-DR2 and narcolepsy, a disorder characterized by sudden and uncontrollable episodes of sleep. As Table 8-2 shows, most of the HLA–disease associations involve the class II MHC genes.

In a few cases the association between MHC alleles and a disease is caused by linkage disequilib-

Table 8-1 ■ Chromosome location and function of major immune response genes

Gene system	Chromosome location	Gene product function
Immunoglobulin heavy chain (C, V, D, and J genes)	14q32	Heavy chain is part of antibody molecule, which binds foreign antigens
Immunoglobulin κ light chain (C, V, and J genes)	2p13	Light chain is the second part of antibody molecule
Immunoglobulin λ light chain (C, V, and J genes)	22q11	Light chain is the second part of the antibody molecule (either κ or λ may be used)
T-cell receptor α	14q11	One chain of the T-cell receptor, which recognizes antigen with MHC molecule
T-cell receptor β	7q35	The other chain of the α-β T-cell receptor
T-cell receptor γ	7p15	One chain of the γ-δ T-cell receptor
T-cell receptor δ	14q11	The second chain of the γ-δ T-cell receptor
MHC (class I, II, and III); includes TAP1 and TAP2	6p21	Cell-surface molecules that present peptides to T-cell receptors; TAP1 and TAP2 are transporter molecules that process foreign peptides and carry them to the endoplasmic reticulum
β2-microglobulin	15q21-22	Forms second chain of the class I MHC molecule
RAG1, RAG2	11p13	Recombinases that participate in VDJ somatic recombination

Table 8-2 ■ Some examples of MHC–disease associations*

Disease	MHC (HLA) associated allele	Approximate relative risk†
Type I diabetes	DR3 and DR4	~5 for DR3 or DR4 alone; 20–40 for DR3/DR4 heterozygotes
Ankylosing spondylitis	B27	90
Narcolepsy	DR2	>100
Celiac disease	DR3, DR7	10
Rheumatoid arthritis	DR1, DR4	5
Myasthenia gravis	DR3, DR7	2.5
Multiple sclerosis	DR2	4
Pemphigus vulgaris	DR4	24
Systemic lupus erythematosus	DR2, DR3	1–3
Hemochromatosis	A3	20
Malaria	Bw53	0.59
Squamous cell cervical carcinoma	DQw3	7

*From Bell et al: The molecular basis of HLA–disease association, Adv Hum Genet 18:1–41, 1989; Langdon et al: Genetic markers in narcolepsy, Lancet 2:1178–1180, 1984; Wank and Thomssen: High risk of squamous cell carcinoma of the cervix for women with HLA-DQw3, Nature 352:723–725, 1991; and Hill et al: Common West African HLA antigens are associated with protection from severe malaria, Nature 352:595–600, 1991.

†Relative risk can be interpreted loosely as the odds that an individual who has a risk factor (in this case, an MHC antigen) will develop the disease, compared with an individual who lacks the risk factor. Thus a relative risk of 4 for DR2 and multiple sclerosis means that persons with DR2 are four times more likely to develop multiple sclerosis than are those without DR2. A relative risk less than 1 (as seen for malaria and Bw53) indicates that the factor is *protective* against the disease.

rium. For example, the hemochromatosis locus is closely linked to HLA-A, and significant associations occur between HLA-A3 and the hemochromatosis disease gene (see Chapter 7). There is no known causal link between HLA-A3 and this disorder, however. More likely the association represents a past event in which the hemochromatosis mutation arose on a chromosome that had the HLA-A3 allele (similar to the myotonic dystrophy example discussed in Chapter 7).

In other cases a causal association may exist. Some MHC–disease associations may involve **autoimmunity**, a puzzling situation in which the body's immune system attacks its own normal cells. For example, type I diabetes is characterized by T-cell infiltration of the pancreas and subsequent T-cell destruction of the insulin-producing β cells. The biologic basis of autoimmunity remains poorly understood, but it is significant that autoimmunity is often seen when class II molecules are inappropriately expressed on the surfaces of cells *not* involved in the immune response. It is thought that such cells may be interpreted by T cells as viral peptides in association with MHC molecules, triggering an immune response. There is also evidence for such "molecular mimicry" in ankylosing spondylitis, another autoimmune disease. Infections of HLA-B27-positive individuals with specific microbes, such as *Klebsiella,* may lead to a **cross-reaction** in which the immune system mistakes the body's normal B27-bearing cells for the microbe.

A significant number of diseases are associated with specific MHC alleles. Some of these associations are the result of linkage disequilibrium, but most are likely to result from causal associations involving autoimmunity.

■ THE ABO AND RH BLOOD GROUPS

Another component of the immune system involves red cell surface molecules that can cause an immune reaction during blood transfusions. The ABO and Rh red cell antigen systems were discussed in Chapter 3 as early examples of polymorphic marker loci. They are also the most important systems determining transfusion compatibility.

ABO System

There are four major ABO blood types: A, B, AB, and O. The first three groups, respectively, represent individuals who carry the A, B, and A and B antigens on their erythrocyte surfaces. Those with type O have neither the A nor the B antigen. Individuals who have a given antigen on their erythrocyte surfaces possess naturally occurring antibodies against all other ABO antigens in their bloodstream. Thus if a type B individual received type A or AB blood, his or her anti-A antibodies would produce a severe and possibly fatal reaction. Type O individuals, who have neither antigen and both anti-A and anti-B antibodies, would react strongly to blood of the other three types (A, B, and AB). It was once thought that type O persons, because they lack both types of antigens, could be "universal donors" (anybody could accept their blood). Similarly, type AB persons were termed "universal recipients" because they lacked both anti-A and anti-B antibodies. However, when transfusions of whole blood containing large volumes of serum are conducted, the *donor's* antibodies can react with the *recipient's* erythrocyte antigens, and a reaction can result. Hence, complete matching is always done for blood transfusions.

The ABO system is an important blood group that can cause a transfusion reaction if donors and recipients are not properly matched.

Rh System

The Rh blood group is encoded by two tightly linked loci, one of which is labeled D. The other locus produces Rh systems labeled C and E through alternative splicing mechanisms. The D locus is of primary interest because it is responsible for Rh maternal–fetal incompatibility and the resulting disease, hemolytic disease of the newborn (HDN). Persons with the DD or Dd genotype have the Rh antigen on their erythrocytes and are termed "Rh-positive." The recessive homozygotes, with genotype dd, are "Rh-negative" and do not have the Rh antigen. About 85% of North Americans are Rh-positive, and about 15% are Rh-negative.

Unlike the ABO system, in which antibodies are present naturally, anti-Rh antibody production requires a direct stimulus. An Rh-negative person does not begin to produce anti-Rh antibodies unless he or she is exposed to the Rh antigen, usually through a blood transfusion or during pregnancy. Maternal–fetal incompatibility results when an Rh-positive man and an Rh-negative woman produce children. If the man's genotype is DD, all of their offspring will be Rh-positive and will have Rh antigens on their erythrocytes. If the man is a heterozygote, with genotype Dd, half of their children will be Rh-positive, on the average.

There are usually no difficulties with the first Rh-incompatible child because few of the fetus's red blood cells cross the placental barrier during gestation. When the placenta detaches at birth, a large number of fetal red blood cells typically enter the mother's bloodstream. These cells, carrying the Rh antigens, stimulate production of anti-Rh antibodies by the mother. These antibodies persist in the bloodstream for a long time, and if the next offspring is again Rh-positive, the mother's anti-Rh antibodies enter the fetus's bloodstream and destroy its red blood cells. As this destruction proceeds, the fetus becomes anemic and begins to release many **erythroblasts** (immature nucleated red cells) into its bloodstream. This phenomenon is responsible for the descriptive term erythroblastosis fetalis. The anemia can lead to a spontaneous abortion or stillbirth. Because the maternal antibodies remain in the child's circulatory system after birth, destruction of red cells can continue if the fetus survives to term. This causes a buildup of **bilirubin** and a jaundiced appearance shortly after birth. Without replacement transfusions, in which the child receives Rh-negative red cells, the bilirubin is deposited in the brain, producing cerebral damage and usually death. Those infants who do not die may suffer from mental retardation, cerebral palsy, and/or high-frequency deafness.

In North American whites, approximately 13% of all matings are Rh-incompatible. Fortunately a simple therapy now exists to avoid Rh sensitization of the mother. During and after pregnancy, an Rh-negative mother is given injections of Rh immune globulin, which consists of anti-Rh antibodies. These antibodies destroy the fetal erythrocytes before they stimulate production of maternal anti-Rh antibodies. Because the injected antibodies do not remain in the mother's bloodstream for long, they do not affect subsequent offspring. To avoid sensitization these injections must be administered with each pregnancy. The mother also must be especially careful not to receive a transfusion containing Rh-positive blood because this would also stimulate production of anti-Rh antibodies.

Maternal–fetal Rh incompatibility (Rh-negative mother and Rh-positive fetus) can produce hemolytic disease of the newborn if the mother's Rh antibodies attack the fetus. Administration of Rh immune globulin prevents this reaction.

A rarer form of maternal–fetal incompatibility can result when a mother with type O blood carries a fetus with type A or B blood. The HDN produced by this combination is usually so mild that it does not require treatment. Interestingly, if the mother is also Rh-negative and the child is Rh-positive, the ABO incompatibility *protects* against the more severe Rh incompatibility. This is because any fetal red blood cells entering the mother's circulatory system are quickly destroyed by her anti-A or anti-B antibodies before she can form anti-Rh antibodies.

■ IMMUNODEFICIENCY DISEASES

Immunodeficiency disease results when one or more components of the immune system is missing or fails to function normally. **Primary immunodeficiency diseases** are caused by defects in cells of the immune system and are usually produced by genetic defects. **Secondary immunodeficiency** occurs when components of the immune system are altered or destroyed by other factors, such as radiation, infection, or drugs. For example, the HIV virus, which causes AIDS, attacks the CD4 T lymphocytes, a central component of the immune system. The result is increased susceptibility to a multitude of opportunistic infections rarely seen in healthy individuals.

B-cell immunodeficiency diseases render the patient especially susceptible to recurrent bacterial infections, such as *Streptococcus pneumoniae*. An important example of a B-cell immunodeficiency is X-linked agammaglobulinemia (XLA). Patients with this disorder, the overwhelming majority of whom are males, lack B cells completely and have no IgA, IgE, IgM, or IgD in their serum. Because IgG crosses the placenta during pregnancy, individuals with XLA have some B-cell immune response for the first several months of life. However this supply is soon depleted, and they develop recurrent bacterial infections. They are treated with large administrations of γ-globulin.

T-cell immunodeficiency diseases directly affect T cells, but they also affect the humoral immune response because B-cell proliferation is largely dependent on helper T cells. Thus these patients develop severe combined immune deficiency (SCID) and are susceptible to many opportunistic infections, including *Pneumocystis carinii* (a protozoan that commonly affects AIDS patients). Without bone marrow transplants, these patients usually die within the first several years. About half of SCID cases are caused by an X-linked recessive gene. About 25% are caused by adenosine deaminase (ADA) deficiency, an autosomal recessive disorder of purine metabolism that results in a buildup of metabolites that are toxic to B and T cells. ADA deficiency is sometimes treated by bone marrow transplants, and it is now being treated successfully with gene therapy (see Chapter 11). Other T-cell immunodeficiency disorders are listed in Table 8-3

Chronic granulomatous disease (CGD) is a primary immunodeficiency disorder in which phagocytes can ingest bacteria and fungi but are then unable to kill them. This brings about a persistent cellular immune response to the ingested microbes, and granulomas (tumorlike masses or nodules of tissue) form, giving the disease its name. These patients develop pneumonia, lymph node infections, and abscesses of the skin, liver, and other sites. The most common cause of CGD is an X-linked gene, but there are also at least three autosomal recessive genes that can cause CGD. Incidentally, X-linked CGD was the first disease gene to be isolated through positional cloning.

Table 8-3 ■ Some examples of primary immunodeficiency diseases

Condition	Mode of inheritance*	Brief description
X-linked agammaglobulinemia	XR	Absence of B cells leads to recurrent bacterial infections
Severe combined immune deficiency (SCID)	XR, AR	T-cell deficiency leading also to impairment of humoral immune response; fatal unless treated by bone marrow transplants or gene therapy
DiGeorge syndrome	AD, sporadic	Congenital malformations include abnormal facial features, congenital heart disease, and thymus abnormality leading to T-cell deficiency
Ataxia telangiectasia	AR	DNA repair defect characterized by abnormal gait (ataxia), telangiectasia (dilated capillaries), and thymus abnormality producing T-cell deficiency
Wiskott-Aldrich syndrome	XR	Small, abnormal platelets, eczema, and abnormal T-cells causing susceptibility to opportunistic infections
Chronic granulomatous disease	XR, AR	Phagocytes ingest microbes but cannot kill them; leads to formation of granulomas and recurrent infections

*AD = autosomal dominant; AR = autosomal recessive; XR = X-linked recessive

Primary immunodeficiency diseases involve intrinsic defects of immune response cells (e.g., B cells, T cells, or phagocytes) and are usually genetically determined. Secondary immunodeficiency disorders, of which AIDS is an example, are caused by external factors.

■ STUDY QUESTIONS

1. Compare the functions of class I and class II MHC molecules.

2. MHC molecules and immunoglobulins both display a great deal of diversity, but in different ways. How and why do these types of diversity differ?

3. In what ways are T-cell receptors and immunoglobulins similar? In what ways are they different?

4. If there are 200 V segments, 6 J segments, and 30 D segments that can encode an immunoglobulin heavy chain of one particular class, how many different immunoglobulins can be formed on the basis of somatic recombination alone?

5. In matching donors and recipients for organ transplants, siblings are often desirable donors because they are more likely to be HLA-compatible with the recipient. If we assume no crossing over within the HLA loci, and assuming four distinct HLA haplotypes among the parents, what is the probability that a transplant recipient will be HLA-identical with a sibling donor?

6. What types of matings will produce Rh maternal–fetal incompatibility?

■ ADDITIONAL READING

Flajnik MF: Advances in immunology, Bioessays 16:671–675, 1994.

Fugger L, Tisch R, Libau R, van Endert P, McDevitt HO: The role of human major histocompatibility complex (HLA) genes in disease. In: Scriver CR, Beaudet AL, Sly WS, Valle D, editors: The Metabolic and Molecular Bases of Inherited Disease, ed 7, Vol. 1, New York, 1995, McGraw-Hill

Gellert M: Molecular analysis of V(D)J recombination, Annu Rev Genet 22:425–446, 1992.

Germain RN: MHC-dependent antigen processing and peptide presentation: providing ligands for T lymphocyte activation, Cell 76:287–299, 1994.

Janeway CA: How the immune system recognizes invaders, Sci Am 269:73–79, 1993.

Janeway CA and Bottomly K: Signals and signs for lymphocyte responses, Cell 76:275–285, 1994.

Kostyu DD: The HLA gene complex and genetic susceptibility to disease, Curr Opin Genet Dev 1:40–47, 1991.

Leder P: The genetic basis of antibody diversity. In Leder P, Clayton DA, Rubenstein E, editors: Introduction to Molecular Medicine, New York, 1994, Scientific American.

Maizels N: Somatic hypermutation: how many mechanisms diversify V region sequences? Cell 83:9–12, 1995.

Milner CM and Campbell RD: Genes, genes and more genes in the human major histocompatibility complex, BioEssays 14:565–571, 1992.

Nepom GT and Erlich H: MHC class-II molecules and autoimmunity, Annu Rev Immunol 9:493–525, 1991.

Nossal GJV: Life, death and the immune system. Sci Am 269:53–62, 1993.

Roitt I, Brostoff J, and Male D: Immunology, ed 3, St Louis, 1993, Mosby.

Strominger JL, Wiley DC: The class I and class II proteins of the human major histocompatibility complex, JAMA 274:1074–1076, 1995.

Trowsdale J: Genomic structure and function in the MHC, Trends Genet 9:117–122, 1993.

Unanue ER: The concept of antigen processing and presentation, JAMA 274:1071–1073, 1995.

Zouali M: Unravelling antibody genes, Nature Genetics 7: 118-120, 1994.

$\mathscr{9}$ Cancer Genetics

Present evidence indicates that approximately 30-40% of us will die of cancer. Largely due to the increasing proportion of our population in older age groups, cancer is increasing in frequency. As shown in this chapter, the causes of cancer are a mixture of genetic and environmental components. Dramatic advances in molecular biology and genetics have now clarified the basic molecular elements of cancer and provide a schematic outline of the cellular events leading to cancer. This understanding will be crucially important in the control of cancer, providing the beginnings of a base of knowledge that should lead to significantly improved therapies and possibly prevention.

Cancer is a collection of disorders that share the common feature of uncontrolled cell growth. This leads to a mass of cells termed a **neoplasm** (Greek for "new formation"), or **tumor**. **Malignant** neoplasms can invade nearby tissues and eventually **metastasize** (spread) to more distant sites in the body. The capacity to invade and metastasize distinguishes malignant from **benign** neoplasms. Tumors can be classified according to the tissue type in which they arise. Major types of tumors include those of epithelial tissue (**carcinomas**), connective tissue (**sarcomas**), lymphatic tissue (**lymphomas**), glial cells of the central nervous system (**gliomas**), and hematopoietic organs (**leukemias**). The cells composing a tumor are usually derived from a single ancestral cell, making them a single clone (**monoclonal**).

The basic biologic features of **carcinogenesis** (cancer development) are clear. Throughout our lives, many of our cells continue to grow and differentiate. These form, for example, the epithelial layers of our lungs and colons and the precursors of the cells of our immune systems. Relatively undifferentiated stem cells produce large numbers of progeny cells to repopulate and renew our worn defensive layers. Through integration of information provided by a complex array of biochemical signals, the new cells are designed to commit themselves to stop growing and differentiate into a cell type appropriate for their heritage and circumstances (Fig. 9-1).

Occasionally one of these cells loses its ability to respond appropriately to environmental and internal signals. It fails to differentiate, continuing to divide without restraint. The descendants of these cells become the founders of neoplasms, capable of further evolution into invasive, metastatic cancer. Our goals are to understand in detail what has gone wrong in such rogue cells, to detect them very early in their careers and, ultimately to intervene in their development, eliminating them from their host systems.

> **All cells in the body are "programmed" to develop, grow, differentiate, and die in response to a complex system of biochemical signals. Cancer results when any cell is freed from these constraints and its abnormal progeny are allowed to proliferate.**

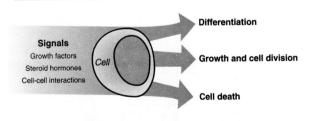

Figure 9-1 ■ In response to environmental signals, a cell may continue to divide, differentiate, or die (apoptosis).

■CAUSES OF CANCER
Genetic Considerations

Genetic events are the primary basis of carcinogenesis. We can create cancer in animal models by damaging specific genes. In cell culture systems, we can reverse a cancer phenotype by introducing normal copies of the damaged genes into the cell. Most of the genetic events that cause cancer occur during the lifetime of the individual, in his or her somatic tissues. The frequency of these events can be altered by exposure to mutagens, thus establishing the link to environmental carcinogens. Because these genetic events occur in somatic cells, they are not transmitted to future generations. Even though they are *genetic* events, they are not *inherited*. It is possible, however, for cancer-predisposing mutations to occur in germline cells. This results in the transmission of cancer-causing genes from one generation to the next, producing families that have a high frequency of specific cancers (Fig. 9-2).

Such "cancer families," although rare, demonstrate that inheritance of a damaged gene can cause cancer. In these families inheritance of one mutant allele seems sufficient to cause a specific form of cancer: almost all individuals who inherit the mutant allele will develop the tumor. The childhood cancer of the eye, retinoblastoma, is a good example. As discussed in Chapter 4, those who inherit a mutant version of the retinoblastoma gene have approximately a 90% chance of developing one or more retinoblastoma tumors.

Although the transmission of cancer as a single gene disorder is relatively uncommon, there is good evidence for a more general pattern of clustering of some cancer types in families. For many kinds of cancer, such as breast and colon, the diagnosis of the cancer in a first-degree relative results in a severalfold increase in one's own risk of developing the cancer. The genetic basis for this apparent familiality of cancer remains obscure. However, it is possible that genetic transmission of altered forms of specific genes is responsible.

The extent to which each of these mechanisms —germline (inherited) mutations versus mutations occurring in somatic cells—contributes to human cancer is an important question. If inherited predispositions are significant determinants of an individual's risk of acquiring a specific form of cancer, it should ultimately be possible to identify at-risk individuals. More intensive screening of defined high-risk populations could result in early detection and intervention, leading to better prognoses for individuals and lowered morbidity and mortality in the population.

> **The basic cause of cancer is damage to specific genes. Usually mutations in these genes accumulate in somatic cells over the years, until a cell loses a critical number of growth control mechanisms and initiates a tumor. If damage occurs in cells of the germline, however, an altered form of one of these genes can be transmitted to progeny and predispose them to cancer.**

Environmental Considerations

What is the role of the environment in carcinogenesis? At the level of the cell, cancer is intrinsically genetic. Tumor cells arise when certain changes, or mutations, occur in genes that are responsible for regulating the cell's growth. However, the frequency and consequences of these

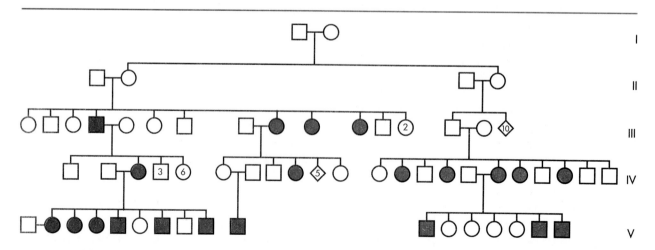

Figure 9-2 ■ A familial colon cancer pedigree. Darkened symbols represent individuals diagnosed with colon cancer.

mutations can be altered by a large number of environmental factors. It is well documented, for example, that many chemicals that cause mutation in experimental animals also cause cancer and are thus **carcinogens**. Thus, neither genetics nor environment is the sole determinant of carcinogenesis; both play key roles in this process.

Two additional lines of argument support the idea that exposure to environmental agents can significantly alter an individual's risk of cancer. The first is that a number of environmental agents with carcinogenic properties have been identified. For example, cigarette smoke has been shown, both epidemiologically and in laboratory experiments, to cause lung cancer. Roles for other environmental agents in specific cancers are also well documented (e.g., uranium dust in lung cancer among miners and asbestos exposure in lung cancer and mesothelioma).

The second line of argument is based on epidemiologic comparisons among populations with differing lifestyles. Many kinds of cancer have different frequencies in different populations. Breast cancer, for example, is prevalent among northern Europeans and Americans but relatively rare among women in developing countries. It is usually difficult, however, to determine whether such dissimilarities reflect differences in lifestyle or in gene frequencies.

Examination of genetically similar populations under differing lifestyles provides an opportunity to evaluate the genetic and environmental components of cancer. Epidemiologic studies among migrant Japanese populations, for example, have yielded important findings with respect to colon cancer. This type of cancer is relatively rare in the Japanese population living in Japan but is the second most common form of cancer in the United States. Stomach cancer, conversely, is frequent in Japan, but relatively rare in the United States. These statistics in themselves cannot distinguish environmental from genetic influences in the two populations. However, because large numbers of Japanese have emigrated, first to Hawaii and then to the U.S. mainland, we can observe what happens to the rates of stomach and colon cancer among the migrants. Importantly, the Japanese emigres have maintained a genetic identity, marrying largely among themselves.

In the U.S. population as a whole, the lifetime risk of colon cancer is approximately 5%; in Japan that risk is 10-fold lower, only 0.5%. Among the first-generation Japanese in Hawaii, the frequency of colon cancer rises severalfold, not yet as high as

in the U.S. mainland, but higher than in Japan. Among second-generation Japanese on the U.S. mainland, the colon cancer rates are 5%, equal to the U.S. average. At the same time, stomach cancer has become relatively rare among Japanese-Americans. These observations strongly indicate an important role for environment or lifestyle in the etiology of colon cancer.

Are we then to assume that genetic factors play no role in colon cancer? The fact remains that in the North American environment some individuals will get colon cancer and others will not. This distinction can result from differences within this environment (e.g., dietary variation) as well as differences in genetic predisposition: inherited genes that increase the individual's probability of developing cancer. To account for the difference in colon cancer frequency between Japanese living in the United States and in Japan, however, we argue that environmental features in Japan render the predisposing genes less penetrant. Furthermore, a genetic component is strongly suggested by the severalfold increase in risk to an individual when a first-degree relative has colon cancer. It is likely, then, that cancer risk is a composite of both genetics and environment, with interaction between the two components.

> **Environmental factors are known to play important roles in carcinogenesis. Because some individuals within the same environment develop cancer and some do not, cancer risk evidently depends upon interaction between inherited factors and environmental components.**

■ INHERITED CANCER GENES
Genetic Control of Cell Growth and Differentiation

Cancers form when the growth and differentiation of cells are deregulated. The past two decades have witnessed the identification of more than 100 cancer-causing genes that encode substances that normally regulate the cellular processes of growth and differentiation. Characterization of the biochemical activities and interactions of these gene products have revealed an increasingly detailed picture of the normal regulation of cell growth and differentiation and the ways in which these processes become deregulated by the events of carcinogenesis.

The fundamental features of this process are now well understood (Fig. 9-3). First, much of cell regulation is mediated by external signals coming

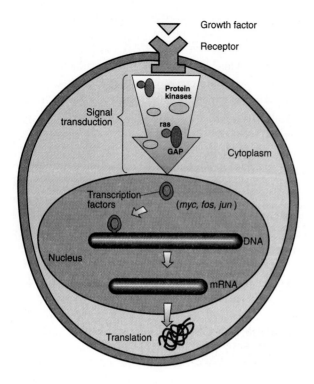

Figure 9-3 ■ The major features of cellular regulation: external growth factors (proteins and steroid hormones such as epidermal growth factor) bind to membrane-spanning growth factor receptors on the cell surface. These activate signal transduction pathways, in which genes such as *ras* participate. Components of the signal transduction pathway in turn interact with nuclear transcription factors, such as *myc* and *fos*, which can bind to regulatory regions in DNA.

to the cell through polypeptide **growth factors** (e.g., platelet-derived growth factor, epidermal growth factor, steroid hormones, and others) produced in other cells. Each growth factor interacts with a specific **growth factor receptor** located on the cell surface. Binding of a growth factor activates the receptor, triggering molecules that send messages to the cell's nucleus in a process termed **signal transduction**. These signal transduction molecules include **protein kinases**, enzymes which can alter the activity of target proteins by phosphorylating them. The ultimate stage of the signal transduction pathway is regulation of DNA transcription in the nucleus. Components of the signal transduction cascade interact with nuclear DNA-binding proteins (**transcription factors**) that regulate the activity of specific genes that influence cellular growth and proliferation. Genes that encode these nuclear DNA-binding proteins include *myc*, *fos*, and *jun*.

The regulation of cell growth is accomplished by substances that include: (1) polypeptide growth factors that transmit signals from one cell to another, (2) growth factor receptors on the cell surface, (3) signal transduction molecules that activate a cascade of phosphorylating reactions within the cell, and (4) nuclear transcription factors.

After several rounds of cell division, cells normally receive extracellular signals that tell them to stop growing and to differentiate into specialized cells. The signals may come by way of polypeptides, steroid hormones, or from direct contact with adjacent cells. The signals are transduced to the nucleus of the recipient cell where, by altering the transcription patterns among genes that govern the steps of the cell cycle, they initiate progression down a differentiation pathway.

The cell, then, is capable of integrating and interpreting the host of signals it receives from its environment. Decisions to grow and divide, or to stop growing and differentiate, result from processing of the signals. The pattern of events occurring in a specific cell is determined by its history and location, which dictate the cell's instantaneous production of gene products.

A cancer cell may emerge from within a population of growing cells, through the accumulation of several independent mutations in the genes that encode the factors we have been discussing. Although these events occur only rarely, the affected cells fail to respond to differentiation signals and continue to grow. Furthermore, cancers seem usually to result from a *progressive* series of events that incrementally increase the extent of deregulation within a cell lineage; eventually, a cell emerges whose descendants multiply without appropriate restraints. Further changes give these cells the capacity to invade adjacent tissues and form metastases. The requirement for more than one mutation has been characterized as the "**multihit concept of carcinogenesis.**" An example of this concept is given by colorectal cancer, in which a number of genetic events are required to complete the progression from a benign growth to a malignant neoplasm (Fig. 9-4).

Mutations may occur in any of the steps involved in regulating cell growth and differentiation. When such mutations accumulate within a cell lineage, the progressive deregulation of growth eventually produces a cell whose progeny form a tumor.

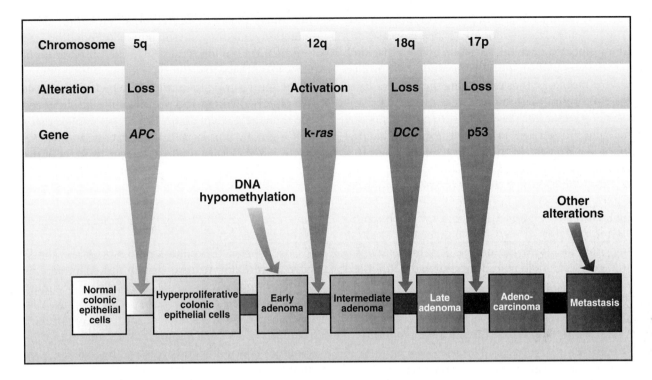

Figure 9-4 ■ The pathway to colon cancer. Loss of the *APC* gene (adenomatous polyposis coli) transforms normal epithelial tissue lining the gut to hyperproliferating tissue. Hypomethylation of DNA, activation of the k-ras proto-oncogene, and loss of the *DCC* (deleted in colon cancer) gene are involved in the progression to a benign adenoma. Loss of the *p53* gene and other alterations are involved in the progression to malignant carcinoma and metastasis. (Adapted from Vogelstein B and Kinzler KW: Trends Genet 9:138-141, 1993.)

The Inherited Cancer Gene Versus the Somatically Altered Gene

Although cancer families have long been recognized, it was not until the early 1970s that we began to understand the relationship between the inherited genetic aberrations and the carcinogenic events that occur in somatic tissue. In 1971 A.G. Knudson's analysis of retinoblastoma, a disease already mentioned as a model of inherited cancer, led him to a hypothesis that opened a new window into the mechanism of carcinogenesis. In the genetic form of retinoblastoma (see Chapter 4), a parent is likely to be affected and, if so, there is a 50% chance of genetic transmission to each of the offspring. In the "sporadic" form, neither parent is affected and there is no additional risk to other progeny. A key distinguishing feature between the two forms is that inherited retinoblastoma is usually bilateral (affects both eyes), whereas sporadic retinoblastoma usually involves only a single tumor and, therefore, only one eye (unilateral).

Knudson reasoned that at least two mutations may be required to create a retinoblastoma. One of the mutations would alter the retinoblastoma gene;

if this happened in the germline, it would be present in all cells of a child receiving the mutant allele. The second mutation would be an additional, unspecified genetic event in an already altered cell. The hypothesis of a second event was required to explain why only a tiny fraction of the retinoblasts of an individual who has inherited a mutant retinoblastoma gene actually gives rise to tumors. Knudson's hypothesis is known as the **two-hit model of carcinogenesis.**

Inherited retinoblastoma would thus be caused by the inheritance of one of the genetic "hits" as a **constitutional** mutation (i.e., a mutation present in all cells of the body). Individuals who inherited one hit would require only one additional mutational event in a single retinoblast for that cell to seed a tumor clone. In sporadic (noninherited) cases, both mutations would have to occur independently within the same retinoblast, a highly improbable combination of rare events even in the million or so cells of the target tissue. The child who developed a retinoblastoma by this two-hit *somatic* route, therefore, was unlikely to develop more than one tumor. The individual *inheriting* a mutant retinoblastoma gene, however, needed only a single, additional genetic hit to a retinoblast for a tumor clone to develop. Knudson argued that such an event was likely to occur in several of the million or so retinoblasts, thus explaining the bilaterality of inherited retinoblastoma.

An important corollary of this hypothesis is that the genes inherited in mutant form in familial tumor syndromes are the same genes as those that generate cancer by somatic mutation. *By understanding the nature of the mutant alleles inherited in rare cancer families, therefore, we will come to understand more about the somatic pathway to common cancer as well.* The converse is likewise true: understanding the nature of somatically mutated genes can help in understanding the inherited versions.

Alfred Knudson's two-hit theory of carcinogenesis in retinoblastoma became the paradigm for a model to describe how inheritance of an altered gene predisposes the gene carrier to cancer. The theory states that a cell can initiate a tumor only when it contains two damaged alleles; therefore a person who inherits one copy of a mutant retinoblastoma gene must experience a second, somatic mutation in one or more retinoblasts to develop one or more retinoblastomas. Two somatic mutations can also occur in a single retinoblast of a non-predisposed fetus, producing sporadic retinoblastoma.

The Retinoblastoma Gene and Tumor Suppressors

What is the nature of the second hit? Again with retinoblastoma as the paradigm, two possibilities seemed plausible at first: (1) the second mutation could affect the function of a gene distinct from the retinoblastoma gene, and the presence of two mutant genes in the same cell would result in the tumor; or (2) the second event could inactivate or alter the remaining (normal) copy of the retinoblastoma gene. The second hit might sometimes involve the consistent loss of a chromosome or an extensive deletion of a specific chromosome region that contains the retinoblastoma gene. Such large-scale chromosomal losses should be detectable with DNA markers if the second possibility is correct.

Losses of marker DNA near the retinoblastoma gene *(RB),* now identified and known to lie on chromosome 13, occur in more than 50% of retino-

blastomas. Several mechanisms, including point mutation, deletion, and somatic recombination, can produce such a loss (Fig. 9-5). The observation of DNA loss shows that the second hit, which occurs in the fetus during the period in which retinoblasts are rapidly dividing and proliferating, has removed the remaining allele of this gene. This implies that a cell with one mutant *RB* allele and one normal *RB* allele cannot form a tumor. Thus the product of the normal gene, even when present only in a single copy, prevents tumor formation. The term **tumor suppressor** has been coined to describe the *RB* gene and a growing list of other cancer-associated genes (Table 9-1).

Characteristic of tumor suppressors is the somewhat perplexing feature that inherited mutations are *dominant* alleles at the level of the individual (heterozygous individuals usually develop the disease) but *recessive* alleles at the level of the cell (heterozygous cells do not form tumors). This apparent contradiction is resolved by realizing that only a single tumor cell is required, from a population of millions of normal cells, to initiate a tumor in the individual. Thus in individuals who have inherited the first hit, a second hit that occurs in any one cell will cause a tumor. Because of the large size of the target retinoblast population, heterozygous individuals form, on the average, several retinoblasts homozygous for an *RB* mutation, each of which leads to a retinoblastoma.

The discovery that retinoblastoma results when both alleles of the same locus on chromosome 13 are inactivated in the same retinoblast led to the concept of tumor suppressor genes. The products of such genes suppress tumor formation by controlling cell growth, and can do so even if a cell contains only one normal version of the gene.

Because of the pivotal role of tumor suppressors in the prevention of tumor formation, their study is of considerable medical significance. By understanding how cancer is naturally suppressed by the body, we can ultimately develop more effective medical therapies for tumor prevention and treatment.

Another Class of Cancer Genes, the Oncogenes

A second specific class of genes that can cause cancer is termed **oncogenes** (i.e., cancer genes). Most oncogenes originate from **proto-oncogenes**, which are genes that are involved in the four basic mechanisms of cell growth regulation mentioned

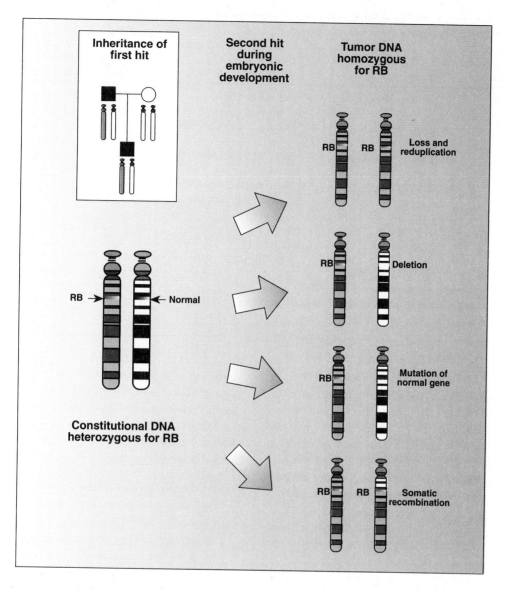

Figure 9-5 ■ **Persons inheriting an *RB* mutation are heterozygous for the mutation in all cells of their body. The second hit occurs during embryonic development and may consist of a point mutation, deletion, loss of the normal chromosome and duplication of the abnormal one, and somatic recombination. Each process leads to homozygosity for the mutant *RB* allele and thus tumor development.** (Adapted from Cavanee, Dryja, Phillips, et al: Nature 305:779–784, 1983.)

above (i.e., growth factors and their receptors, signal transduction molecules, and nuclear transcription factors). When a mutation occurs in a proto-oncogene, it can become an oncogene, a gene whose product can upset normal cell growth and differentiation. When an oncogene causes a cell to proceed from regulated to unregulated growth, the cell is said to have been **transformed**. Unlike most tumor suppressors, oncogenes are usually dominant at the cellular level: only a single copy of a mutated oncogene is required to contribute to the multistep process of tumor progression. In this section we review three approaches that have been used to identify specific oncogenes.

Retroviral Definition

Retroviruses, a type of RNA virus, are capable of using reverse transcriptase to transcribe RNA into DNA. In this way a retrovirus can insert its genes into the DNA of a host cell. The first oncogenes to be identified came from the study of retroviruses that cause cancer in animal systems. These retroviruses carry altered versions of growth-promoting genes into cells. In an earlier cycle of infection, a retrovirus may have incorporated an oncogene from the genome of its host. When the retrovirus invades a new cell, it can transfer the oncogene into the genome of the new host, thus transforming the cell.

Table 9-1 ■ A partial list of tumor supressor genes

Gene	Chromosome location	Proposed function	Disease caused by germline mutation	Tumors caused by somatic mutation
RB	13q14	Nuclear transcription factor	Retinoblastoma, osteosarcoma	Retinoblastoma, osteosarcoma, breast, lung, prostate, bladder carcinoma
APC	5q21	Possibly involved in cell adhesion	Adenomatous polyposis coli	Colon, pancreatic, stomach carcinoma
NF1	17q11	GTPase-activating protein	Neurofibromatosis type 1	Neuroblastoma, malignant melanoma, colon carcinoma
NF2	22q	Cell membrane–cytoskeletal link	Neurofibromatosis type 2 (bilateral acoustic neuromas)	Central schwannomas and meningiomas
p53	17p13	Transcription/cell cycle regulation	Li-Fraumeni syndrome	Soft tissue sarcoma, breast and colon carcinoma, leukemia, and others
VHL	3p25	Possibly involved in cell adhesion and signal transduction	von Hippel-Landau disease	Renal cell carcinoma hemangioblastoma, pheochromocytoma
WT1	11p13	Nuclear transcription factor	Wilms tumor (childhood kidney tumor)	Nephroblastoma

A number of gene products that receive and interpret extracellular signals for growth or differentiation have been identified through oncogenes carried by transforming retroviruses. For example, the *sis* oncogene, carried by the *si*mian *s*arcoma virus, has been identified as an altered version of the human gene that encodes platelet-derived growth factor (PDGF). Retrovirus studies have likewise identified the gene encoding the receptor molecule for another of the growth factors, epidermal growth factor (EGF), through the *Erb*B oncogene. The *ras* (*ra*t *s*arcoma) oncogenes, Harvey and Kirsten, were first identified through trans-

forming retroviruses. More recently, transforming retroviruses have identified the nuclear transcription factor genes, *myc, jun,* and *fos,* as other molecular components capable of initiating cell transformation (see Table 9-2 for a partial summary of proto-oncogenes).

Proto-oncogenes encode products that control cell growth and differentiation. When mutated, they may become oncogenes, which can cause cancer. Most oncogenes act as dominant mutations and cause cellular growth rates to increase. Retroviruses are

Table 9-2 ■ A partial list of proto-oncogenes

Oncogene	Chromosome location	Function
Growth factors		
*hst*l	11q13	Heparin-binding growth factor
sis	22q12-q13	Subunit of platelet-derived growth factor (PDGF)
Growth factor receptors		
erbA	17q11	Thyroid hormone receptor
src	20q11	Tyrosine kinsase
*raf*1	3p25	Cytoplasmic serine kinase
Signal transduction proteins		
H-ras	11p15	GTP-binding protein
abl	9q34	Protein kinase
trk	1q32	Protein kinase
Nuclear DNA-binding proteins		
myb	6q22	Binds DNA
fos	14q24-q31	Interacts with *jun* proto-oncogene to regulate transcription
myc	8q24	Binds DNA

capable of inserting oncogenes into the DNA of a host cell, thus transforming the host into a tumor-producing cell. The study of such retroviral transmission has identified a number of specific proto-oncogenes through their oncogenic variants.

Transfection Experiments

The identification of cellular genes involved in carcinogenesis was complemented by experiments in which mutated forms of cellular proto-oncogenes were transferred from tumor cells to non-tumor cells (**transfection**), causing transformation of the recipients. The prototype experiment was the transfer of DNA from a human bladder cancer cell line into mouse cells. A few recipient cells became fully transformed; cloning and examination of the human-specific DNA sequences present in the transformed mouse cells revealed that the transforming gene was a mutant allele of the same Harvey *ras* oncogene previously identified by retroviral studies.

Characterization of the protein product of mutant forms of *ras* has revealed an important mechanism for the regulation of signal transduction. The normal *ras* (proto-oncogene) protein product interacts with guanine nucleotide cofactors. The *ras* protein normally cycles between an *active* form bound to **guanosine triphosphate (GTP)**, and an *inactive* form bound to **guanosine diphosphate (GDP)**. The biochemical consequence of *ras* mutations is a *ras* protein unable to shift from the active GTP form (which stimulates growth) to the inactive GDP form. The mutant *ras* protein cannot quench its growth signal.

The transfection of oncogenes from tumor cells to normal cells can cause transformation of the normal cells. This helps to confirm the role of oncogenes in carcinogenesis.

Mapping in Tumors

The association of specific chromosomal translocations with human tumors provides a third method for observing the functions of oncogenes. As discussed in Chapter 6, specific chromosomal rearrangements are characteristic of some tumor types. A well-known example is the Philadelphia chromosome, in which a translocation between chromosomes 9 and 22 activates the *abl* proto-oncogene and produces chronic myelogenous leukemia (*SOL* 70). Recently, close examination of the site on chromosome 17 of the t(15;17)(q22;q11.2–12) translocation characteristic of acute promyelocytic

leukemia (APL) has revealed the presence of the gene encoding retinoic acid receptor alpha (*RARA*). Interestingly, retinoic acid was already known as a therapeutic agent for APL. It has been suggested that retinoic acid may be a differentiation signal and that disruption of the receptor by the translocation may encourage tumor formation by preventing transduction of this signal.

Some oncogenes have been identified when specific rearrangements of chromosomal material were found to be associated with certain cancers. As translocation of genetic material in these cases is likely to have disrupted genes vital to growth control in those cell types, the sites of such rearrangements can be investigated to identify new proto-oncogenes.

■IDENTIFICATION OF INHERITED CANCER GENES

Although the methods described in the previous section were successful in identifying many oncogenes, they did not identify those tumor suppressor genes that transmit inherited forms of cancer. This may have been because these methods require dominant expression of the mutant phenotype, whereas the mutant tumor suppressor alleles seem to have a primarily recessive phenotype at the level of the cell. An alternative approach to the identification of these genes was necessary.

When genes responsible for genetically transmitted diseases cannot be identified through known biochemical behavior, they become candidates for investigations based on gene mapping and detection of mutations in patients, as described in Chapter 7. There are two avenues for the initial mapping of tumor genes. The primary and most general route is through linkage mapping in families, where the pattern of inheritance of the cancer phenotype defines the genetic transmission of an altered allele. The chromosomal segment bearing this mutation can in turn be defined by linkage with polymorphic markers.

The second basis for mapping takes advantage of chromosomal losses associated with revealed tumor suppressor genes. As already described, the genetically transmitted mutation is a recessive allele at the cellular level; it does not reveal its tumor phenotype unless both normal copies of the gene are lost. Often an inherited mutant allele is unmasked by a deletion of part or all of the homologous chromosome carrying the normal allele. Therefore the microscopic observation that a specific chromosome has been lost in a tumor suggests a map location for the inherited mutation. Small deletions can be helpful in pinpointing the sub-chromosomal location of the gene being sought. As mentioned in Chapter 7, the detection of deletions on chromosome 13q in retinoblastoma patients was an important step in finding the retinoblastoma gene.

In some cases the portion of the chromosome that is lost or altered may be too small to be observed under a microscope. These cases are especially important because they define a relative-ly small region in which the cancer-causing gene is located. These regions are sometimes pinpointed by examining a series of closely linked marker polymorphisms in the region and determining that all of them are homozygous in tumor DNA but *not* in constitutional DNA. This **loss of heterozygosi-ty** in tumor DNA indicates that the normal tumor suppressor gene, as well as polymorphic markers surrounding it, have been lost, leaving only the abnormal copy or copies of the tumor suppressor gene (see Fig. 9-5). This approach was used, for ex-ample, to help narrow the locations of the retinoblas-toma gene on the long arm of chromosome 13 and a gene for Wilms tumor (nephroblastoma) on 11p.

Although gene mapping studies can often define a region in which an inherited cancer gene is located, they cannot alone identify the disease gene. As discussed in Chapter 7, detection of mutations carried in DNA from patients with the disease is crucial for identifying the specific di-sease-causing gene.

> **Map locations of tumor-associated genes can be detected through linkage analysis or by showing that one homolog of a chromo-some (or a part of it) is missing in DNA from a tumor. Confirmation of the etiologic role of a possible cancer-causing gene is obtained by showing the consistent presence of muta-tions in the gene in DNA from patients.**

The *RB* Gene

As previously described, the *RB* gene was mapped to chromosome 13q14 by deletion map-ping, linkage analysis, and loss of heterozygosity studies. This in turn led to the cloning and se-quencing of this gene. Subsequent analyses of the normal gene product, pRB, have shown that it is a phosphorylated nuclear protein with DNA-binding properties. pRB binds to and potentially inactivates the E2F transcription complex, which is involved in cell cycle regulation. This binding is inhibited by phosphorylation of the pRB protein just before S-phase in the cell cycle. The release of the E2F transcription complex from pRB control allows the cell cycle to proceed. Because of the key role played by pRB in cell cycle regulation, loss of the *RB* gene through mutation may contribute to un-controlled cell division and thus to tumor develop-ment.

> **The normal product of the *RB* gene appears to be an inhibitory component of the E2F transcription complex. Loss of both copies of the *RB* gene leads to deregulation of the cell cycle and uncontrolled cell division.**

Neurofibromatosis Type I (NFl)

The initial evidence for mapping of the *NF1* gene to chromosome 17 came from linkage studies in families. Subsequently, chromosomal transloca-tions were discovered in the karyotypes of two unrelated neurofibromatosis patients, each with a breakpoint on chromosome 17q at a location indis-tinguishable from the map location of the *NF1* gene. Located only 50 kb apart, the breakpoints provided the physical clues necessary to define several candidate genes that were screened for mutations in NF1 patients (Fig. 9-6).

The nucleotide sequence of the *NF1* gene provid-ed an early clue to function when its predicted amino acid sequence was compared with amino acid sequences of known gene products found in computerized data bases. Extended similarities were observed with the mammalian GTPase-activa-ting protein (GAP). This was an important finding because at least one function of GAP is to increase the rate of hydrolysis of GTP bound to ras protein. Because the ras protein is a key component of the signal transduction pathway, this indicates that the NF1 gene product also plays a role in signal trans-duction.

By identifying the *NF1* gene product as a compo-nent in signal transduction, a picture began to form of how the inheritance of mutation in one *NF1* allele might contribute to the development of neurofibromas and *café-au-lait* spots. It is possible that the *NF1* gene participates in transducing the ras GTP signal. If so, then reduced activity of the *NF1* gene might lower that signal sufficiently to permit the cell to escape from differentiation and continue its growth. Loss of the remaining allele might further encourage unchecked growth. It is likely that discovery of the *NF1* gene has led to identification of a key agent in the fundamental process of signal transduction.

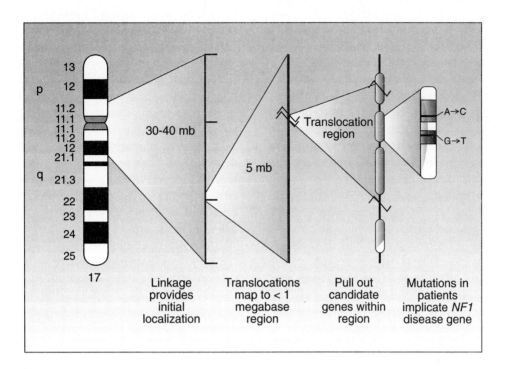

Figure 9-6 ■ Localization of the *NF1* gene on chromosome 17q involved linkage analysis and identification of two translocation breakpoints that interrupted the disease gene. Candidate genes were isolated from this region and tested for mutations in NF1 patients and normal controls.

The gene responsible for NF1 was mapped to chromosome 17q by linkage in families and identified through translocations and point mutations in patients. DNA sequencing of the gene predicted a protein product with a domain related to GAP, and a similar role in signal transduction was confirmed by biochemical experiments.

The p53 Gene

Somatic mutations in the *p53* gene are found in approximately 50% of all human tumors, making this the most commonly altered cancer gene. Mutations in the *p53* gene occur in more than 50 different types of tumors, including those of the bladder, brain, breast, cervix, colon, esophagus, larynx, liver, lung, ovary, pancreas, prostate, skin, stomach, and thyroid. Mutations of this gene are found in approximately 40% of breast cancers, 50% of lung cancers, and 70% of colorectal cancers.

Initially, chromosomal losses and deletions of the short arm of chromosome 17 had been shown to be characteristic of colon carcinoma. Overlapping deletions defined a segment of 17p commonly altered in tumor DNAs. Examination of the genes that had been mapped to this region revealed that the *p53* gene was among them. The numerous mutations found in *p53* in colonic tumors indicate a significant role for this gene in colon tumori-

genesis. Furthermore, the mutations tend to cluster in several specific, highly conserved regions of the gene. Unlike the *RB* and *APC* genes (see below), in which most mutations are of the nonsense type, 80% to 90% of *p53* alterations are missense mutations.

Although tumor-causing *p53* mutations have been observed primarily in somatic cells, germline mutations of *p53* are responsible for an inherited cancer condition known as the Li-Fraumeni syndrome (LFS). This rare syndrome is transmitted in autosomal dominant fashion and involves breast and colon carcinomas, soft tissue sarcomas, osteosarcomas, brain tumors, leukemia, and adrenocortical carcinomas. These tumors usually develop at early ages in LFS family members, and multiple primary tumors are commonly seen in an affected individual. The demonstration of consistent *p53* mutations in the constitutional DNA of LFS patients confirmed the causative role of this gene. As in retinoblastoma, the inheritance of a mutated *p53* gene greatly increases the individual's susceptibility to subsequent cell transformation and tumor development. Among LFS family members who inherit an abnormal *p53* gene, approximately 50% will develop invasive cancer by age 30, and more than 90% will develop invasive cancer by age 70. However, the penetrance with regard to any *specific* tumor type is much lower. Colon cancer, for example, is seen in only a small proportion of individuals who inherit a *p53* mutation.

The genetics of mutant *p53* alleles is intriguing. Alleles seem variably to function as dominant oncogenes or, in a cell-recessive fashion, as tumor suppressors. The mode of action appears to depend on the specific type of mutation and, perhaps, on the cell or tissue in question. The type of mutation observed in *p53* can provide clues regarding the carcinogen that produced the mutation. For example, dietary ingestion of aflatoxin B_1, which can produce liver cancer, is associated with a G→T mutation that produces an arginine→serine substitution at position 249 of the *p53* gene product. Cigarette smoke exposure is correlated with a G→T mutation seen in carcinomas of the lung, head, and neck. Thus examination of the type of *p53* mutation seen in a tumor may provide clues about the identity of the causative carcinogenic agent.

Like the *RB* gene, *p53* encodes a phosphorylated nuclear protein with DNA-binding properties. It acts as a transcription factor and interacts with a number of other genes. For example, it has been shown recently to activate a gene called *WAF1* (also called *p21*), whose protein product halts the cell cycle in the G1 phase, before DNA replication occurs. This provides the cell with time in which to repair damaged DNA. If *p53* is mutated, cells may replicate damaged DNA. In addition, *p53* is involved in the programmed death **(apoptosis)** of abnormal or damaged cells.

p53 is medically important in at least two ways. First, the presence of *p53* mutations in tumors, particularly those of the breast and colon, signals a more aggressive cancer with relatively poorer survival prospects. Second, *p53* could ultimately prove important in tumor prevention. Laboratory experiments show that the insertion of a normal *p53* gene into tumor cells results in a significant decrease in tumorigenesis. This indicates that the insertion of normal *p53* into cancer patients' tumors using gene therapy approaches (see Chapter 11) could become an effective cancer treatment.

Mutant forms of the *p53* gene on chromosome 17p are found in about 50% of tumors. Mutant alleles sometimes seem to fit the dominant oncogene model and at other times the recessive tumor suppressor model. Normal *p53* helps to regulate the cell cycle and may be involved in the programmed death (apoptosis) of damaged cells.

Familial Polyposis Gene

Familial polyposis (adenomatous polyposis coli, APC) is characterized by the appearance, early in life, of multiple adenomas, or polyps, of the colon. Colonic adenomas are now understood to be the immediate precursors to colon cancer. The multiple adenomas of the APC patient, therefore, present a grave risk of early malignancy. Because early detection and removal of adenomatous polyps can significantly reduce the occurrence of colon cancer, it is important to understand the causative gene and its role in development of polyps (Clinical Commentary 9-1).

The *APC* gene was initially placed on the map of the long arm of chromosome 5 by linkage analysis in families, after a cytogenetically visible chromosomal deletion in a patient with this syndrome provided an important clue to its location. Later discovery of small, overlapping deletions in two unrelated patients provided the key to isolation of the gene. Among the genes that lay within the 100-kb region that was deleted in both patients, one was found that showed apparent mutations in other patients. One of these was a new mutation in a patient whose parents were unaffected with *APC*; that observation confirmed the identification of the *APC* gene. A second gene in this region, termed *MCC* (mutated in colon cancer), is also frequently mutated in colon tumors, but it is not responsible for inherited predispositions to colorectal cancer.

The *APC* gene encodes a protein product that bears little resemblance to other known proteins. Thus it has been somewhat difficult to determine its function. Recent studies have shown, however, that the *APC* protein product interacts with b-catenin, a molecule involved in cell adhesion. This may be an important finding because abnormalities in cell–cell adhesion are characteristic of tumors.

An important feature of the genetics of the *APC* gene is that, with the exception of several large deletions and one serine→cysteine amino acid substitution, all of the mutations found in *APC* thus far have produced either stop codons (nonsense mutations) or frameshifts in the nucleotide sequence of the gene. Alleles altered in either of these ways would be expected to encode an inactive gene product. Because nonsense mutations should be relatively rare in comparison with missense mutations, the latter probably occur without creating a recognizable polyposis phenotype. An intriguing interpretation is that missense mutations produce a distinct phenotype that is relatively subtle, with low expressivity and/or reduced penetrance.

Clinical Commentary 9-1. The APC Gene and Colorectal Cancer

About one in 20 Americans will be diagnosed with colorectal cancer. Currently the mortality rate for this cancer is approximately one third. Genetic and environmental factors, such as dietary fat and fiber, are known to influence the probability of occurrence of colorectal cancer.

As indicated in the text, familial polyposis coli is an autosomal dominant subtype of colon cancer characterized by a large number (usually >100) of early-onset adenomatous polyps (Fig. 9-7). Germline mutations in the *APC* gene are consistently identified in family members affected with familial polyposis coli. Approximately one third of these cases are the result of new mutations in this gene. Because of the large size of the gene and the large number of disease-causing mutations, it is difficult and expensive to test family members for germline mutations to determine whether they inherited the disease gene. However, a new test takes advantage of the fact that most *APC* mutations are nonsense or frameshift mutations that yield a truncated protein product. The test involves the in vitro manufacture of a protein product from *APC* DNA to determine whether the at-risk individual has inherited an *APC* mutation. This is important for family members because it alerts them to the necessity of frequent surveillance and possible colectomy.

Familial polyposis coli, however, is relatively rare, affecting only about one in 8000 individuals. The broader significance of the *APC* gene derives from the fact that *somatic* mutations in *APC* are seen in approximately 60% of all colon cancers. Furthermore, *APC* mutations occur early in the development of colorectal malignancies. A better understanding of the *APC* gene product, how it interacts with other proteins, and how it may interact with environmental factors, such as diet, may provide important clues for the prevention and treatment of common colon cancer. In this way, the mapping and cloning of a gene responsible for a relatively rare cancer syndrome may have widespread clinical implications.

Treatment for colorectal cancer usually involves surgical resection of the colon. However, because colorectal carcinoma is preceded by the appearance of benign polyps, it is one of the most preventable of cancers. The National Polyp Study Workgroup estimates that colonoscopic removal of polyps could reduce the nationwide incidence of colon cancer by as much as 90%. The importance of early intervention and treatment further underscores the need to understand early events in colorectal cancer, such as somatic mutations in the APC gene.

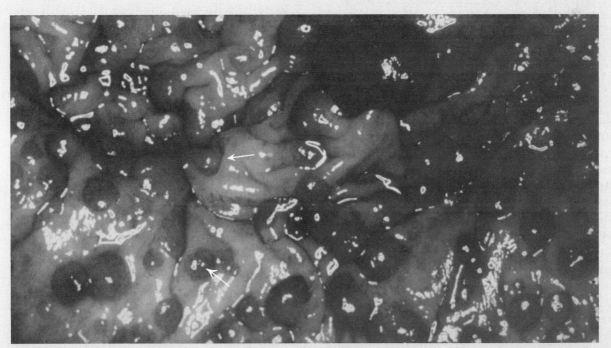

Figure 9-7 ■ A portion of a colon removed from a patient with familial polyposis coli, illustrating a large number of adenomatous polyps covering the colon. Each of these benign neoplasms has the potential to become a malignant tumor. (Courtesy of Dr. Randall Burt, University of Utah Health Sciences Center).

This hypothesis is interesting because pedigree analyses have suggested that there may be common alleles that predispose carriers to development of one to several polyps that appear relatively late in life. If such alleles exist, they may define a significant fraction of our population as predisposed to colon cancer, and frequent screening of these people for polyps would be merited. Support for this hypothesis comes from the characterization of several pedigrees that transmit an *APC* allele that causes an intermediate polyp phenotype. Within each of these families, individuals inheriting the mutant allele can exhibit a variable number of polyps, from one or none to more than a hundred, but with an average of only 10 to 20. Therefore alleles with markedly reduced expressivity do exist at the polyposis locus. The remaining question, crucial for a hypothesis that would assign them an important role in common colon cancer, is their frequency in the population.

> **The familial polyposis gene (APC) on chromosome 5q was ultimately identified by mutations in patients. Most of the known mutations in APC patients encode inactive gene products, but less damaging mutations might exist in the general population. If they do, they might contribute to the etiology of common colon cancer: inheritance of an "attenuated" allele could predispose many individuals to the isolated colonic polyps that may progress to carcinoma.**

Other Inherited Cancer Genes

Several other genes associated with inherited cancer syndromes have been mapped to specific chromosomal locations, and some have subsequently been cloned: multiple endocrine neoplasia type I (*MEN*1) to 11q and *MEN* types 2A and 2B to 10q, neurofibromatosis type 2 to chromosome 22, von Hippel-Lindau disease to 3p, and Weidemann-Beckwith syndrome to 11p. A gene responsible for an inherited, early-onset form of breast cancer has been mapped to 17q. A gene for an inherited predisposition to malignant melanoma has been mapped to 9p. Some of these genes are listed in Table 9-1, and others are discussed in some of the review articles listed at the end of the chapter. With the current generation of genomic resources, such as libraries of yeast artificial chromosomes (YACs) containing human DNA sequences, it is reasonable to expect the identification of more of these genes through positional cloning within the next several years.

■ MOLECULAR BASIS OF CANCER

Each of the identified genes associated with inherited cancer syndromes provides a unique insight into the genetic mechanisms of carcinogenesis. Those that represent important elements in transcriptional regulation of the cell cycle (*RB*, *p53*) and signal transduction (*NF1*) promise to make significant contributions to our understanding of these processes. Those genes not yet cloned and characterized promise to be equally revealing.

It is striking that all of the inherited tumor-causing genes described to date seem to have cell-recessive properties, at least at the level of the carcinoma. This observation suggests that an inherited allele that produces a disease phenotype in the heterozygous state would not be tolerated during development. That view is supported by the nearly ubiquitous tissue distribution of the products of these genes. As they are expressed in many if not all cell types, they may each play a fundamental role during embryonic development.

From a medical perspective, the characterization of inherited tumor genes can be fruitful. Presymptomatic diagnosis of at-risk individuals in cancer families may specify those who must undergo close surveillance or even intervention, and it can lift a major medical and psychological burden from those who have not inherited the family's mutant allele. If more subtle, predisposing alleles prove to be important in the incidence of cancer in general, the ability to define an at-risk population might reduce the overall cost of cancer surveillance in the population as a whole. In the future, greater understanding of these genes and their functions will offer hope for the ultimate prevention of tumorigenesis, as these genes are clearly rate-limiting for tumor formation. If their mutant alleles serve as indicators for the appearance of nascent tumors, or if their normal functions can be restored by medical intervention, they will have served an important role in cancer prevention.

> **The continued mapping and cloning of genes for cancer syndromes will provide valuable insights into mechanisms of carcinogenesis and into fundamental biologic processes. Presymptomatic diagnosis of family members at risk for cancer, and ultimately the use of genetic interventions, are other important goals and potential rewards of such studies.**

■ IS GENETIC INHERITANCE IMPORTANT IN COMMON CANCERS?

The role, or even the significance, of inherited predisposition in the common cancers, such as carcinomas of breast, colon, or prostate, is not yet certain. An apparently increased frequency of common cancers in some families has led some to suggest that common cancer-causing alleles may exist. Familial clustering translates into an increased relative risk of breast cancer, for example, among women with first-degree relatives who have had breast cancer. The genetic basis of this increased risk has not yet been demonstrated. However, recent evidence indicates that approximately 40% of premenopausal breast cancer cases are associated with a predisposing gene located on the short arm of chromosome 17. In addition, statistical analysis of large pedigrees has provided support for a genetic component in common colon cancer.

How will we ultimately determine whether common "cancer alleles" exist in the population? One way, perhaps, could be to exploit new approaches of gene mapping that identify genes involved in cellular pathways to cancer. Each of these becomes a candidate gene which, we hypothesize, may confer a predisposition to cancer. The most critical test of the candidate gene hypothesis will be to determine whether there are mutations in the gene among cancer patients. Finding them will validate the genetic hypothesis. If no mutations are found, however, we will remain uncertain because a genetic predisposition could still be conferred by an allele of a gene not yet identified and tested.

Another consideration is the potential action of genes whose role is to repair damage to DNA. Several inherited disorders, such as xeroderma pigmentosum (XP) and ataxia telangiectasia (AT), discussed in Chapter 6, result in greatly increased sensitivity to agents known to damage DNA. Increased frequencies of cancers are also seen in patients with these syndromes. Primarily because radiation-sensitive mutant strains of bacteria show an increased rate of random mutation that has been traced to failure of DNA repair systems, it has been popular to hypothesize that the mutant human alleles that confer radiation sensitivity in XP and AT might also experience elevated rates of random mutation. An increased frequency of random mutation in the cells of affected individuals could readily translate into a greater likelihood that mutations will occur in genes that are involved in the carcinogenetic pathway.

This hypothesis is gaining currency with the discovery that approximately 90% of hereditary nonpolyposis colorectal cancer (HNPCC) cases are caused by mutations at one of two genes, *hMLH1* and *hMSH2*. Both of these genes are involved in the recognition and repair of DNA **mismatches** (i.e., incorrect complementary base pairing, such as the pairing of G with T instead of G with C). Mutations in *hMLH1* or *hMSH2* may allow mismatches to persist in cells, contributing to the progression of colorectal cancer.

The question of whether common cancer alleles exist in the population may be approached by seeking mutations among the growing number of identified genes known to be involved in cellular mechanisms leading to cancer. Other candidate genes might include those that function to repair damage to DNA. Recent examples include two DNA mismatch repair genes involved in colorectal cancer.

A detailed description of the genes and genetic events underlying cancer is rapidly emerging. Although the identified genes fall into two relatively distinct categories, with the mutant oncogenes acting as promoters of cell growth and the mutant tumor suppressors often failing to inhibit cell growth, they share a commonality in that each affects the genetic regulation of cell growth and development. Although acting at different points, they regulate the same fundamental cell activities and information pathways. New technologies of molecular biology and genetics are now identifying the specific genes associated with specific tumor types. Significant new information is becoming available to researchers and clinicians and can be expected to create a new generation of highly specific diagnostic and therapeutic tools to reduce the cancer burden.

■ STUDY QUESTIONS

1. The G6PD locus is located on the X chromosome. Studies of G6PD alleles in tumor cells from *women* show that all tumor cells usually express the same single G6PD allele, even though the women are heterozygous at the G6PD locus. What does this finding imply about the origin of the tumor cells?

2. If we assume that the somatic mutation rate at the *RB* locus is 3 mutations per million cells, and that there is a population of 2 million retinoblasts per individual, what is the expected

frequency of sporadic retinoblastoma in the population? What is the expected number of tumors per individual among those who inherit a mutated copy of the RB gene?

3. Compare and contrast oncogenes and tumor suppressor genes. How have the characteristics of these classes of cancer-causing genes affected our ability to detect them?

4. Members of Li-Fraumeni syndrome families nearly always develop tumors by the age of 65 to 70 years, but the probability of developing a specific type of cancer, such as breast or colon carcinoma, is relatively small. Explain this.

■ ADDITIONAL READING

Bates S, Vousden KH: p53 in signaling checkpoint arrest or apoptosis, Curr Opin Genet Dev 6:12–19, 1996.

Bodmer W, Bishop T, and Karran P: Genetic steps in colorectal cancer, Nature Genet 6:217–219, 1994.

Burt RW and Lipkin M: Gastrointestinal cancer. In King RA, Rotter JI, and Motulsky AG, editors: The genetic basis of common diseases, New York, 1992, Oxford University Press.

Cavanee WK, White RL: The genetic basis of cancer, Sci Am 272:72–79, 1995.

Dunlop MG: Mutator genes and mosaicism in colorectal cancer, Curr Opin Genet Dev 6:75–80, 1996.

Fishel R, Kolodner RD: Identification of mismatch repair genes and their role in the development of cancer, Curr Opin Genet Dev 5:382–395, 1995.

Goddard AD and Solomon E: Genetic aspects of cancer, Adv Hum Genet 21:321–376, 1993.

Haffner R, Oren M: Biochemical properties and biological effects of p53, Curr Opin Genet Dev 5:84–90, 1995.

Harris CC and Hollstein M: Clinical implications of the *p53* tumor-suppressor gene, N Engl J Med 329:1318–1327, 1993.

Hartwell LH, Kastan MB: Cell cycle control and cancer, Science 266:1821–1828, 1994.

Kamb A: Cell-cycle regulators and cancer, Trends Genet 11:136–140, 1995.

Knudson AG: Antioncogenes and human cancer, Proc Natl Acad Sci, USA 90:10914–10921, 1993.

Krontiris TG: Oncogenes, N Eng J Med 333:303–306, 1995.

Lasko D, Cavenee W, and Nordenskjöld M: Loss of constitutional heterozygosity in human cancer, Annu Rev Genet 25:281–314, 1991.

Mak YF, Ponder BAJ: RET oncogene, Curr Opin Genet Dev 6:82–86, 1996.

Malkin D, Li FP, Strong LC, et al: Germ line *p53* mutations in a familial syndrome of breast cancer, sarcomas, and other neoplasms, Science 250:1233–1238, 1990.

Olsen JH, Boice JD, Seersholm N, Bautz A, Fraumeni JF: Cancer in the parents of children with cancer, N Eng J Med 333:1594–1599, 1995.

Polakis P: Mutations in the APC gene and their implications for protein structure and function, Curr Opin Genet Dev 5:66–71, 1995.

Powell SM, Petersen GM, Krush AJ, et al: Molecular diagnosis of familial adenomatous polyposis, N Engl J Med 329:1982–1987, 1993.

Vogelstein B and Kinzler KW: The multistep nature of cancer, Trends Genet 9:138–141, 1993.

Weinberg RA: Molecular mechanisms of carcinogenesis. In Leder P, Clayton DA, Rubenstein E, editors: Introduction to Molecular Medicine, New York, 1994, Scientific American.

Weinberg RA: Tumor suppressor genes, Science 254:1138–1146, 1991.

10 Multifactorial Inheritance and Common Diseases

The focus of previous chapters has been on diseases that are caused by single genes or by abnormalities of single chromosomes. Much progress has been made in identifying specific mutations that cause these diseases, leading to better risk estimates and in some cases more effective treatment of the disease. However, these conditions form only a small portion of the total burden of human genetic disease. Most congenital malformations are not caused by single genes or chromosome defects. Many common adult diseases, such as cancer, heart disease, and diabetes, have genetic components, but again they are usually not caused by single genes or by chromosome abnormalities. These diseases, whose treatment collectively occupies the attention of most health care practitioners, are the result of a complex interplay of multiple genetic and environmental factors.

■ PRINCIPLES OF MULTIFACTORIAL INHERITANCE

Basic Model

Traits in which variation is thought to be caused by the combined effects of multiple genes are **polygenic** (many genes). When environmental factors are also believed to cause variation in the trait, which is usually the case, the term **multifactorial** is used. Many **quantitative** traits (those, such as blood pressure, which are measured on a continuous numerical scale) are multifactorial. Because they are caused by the additive effects of many genetic and environmental factors, these traits tend to follow a normal, or "bell-shaped," distribution in populations.

Let us use an example to illustrate this concept. To begin with the simplest case, suppose (unrealistically) that height is determined by a single gene with two alleles, A and a. Allele A tends to make people tall, whereas allele a tends to make them short. If there is no dominance at this locus, then the three possible genotypes, AA, Aa, and aa, will produce three phenotypes: tall, intermediate, and short. Assume that the gene frequencies of A and a are each 0.50. If we look at a population of individuals, we will observe the height distribution depicted in Figure 10-1, A.

Now suppose, a bit more realistically, that height is determined by two loci instead of one. The second locus also has two alleles, B (tall) and b (short), and they affect height in exactly the same way as alleles A and a. There are now nine possible genotypes in our population: aabb, aaBb, aaBB, Aabb, AaBb, AaBB, AAbb, AABb, and AABB. An individual may have zero, one, two, three, or four "tall" alleles, so there are now five distinct phenotypes (Fig. 10-1, B). Although the height distribution in our population is not yet normal, it approaches a normal distribution more closely than in the single-gene case above.

We now extend our example so that many genes and environmental factors influence height, each having a small effect. Then there are many possible phenotypes, each differing slightly, and the height distribution approaches the bell-shaped curve shown in Figure 10-1, C.

It should be emphasized that the individual genes underlying a multifactorial trait such as height follow the mendelian principles of segregation and independent assortment, just like any other gene. The only difference is that many of them *act together* to influence the trait.

Blood pressure is another example of a multifactorial trait. There is a correlation between parents' blood pressures (systolic and diastolic) and those of their children. There is good evidence that this correlation is due in part to genes. But blood pressure is also influenced by environmental factors, such as diet and stress. One of the goals of genetic research is the identification and measurement of the relative roles of genes and environment in the causation of multifactorial diseases.

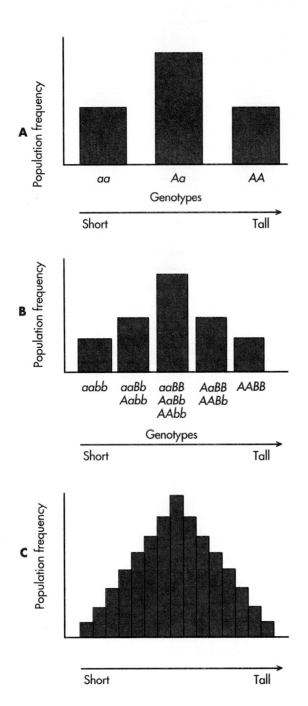

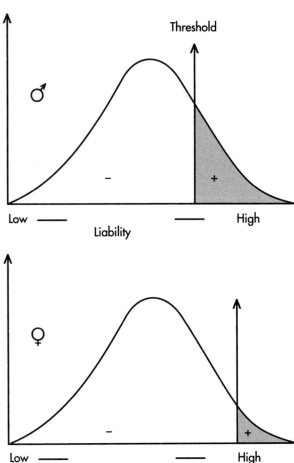

ial. When they can be measured on a continuous scale, they often follow a normal distribution.

Threshold Model

A number of diseases do not follow the bell-shaped distribution. Instead they appear to be either present or absent in individuals. Yet they do not follow the patterns expected of single-gene diseases. A commonly used explanation for such diseases is that there is an underlying **liability distribution** for the disease in a population (Fig. 10-2). Those individuals who are on the low end of the distribution have little chance of developing the disease in question (i.e., they have few of the alleles or environmental factors that would cause the disease). Those who are closer to the high end of the distribution have more of the disease-causing genes and environmental factors and are more

Figure 10-1 ■ *A,* The distribution of height in a population, assuming that height is controlled by a single locus with genotypes *AA, Aa,* and *aa.* *B,* The distribution of height, assuming that height is controlled by two loci. There are now five distinct phenotypes instead of three, and the distribution begins to look more like the normal distribution. *C,* Distribution of height, assuming that multiple factors, each with a small effect, contribute to the trait (the multifactorial model).

Many traits are thought to be influenced by multiple genes as well as environmental factors. These traits are said to be multifactor-

Figure 10-2 ■ A liability distribution in a population for a multifactorial disease. To be affected with the disease, an individual must exceed the threshold on the liability distribution. This figure shows two thresholds, a lower one for males and a higher one for females (as in pyloric stenosis).

likely to develop the disease. For diseases that are either present or absent, it is thought that a **threshold of liability** must be crossed before the disease is expressed. Below the threshold the individual appears normal; above it he or she is affected by the disease.

A disease that is thought to correspond to this threshold model is pyloric stenosis, a disorder that presents shortly after birth and is caused by a narrowing or obstruction of the pylorus, the area between the stomach and intestine. Chronic vomiting, constipation, weight loss, and electrolyte imbalance result from the condition, but it sometimes resolves spontaneously or can be corrected by surgery. The prevalence of pyloric stenosis is about 3 per 1000 live births in whites. It is much more common in males than females, affecting 1 of 200 males and 1 of 1000 females. It is thought that this difference in prevalence reflects *two* thresholds in the liability distribution, a lower one in males and a higher one in females (see Fig. 10-2). A lower male threshold implies that fewer disease-causing factors are required to generate the disorder in males.

The liability threshold concept may explain the pattern of recurrence risks for pyloric stenosis seen in Table 10-1. Notice that males, having a lower threshold, always have a higher risk than females. However, the sibling risk also depends on the sex of the proband. It is higher when the proband is female than when the proband is male. This reflects the concept that females, having a higher liability threshold, must be exposed to more disease-causing factors than males in order to develop the disease. Thus a family with an affected female must have more genetic and environmental risk factors, producing a higher recurrence risk for pyloric stenosis in future offspring. We would expect that the highest risk category would be *male* relatives of *female* probands; Table 10-1 shows that this is indeed the case.

A similar pattern has been observed in a recent

study of infantile autism, a behavioral disorder in which the male–female sex ratio is approximately 4:1. As expected for a multifactorial disorder, the recurrence risk for siblings of male probands (3.5%) was substantially lower than that of siblings of female probands (7%). When the sex ratio for a disease is reversed (i.e., more affected females than males), we would expect a higher recurrence risk when the proband is male.

A number of other congenital malformations are thought to correspond to this model. They include isolated[†] cleft lip and/or cleft palate (CL/P; *SOL* 65, 66), neural tube defects (anencephaly and spina bifida), club foot (talipes), and some forms of congenital heart disease (*SOL* 74, 85-88). In addition, many of the common adult diseases, such as hypertension, coronary heart disease, stroke, diabetes mellitus (types I and II), and some cancers, are caused by complex genetic and environmental factors and can thus be considered multifactorial diseases.

> **The threshold model applies to many multifactorial diseases. It assumes that there is an underlying liability distribution in a population and that a threshold on this distribution must be passed before a disease is expressed.**

Recurrence Risks and Transmission Patterns

Whereas recurrence risks can be given with confidence for single-gene diseases (50% for typical autosomal dominant diseases, 25% for autosomal recessive diseases, etc.), the situation is more complicated for multifactorial diseases. This is because the number of genes contributing to the disease is usually not known, the precise allelic constitution of the parents is not known, and the extent of environmental effects can vary substantially. For most multifactorial diseases, **empirical risks** (i.e., risks based on direct observation of data) have been derived. To estimate empirical risks, a large series of families is examined in which one child has developed the disease (the proband). Then the siblings of each proband are surveyed to calculate the percentage who have also developed the disease. For example, in Great Britain about 5% of siblings of neural tube defect cases also have neural tube defects (Clinical Commentary 10-1). Thus the recurrence risk for parents who have had one child with a neural tube defect is 5% in

---

Table 10-1 ■ Recurrence risk (%) for pyloric stenosis, subdivided by genders of affected probands and relatives*

Relatives	Male probands		Female probands	
	London	Belfast	London	Belfast
Brothers	3.8	9.6	9.2	12.5
Sisters	2.7	3.0	3.8	3.8

*Adapted from Carter: Br Med Bull 32:21–26, 1976. Note that the risks differ somewhat between the two populations.

[†]In this context, the term "isolated" means that this is the only observed disease feature (i.e., the feature is not part of a larger constellation of findings, as in cleft lip/palate secondary to trisomy 13).

Clinical Commentary 10-1. Neural Tube Defects

Neural tube defects (NTDs), which include anencephaly, spina bifida, and encephalocele (as well as several other less common forms), are one of the most important classes of birth defects, with a newborn prevalence of 1 to 3 per 1000. There is considerable variation in the prevalence of NTDs among various populations, with an especially high rate among some British and Irish populations (as high as 5 or more per 1000 births). In the United States, NTDs are 2 to 3 times more common in the eastern than in the western parts of the country. For reasons that are not fully known, the prevalence of NTDs has been decreasing in many parts of the United States and Europe during the past two decades.

Normally the neural tube closes at about the fourth week of gestation. A defect in closure or a subsequent reopening of the neural tube results in an NTD. Spina bifida (Fig. 10-3, *A; SOL* 79, 80) is the most commonly observed NTD and consists of a protrusion of spinal tissue through the vertebral column (the tissue usually includes meninges, spinal cord, and nerve roots). About 75% of spina bifida patients have secondary hydrocephalus (*SOL* 89) which sometimes in turn produces mental retardation. Paralysis or muscle weakness, lack of sphincter control, and club feet are often observed. A recent study conducted in British Columbia showed that survival rates for spina bifida patients have improved dramatically over the past several decades. Fewer than 30% of cases born between 1952 and 1969 survived to age 10, whereas 65% of those born between 1970 and 1986 survived to this age. Anencephaly (Fig. 10-3, *B; SOL* 75-78) is characterized by partial or complete absence of the cranial vault and calvarium and partial or complete

absence of the cerebral hemispheres. At least two thirds of anencephalics are stillborn; term deliveries do not survive more than a few hours or days. Encephalocele (Fig. 10-3, *C; SOL* 81, 82) consists of a protrusion of the brain into an enclosed sac. It is seldom compatible with survival.

NTDs are thought to arise from a combination of genetic and environmental factors. In most populations surveyed thus far, empirical recurrence risks for siblings of affected cases range from 2% to 5%. Consistent with a multifactorial model, the recurrence risk increases with additional affected siblings. Studies conducted in Great Britain showed that the sibling recurrence risk was approximately 5% when one sibling was affected and 10% when two were affected. A recent Hungarian study showed that the overall prevalence of NTDs was 1 in 300 births and that the sibling recurrence risks were 3%, 12%, and 25% after one, two, and three affected offspring, respectively. Recurrence risks tend to be slightly lower in populations with lower NTD prevalence rates, as predicted by the multifactorial model. Recurrence risk data support the idea that the major forms of NTDs are caused by similar factors. An anencephalic conception increases the recurrence risk for subsequent spina bifida conceptions, and vice-versa.

NTDs can usually be diagnosed prenatally, sometimes by ultrasound and usually by an elevation in alpha-fetoprotein (AFP) in the maternal serum or amniotic fluid (see Chapter 11). A spina bifida lesion can be either open or closed (i.e., covered with a layer of skin). Fetuses with open spina bifida are more likely to be detected by AFP assays.

A major recent epidemiologic finding is that mothers who supplement their diet with folic acid at the time of conception are less likely to produce children with NTDs. This result has been replicated in several

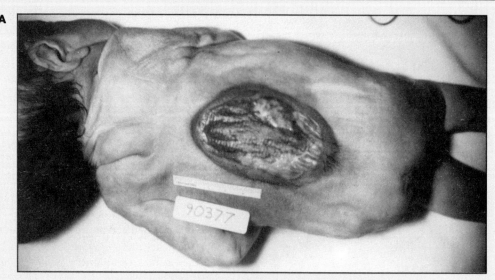

A

Continued.

B

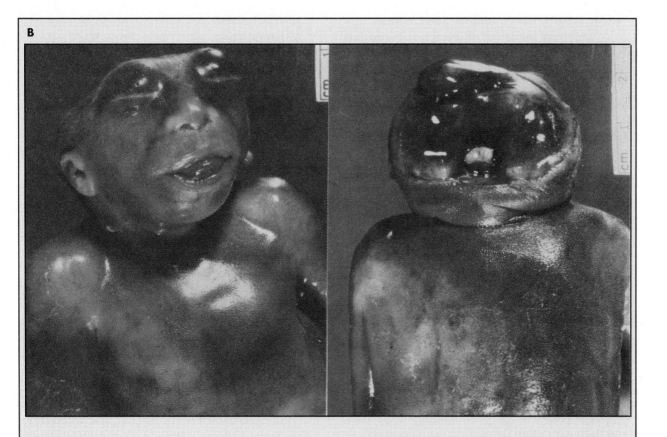

different populations and thus appears to be well confirmed. It has been estimated that as many as 50% of NTDs can be avoided simply by dietary folic acid supplementation. (Traditional prenatal vitamin supplements would not have much effect, because administration does not usually begin until well after the time that the neural tube closes.) Because mothers would be likely to ingest similar amounts of folic acid from one pregnancy to the next, folic acid deficiency could well account for at least part of the elevated sibling recurrence risk for NTDs. This is an important example of a *nongenetic* factor that contributes to familial clustering of a disease.

C

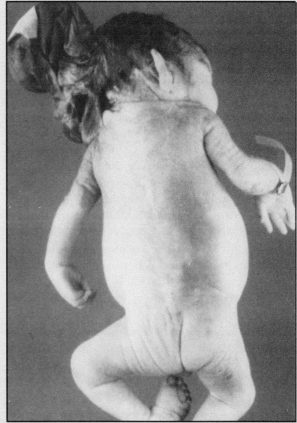

Figure 10-3 ▪ The major neural tube defects (NTDs). *A,* An infant with an open spina bifida (meningomyelcele). *B,* A fetus with anecephaly. Note the abnormalities of the orbits of the eye and the cranial defect. *C,* An occipital encephalocele. (All NTD photographs courtesy of Dr. Edward Klatt, University of Utah Health Sciences Center.)

in Great Britain. For conditions such as cleft lip/palate, which are not lethal or severely debilitating, recurrence risks can also be estimated for the offspring of affected parents. Empirical recurrence risks are specific for each multifactorial disease.

In contrast to most single-gene diseases, recurrence risks for multifactorial diseases can change substantially from one population to another (notice the differences between the London and Belfast populations shown in Table 10-1). This is because gene frequencies as well as environmental factors can differ among populations. For example, the empirical risk for neural tube defects in North America is about 2% to 3%, somewhat lower than that of the British population.

> **Empirical recurrence risks for multifactorial diseases are based on studies of large collections of families. These risks are specific to a given population.**

It is sometimes difficult to distinguish polygenic or multifactorial diseases from single-gene diseases that have reduced penetrance or variable expression. Large data sets and good epidemiologic data are necessary to make the distinction. Several criteria are usually used to define multifactorial inheritance:

1. *The recurrence risk becomes higher if more than one family member is affected.* For example, the sibling recurrence risk for a ventricular septal defect (VSD, a type of congenital heart defect) is 3% if one sibling has had a VSD but increases to approximately 10% if two siblings have had VSDs. In contrast, the recurrence risk for single-gene diseases remains the same regardless of the number of affected siblings. It should be emphasized that this increase does not mean that the family's risk has actually *changed*. Rather, it means that we now have more information about the family's true risk: because they have had two affected children, they are probably located higher on the liability distribution than a family with only one affected child. In other words, they have more risk factors (genetic and/or environmental) and are more likely to produce an affected child.

2. *If the expression of the disease in the proband is more severe, the recurrence risk is higher.* This is again consistent with the liability model because a more severe expression indicates that the affected individual is at the extreme tail of the liability distribution (see Fig. 10-2). His or her relatives are thus at a higher risk to inherit

disease genes. For example, the occurrence of a bilateral (both sides) cleft lip/palate confers a higher recurrence risk on family members than does the occurrence of a unilateral (one side) cleft.

3. *The recurrence risk is higher if the proband is of the less commonly affected sex* (see the above discussion of pyloric stenosis). This is because an affected individual of the less susceptible sex is usually at a more extreme position on the liability distribution.

4. *The recurrence risk for the disease usually decreases rapidly in more remotely related relatives* (Table 10-2). While the recurrence risk for single-gene diseases decreases by 50% with each degree of relationship (e.g., an autosomal dominant disease has a 50% recurrence risk for siblings, 25% for uncle–nephew relationships, 12.5% for first cousins), it decreases much more quickly for multifactorial diseases. This reflects the fact that many genes and environmental factors must combine to produce a trait. All of the necessary risk factors are unlikely to be present in less closely related family members.

5. *If the prevalence of the disease in a population is f, the risk for offspring and siblings of probands is approximately* $\sqrt{f}$. This does not hold true for single-gene traits because their recurrence risks are independent of population prevalence. It is not an absolute rule for multifactorial traits either, but many such diseases do tend to conform to this prediction. Examination of the risks given in Table 10-2 shows that the first three diseases follow the prediction fairly well. However, the observed sibling risk for the fourth disease, infantile autism, is substantially higher than predicted by $\sqrt{f}$.

> **Risks for multifactorial diseases usually increase if (1) more family members are affected, (2) the disease has more severe expression, and (3) the affected proband is a member of the less commonly affected sex. Recurrence risks decrease rapidly with more remote degrees of relationship. In general the sibling recurrence risk is approximately equal to the square root of the prevalence of the disease in the population.**

Multifactorial versus Single-Gene Inheritance

It is important to clarify the difference between a multifactorial disease and a single-gene disease in which there is locus heterogeneity. In the former case, a disease is caused by the simultaneous opera-

Table 10-2 ▪ Recurrence risk (%) for first-, second-, and third-degree relatives

Disease	First-degree	Second-degree	Third-degree	General population
Cleft/lip palate	4	0.7	0.3	0.1
Club foot	2.5	0.5	0.2	0.1
Congenital hip dislocation	5	0.6	0.4	0.2
Infantile autism	4.5	0.1	0.05	0.04

tion of multiple genetic and environmental factors, each of which has a relatively small effect. In contrast, a disease with locus heterogeneity, such as osteogenesis imperfecta, requires only a single mutation for its causation. Because of locus heterogeneity, a chromosome 7 mutation may cause the disease in one family, whereas a chromosome 17 mutation may cause the disease in another family. There is thus more than one gene that can cause the disease, but *in a given individual* a single gene causes the disease.

In some cases a trait may be influenced by the combination of both a single gene with large effects and a multifactorial "background" in which additional genes and environmental factors have individually small effects. This concept is illustrated in Figure 10-4. Imagine that variation in height, for

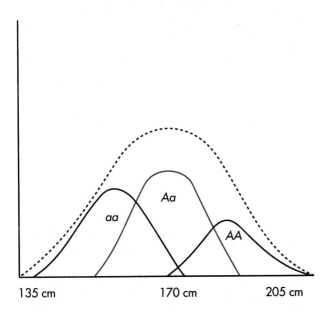

135 cm   170 cm   205 cm

Figure 10-4 ▪ The distribution of height, assuming the presence of a major gene (genotypes *AA, Aa,* and *aa*) combined with a multifactorial background. The multifactorial background causes variation in height among individuals of each genotype. If the distributions of each of the three genotypes are superimposed, then the overall distribution of height is approximately normal, as shown by the dotted line.

example, is caused by a single locus (termed a **major gene**) and a multifactorial component. Individuals with the *AA* genotype will tend to be taller, those with the *aa* genotype will tend to be shorter, and those with *Aa* will tend to be intermediate. But additional variation is caused by other factors (the multifactorial component). Thus those with the *aa* genotype will vary in height from 130 to about 170 cm, those with the *Aa* genotype will vary in height from 150 to 190 cm, and those with the *AA* genotype will vary from 170 to 210 cm. There is substantial overlap among the three major genotypes because of the influence of the multifactorial background. The total distribution of height, which is bell-shaped, is caused by the superposition of the three distributions about each genotype.

Many of the diseases to be discussed next appear to have both major gene and multifactorial components in populations. Thus there are subsets of the population in which diseases, such as colon cancer, breast cancer, or heart disease, are inherited as single-gene disorders (with additional variation in disease susceptibility contributed by other genetic and environmental factors). These subsets usually account for only a small percentage of the total number of disease cases. It is nevertheless important to identify the responsible major genes, because their function can provide important clues to the pathophysiology and treatment of the disease.

Multifactorial diseases can be distinguished from single-gene disorders caused by mutations at different loci (locus heterogeneity). Sometimes a disease may have both single-gene and multifactorial components.

▪ NATURE AND NURTURE: DISENTANGLING THE EFFECTS OF GENES AND ENVIRONMENT

Family members share genes and a common environment. Family resemblance in traits such as blood pressure reflects both genetic and environmental commonality ("nature" and "nurture," respectively). For centuries, people have debated the relative importance of these two types of factors. It is a mistake, of course, to view them as mutually exclusive. Few traits are influenced *only* by genes or *only* by environment. Most are influenced by both. It is useful to try to determine the *relative* influence of genetic and environmental factors. This can lead to a better understanding of disease etiology. It can also help to plan public health strategies. A disease in which the genetic influence is relatively small, such as lung cancer, may be prevented most effectively through emphasis on lifestyle changes (avoidance of tobacco). When a disease has a relatively larger genetic component, as in breast cancer, examination of family history should be emphasized in addition to lifestyle modification.

Here we will review two research strategies that are often used to estimate the relative influence of genes and environment: twin studies and adoption studies. We will then discuss a method that aims to delineate the individual genes responsible for multifactorial diseases.

Twin Studies

Twins occur with a frequency of about 1 in 100 births in white populations. They are a bit more common in Africans and a bit less common among Asians. **Monozygotic** (MZ, or "identical") twins originate when, for unknown reasons, the developing embryo divides to form two separate but identical embryos. Because they are genetically identical, MZ twins are an example of natural clones. Their physical appearances can be strikingly similar (Fig. 10-5). **Dizygotic** (DZ, or "fraternal") twins are the result of a double ovulation followed by the fertilization of each egg by a different sperm.* Thus dizygotic twins are genetically no more similar than siblings. Because two different sperm cells are required to fertilize the two eggs, it is possible for each DZ twin to have a different father.

Because MZ twins are genetically identical, any differences between them should be due only to environmental effects. MZ twins should thus resemble one another very closely for traits that are strongly influenced by genes. DZ twins provide a convenient comparison, because their environmental differences should be similar to those of MZ twins, but their genetic differences are as great as those between siblings. Twin studies thus usually consist of comparisons between MZ and DZ twins.

If both members of a twin pair share a trait (e.g., a cleft lip), they are said to be **concordant**. If they do not share the trait, they are **discordant**. For a trait determined totally by genes, MZ twins should always be concordant, while DZ twins should be concordant less often because they, like siblings, share only 50% of their genes. Concordance rates may differ between opposite-sex DZ twin pairs and same-sex DZ pairs for some traits, such as those that have different frequencies in males and females. For such traits, only same-sex DZ twin pairs should be used when comparing MZ and DZ concordance rates because MZ twins are necessarily of the same sex.

A concordance estimate would not be appropriate for quantitative traits, such as blood pressure or height. Here the **intraclass correlation coefficient** is used. This statistic varies between -1.0 and 1.0 and measures the degree of similarity in two quantities in a population. The quantities could be height measurements in each member of a twin pair. The measurements are made in a collection of twins, and correlation coefficients are estimated separately for the MZ sample and the DZ sample. If a trait were determined entirely by genes, we would expect the correlation coefficient for MZ pairs to be 1.0. A correlation coefficient of 0.0 would mean that there is no similarity between MZ twins for the trait in question. Because DZ twins share half of their genes, we would expect a DZ correlation coefficient of 0.50 for a trait determined entirely by genes.

Monozygotic (identical) twins are the result of an early cleavage of the embryo, whereas dizygotic (fraternal) twins are caused by the fertilization of two eggs by two sperm cells. Comparisons of concordance rates and correlations in MZ and DZ twins help to determine the extent to which a trait is influenced by genes.

Concordance rates and correlation coefficients for a number of traits are given in Table 10-3 (page 194). Notice that the concordance rates for contagious diseases, such as measles, are similar in MZ and DZ twins. This is expected because a contagious disease is unlikely to be influenced markedly by genes. However, the concordance rates are dissimilar for schizophrenia and bipolar affective disorder, indicating a sizable genetic component for these diseases. The MZ correlations for dermatoglyphics (fingerprints), which are determined almost entirely by genes, are close to 1.0.

*Whereas MZ twinning rates are constant across populations, DZ twinning rates vary somewhat. DZ twinning increases with maternal age until about age 40, after which it declines.

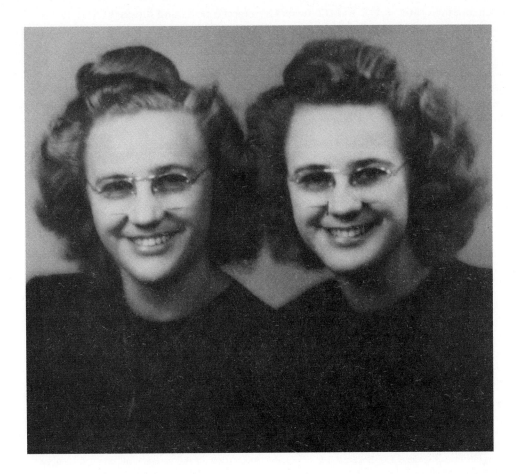

Figure 10-5 ■Monozygotic twins, showing a striking similarity in physical appearance. Both twins developed myopia as teenagers.

Correlations and concordance rates in MZ and DZ twins can be used to measure the **heritability** of multifactorial traits. Essentially, heritability is the percentage of population variation in a trait that is due to genes (statistically, it is the proportion of the total **variance** of a trait that is caused by genes). A simple formula for estimating heritability *(h)* from twin correlations or concordance rates is: $h = 2(c_{MZ} - c_{DZ})$, where c_{MZ} is the concordance rate (or intraclass correlation) for monozygotic twins and c_{DZ} is the concordance rate (or intraclass correlation) for dizygotic twins.* As this formula illustrates, traits that are largely determined by genes will result in a heritability estimate that approaches 1.0 (i.e., c_{MZ} will approach 1.0 and c_{DZ}

will approach 0.5). As the difference between concordance rates becomes smaller, heritability approaches 0. Correlations and concordance rates in other pairs of relatives (e.g., parents and offspring) can also be used to measure heritability.

Like recurrence risks, heritability values are specific for the population in which they are estimated. However, there is usually agreement from one population to another regarding the general range of heritability estimates of most traits (e.g., the heritability of height is nearly always high, whereas the heritability of contagious diseases is nearly always low). The same is true of empirical recurrence risks.

Comparisons of correlations and concordance rates in MZ and DZ twins allow the estimation of heritability, a measure of the proportion of population variation in a disease that can be attributed to genes.

*This formula represents one of the simplest ways of estimating heritability. A description of more complex and accurate approaches can be found in the books by Cavalli-Sforza and Bodmer and Neale and Cardon cited at the end of this chapter.

Table 10-3 ▪ Concordance rates in MZ and DZ twins for selected traits and diseases*

Trait or disease	Concordance rate		Heritability†
	MZ twins	DZ twins	
Affective disorder (bipolar)	0.79	0.24	>1.0
Affective disorder (unipolar)	0.54	0.19	0.70
Alcoholism	>0.60	<0.30	0.60
Autism	0.92	0.0	>1.0
Blood pressure (diastolic)‡	0.58	0.27	0.62
Blood pressure (systolic)‡	0.55	0.25	0.60
Body fat percentage‡	0.73	0.22	>1.0
Body mass index‡	0.95	0.53	0.84
Cleft lip/palate	0.38	0.08	0.60
Club foot	0.32	0.03	0.58
Dermatoglyphics (finger ridge count)‡	0.95	0.49	0.92
Diabetes mellitus	0.45–0.96	0.03–0.37	>1.0
Diabetes mellitus (type I)	0.55	—	—
Diabetes mellitus (type II)	0.90	—	—
Epilepsy (idiopathic)	0.69	0.14	>1.0
Height‡	0.94	0.44	1.0
IQ‡	0.76	0.51	0.50
Measles	0.95	0.87	0.16
Multiple sclerosis	0.28	0.03	0.50
Myocardial infarction (males)	0.39	0.26	0.26
Myocardial infarction (females)	0.44	0.14	0.60
Schizophrenia	0.47	0.12	0.70
Spina bifida	0.72	0.33	0.78

*The data were compiled from a large variety of sources and represent primarily European and U.S. populations.
†Several heritability estimates exceed 1.0. Because it is impossible for >100% of the variance of a trait to be genetically determined, these values indicate that other factors, such as shared environmental factors, must be operating.
‡Because these are quantitative traits, correlation coefficients are given rather than concordance rates.

At one time twins were thought to provide a perfect "natural laboratory" in which to determine the relative influences of genetics and environment. But several difficulties arise. One of the most important is the assumption that the environments of MZ and DZ twins are equally similar. MZ twins are often treated more similarly than DZ twins. The eminent geneticist L.S. Penrose once joked that, if one were to study the clothes of twins, it might be concluded that clothes are inherited biologically. A greater similarity in environment can make MZ twins more concordant for a trait, inflating the apparent influence of genes. In addition, MZ twins may be more likely to seek the same type of environment, further reinforcing environmental similarity. On the other hand, it has been suggested that MZ twins tend to develop personality differences in an attempt to assert their individuality.

Another difficulty is that somatic mutations can occur during mitotic divisions of the cells of MZ twin embryos. Thus the MZ twins may not be quite "identical." Finally, the uterine environments of different pairs of MZ twins can be more or less similar, depending on whether there are 2 amnions and 2 chorions, 2 amnions and 1 shared chorion, or 1 shared amnion and 1 shared chorion.

Of the various problems with the twin method, the greater degree of environmental sharing among MZ twins is perhaps the most serious. One way to circumvent this problem, at least in part, is to study MZ twins who are raised in separate environments. Similarities among these twin pairs should be caused by genetic, rather than environmental, similarities. As one might expect, it is not easy to find such twin pairs. A major effort to do so has been undertaken by Thomas Bouchard of the University of Minnesota. His studies have shown a rather remarkable congruence among MZ twins reared apart, even for many behavioral traits. However, these studies must be viewed with caution because the sample sizes are relatively small and because many of the twin pairs had at least some contact with each other before they were studied.

Although twin studies provide valuable information, they are also affected by certain biases. The most serious is greater environmental similarity among MZ twins than among DZ twins. Other biases include somatic mutations that may affect only one MZ twin and differences in the uterine environments of twins.

Adoption Studies

Studies of adopted children are also used to estimate the genetic contribution to a multifactorial trait. Children born to parents who have a disease but adopted by parents lacking the disease can be studied to determine whether they develop the disease. In some cases such children develop the disease more often than a comparative control population (i.e., adopted children who were born to parents who do *not* have the disease). This provides some evidence that genes may be involved in the causation of the disease since the adopted children do not share an environment with their affected natural parents. For example, about 8% to 10% of adopted children of a schizophrenic parent develop schizophrenia, whereas only 1% of adopted children of normal parents become schizophrenics.

As with twin studies, several precautions must be exercised in interpreting the results of adoption studies. First, prenatal environmental influences could have long-lasting effects on an adopted child. Second, children are sometimes adopted after they are several years old, ensuring that some environmental influence would have been imparted by the natural parents. Finally, adoption agencies sometimes try to match the adoptive parents with the natural parents in terms of background, socioeconomic status, etc. All of these factors could exaggerate the apparent influence of biologic inheritance.

Adoption studies provide a second means of estimating the influence of genes on multifactorial diseases. They consist of comparing disease rates among the adopted offspring of affected parents with rates among adopted offspring of unaffected parents. As with the twin method, certain biases can influence these studies.

These reservations, as well as those summarized for twin studies, underscore the need for caution in basing conclusions upon twin and adoption studies. These approaches do not provide definitive measures of the role of genes in multifactorial disease, nor can they identify specific genes responsible for disease. Instead they serve a useful purpose in providing a preliminary indication of the extent to which a multifactorial disease may be caused by genetic factors.

■ THE GENETICS OF COMMON DISEASES

Having discussed the principles of multifactorial inheritance, we turn next to a discussion of the common multifactorial disorders themselves. Some of these disorders, the congenital malformations, are by definition present at birth. Others, including heart disease, cancer, diabetes, and most psychiatric disorders, are seen primarily in adolescents and adults. Because of their complexity, unraveling the genetics of these disorders is a daunting task. Nonetheless, significant progress is now being made.

Congenital Malformations

Approximately 2% of newborns present with a **congenital** (present at birth) malformation; most of these would be considered "multifactorial" in etiology. Some of the more common congenital malformations are listed in Table 10-4. In general, sibling recurrence risks for most of these disorders range from 1% to 5%.

Some congenital malformations, such as cleft lip/palate and pyloric stenosis, are relatively easy to repair and thus are not considered to be serious problems. Others, such as the neural tube defects, usually have more severe consequences. Although some cases of congenital malformations may occur in the absence of any other problems, it is common for them to be associated with other disorders. For example, hydrocephaly and club foot are often seen secondary to spina bifida, cleft lip/palate is often seen in babies with trisomy 13, and congenital heart defects are seen in many disorders, including Down syndrome.

Table 10-4 ■ Prevalence rates of common congenital malformations in whites

Disorder	Prevalence per 1000 births (approximate)
Cleft lip/palate	1
Club foot	1
Congenital heart defects	4–8
Hydrocephaly	0.5–2.5
Isolated cleft palate	0.4
Neural tube defects	1–3
Pyloric stenosis	3

Box 10-1. Finding the Underlying Genes: The Quantitative Trait Locus Method

As already mentioned, twin and adoption studies are not designed to reveal specific genes that cause multifactorial diseases. Nevertheless, the identification of specific causative genes is an important goal because only then can we begin to understand the underlying biology of the disease and undertake to correct the defect. For complex multifactorial traits, this is a formidable task. Fortunately recent advances in gene mapping and molecular biology promise to make this goal more attainable. The **quantitative trait locus method** is one example of an approach that takes advantage of these advances. It consists basically of the following steps:

1. Breeding experiments are carried out with experimental animals, such as rats, to select progeny that have extreme values of a trait (e.g., those rats that have high blood pressure levels). These are then crossed with normal animals to produce offspring that each have one normal chromosome and one ''affected'' chromosome that presumably contains genes for high blood pressure. These offspring are in turn mated with the normal animals (a ''back-cross''). This produces a third generation in whom one chromosome has only the normal genes and the homologous chromosome has experienced recombinations between the normal and affected chromosomes (as a result of crossovers between the normal and affected chromosomes during meiosis in the parents). This procedure produces progeny that are useful for linkage analysis.

2. High-resolution genetic maps of the experimental organism must be available. This means that polymorphic markers must be identified at regular intervals (ideally, every 10 cM or so) throughout the organism's genome.

3. Linkage analysis (see Chapter 7) is performed, comparing each polymorphic marker against the trait. Because animals with extreme values have been selected, this procedure should uncover markers that are linked to loci that produce the extreme phenotype.

4. Once a linked marker (or markers) has been found, it may be possible to isolate and clone the actual functional gene partially responsible for the trait using the techniques outlined in Chapter 7.

5. When a functional gene has been cloned in the experimental organism, it is used as a probe to search the human genome for a gene with high DNA sequence homology that may have the same function (a candidate gene). This approach is feasible because the DNA sequences of functionally important genes are often similar in humans and experimental animals such as rodents.

This approach has been applied in studies of type I diabetes and hypertension. A limitation of the quantitative trait locus method is that it usually requires an animal model for the disease under study so that selective breeding experiments can be carried out. Another limitation is that this technique only detects individual genes that cause disease in the animal model, but it cannot assess the pattern of *interactions* of these genes. There is evidence that the nature of these interactions may be critically important, and they may well differ in humans and experimental animals. Despite these reservations, this approach demonstrates the way in which new developments in molecular genetics and gene mapping may increase our knowledge of the genes responsible for multifactorial disease.

Some progress has been made in isolating single genes for congenital malformations. For example, an X-linked gene has been found to cause some cases of isolated cleft palate. A gene for Hirschsprung disease (congenital aganglionic megacolon; *SOL* 71) was mapped to chromosome 10 after statistical studies revealed that a more severe presentation of the disease (aganglionosis beyond the sigmoid colon) was caused by a single dominant gene with reduced penetrance. The less severe cases of Hirschsprung disease may be multifactorial in origin, or they may be caused by other, as yet unidentified, single genes.

Environmental factors have also been shown to cause some congenital malformations. An example is thalidomide, a sedative used during pregnancy in the early 1960s. When ingested during early pregnancy this drug often caused phocomelia (severely shortened limbs) in babies. Maternal exposure to retinoic acid, which is used to treat acne, can cause congenital defects of the heart, ear, and central nervous system. Maternal rubella infection can cause congenital heart defects. Other environmental factors that can cause congenital malformations are discussed in Chapter 12.

Congenital malformations are seen in approximately 1 in 50 live births. Most of them are considered to be multifactorial disorders. Specific genes and environmental causes have been detected for some congenital malformations, but the causes of most congenital malformations remain largely unknown.

Multifactorial Disorders in the Adult Population

Until recently, little was known about specific genes responsible for common adult diseases. With more powerful laboratory and analytic techniques, this situation is changing. We next review recent progress in understanding the genetics of the major common adult diseases. Table 10-5 gives approximate prevalence figures for these disorders in the United States.

Coronary Heart Disease

It is well known that coronary heart disease (CHD) is currently the leading killer of Americans, accounting for approximately 25% of all deaths in this country. It is caused by atherosclerosis, a narrowing of the coronary arteries due to the formation of lipid-laden lesions. This narrowing impedes blood flow to the heart and can eventually result in a myocardial infarction (destruction of heart tissue caused by an inadequate supply of oxygen). When atherosclerosis occurs in arteries supplying blood to the brain, a stroke can result. A number of risk factors for heart disease have been identified, including obesity, cigarette smoking, hypertension, elevated cholesterol level, and positive family history (usually defined as having one affected first-degree relative). Many studies have examined the role of family history in CHD, and they show that an individual with a positive family history is 2 to 7 times more likely to suffer from heart disease than is an individual with no family history. Generally these studies also show that the risk increases if: (1) there are more affected relatives, (2) the affected relative(s) is female (the less commonly affected sex) rather than male, and (3) age of onset in the affected relative is early (before age 55). For example, one recent study showed that

men between the ages of 20 and 39 had a threefold increase in CHD if they had one affected first-degree relative. This risk increased to thirteenfold if there were two first-degree relatives affected with CHD before age 55.

What part do genes play in the familial clustering of heart disease? Because of the key role of lipids in atherosclerosis, many current studies are focusing on the genetic determination of various lipoproteins. Undoubtedly the most important advance in this area has been the isolation and cloning of the gene for the LDL (low-density lipoprotein) receptor defects that cause familial hypercholesterolemia (Clinical Commentary 10-2). More than a dozen other genes involved in lipid metabolism and transport have been mapped to specific chromosome locations, including at least nine genes thus far discovered for various apolipoproteins (these are the protein components of lipoproteins) (Table 10-6 page 200). Mapping and functional analysis of these genes are leading to an increased understanding, and eventually more effective treatment, of CHD.

Family studies of rare forms of heart disease are also providing important information on the genetics of heart disease. For example, various forms of inherited cardiomyopathy have been mapped to the X chromosome, the mitochondrion, and to several autosomes. It is especially interesting that one form of familial hypertrophic cardiomyopathy (FHC) is caused by mutations in the β-myosin heavy chain gene on chromosome 14. These mutations may produce abnormal contractile function. Additional mutations responsible for FHC have been found in the genes encoding myosin binding protein-C, α-tropomyosin, and cardiac troponin T.

In addition, recent studies have mapped genes for the autosomal dominant disorder long QT syndrome (describing the characteristically abnormal electrocardiogram profile) to chromosomes 3, 4, 7, and 11. This disorder predisposes affected individuals to severe ventricular fibrillation that can cause death. Because the disorder is difficult to diagnose accurately, linked markers and mutation analysis will enable more accurate diagnosis of affected family members. Two of the LQT genes encode potassium channels, and a third encodes a sodium channel. All three channels are involved in cardiac repolarization, consistent with the disease phenotype. Identification of the disease-causing genes and their products is now guiding the development of drug therapy to activate these channels.

It should be emphasized that environmental factors, many of which are easily modified, are also

---

10-5 ■ Prevalence data for common adult diseases

Disease	No. of affected Americans (approximate)
Alcoholism	10 million
Alzheimer disease	4 million
Bipolar affective disorder	1 million
Cancer (all types)	6 million
Coronary heart disease	5 million
Diabetes (type I)	1 million
Diabetes (type II)	5–10 million
Epilepsy	2 million
Hypertension	25–30 million
Multiple sclerosis	250,000
Obesity*	50 million
Schizophrenia	2 million

*Defined as 20% or more above ideal body weight.

Clinical Commentary 10-2. Familial Hypercholesterolemia

Autosomal dominant familial hypercholesterolemia (FH) is an important cause of heart disease, accounting for approximately 5% of myocardial infarctions in persons under age 60. FH is one of the most common autosomal dominant disorders: in most populations surveyed to date, about 1 in 500 persons is a heterozygote. Plasma cholesterol levels are approximately twice as high as normal (i.e., about 300 to 400 mg/dl), resulting in substantially accelerated atherosclerosis and the occurrence of distinctive cholesterol deposits in skin and tendons called xanthomas, (Fig. 10-6). Data compiled from five studies showed that approximately 75% of men with FH developed coronary disease, and 50% had a fatal myocardial infarction, by age 60. The corresponding percentages for women were lower (45% and 15%, respectively) because women generally develop heart disease at a later age than men.

Consistent with Hardy-Weinberg predictions, about 1 in 1 million births is homozygous for the FH gene. Homozygotes are much more severely affected, with cholesterol levels ranging from 600 to 1200 mg/dl. Most experience myocardial infarctions prior to age 20, and a myocardial infarction at 18 months of age has been reported. If untreated, most FH homozygotes will die before the age of 30.

All cells require cholesterol as a component of their plasma membrane. They can either synthesize their own cholesterol or preferentially they obtain it from the extracellular environment, where it is carried primarily by low-density lipoprotein (LDL). In a proc-

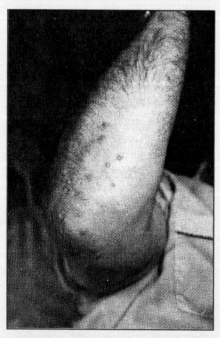

Figure 10-6 ■ Xanthomas (fatty deposits) are often seen in a patient with familial hypercholesterolemia (*SOL* 63, 64).

ess known as **endocytosis**, LDL-bound cholesterol is taken into the cell via LDL receptors on the cell's surface (Fig. 10-7). FH is caused by a reduction in the number of functional LDL receptors on cell surfaces. Lacking the normal number of LDL receptors, cellular cholesterol uptake is reduced, and circulating cholesterol levels increase.

Much of what we know about endocytosis has been learned through the study of LDL receptors. The process of endocytosis and the processing of LDL in the cell are described in detail in Figure 10-7. These processes result in a fine-tuned regulation of cholesterol levels within cells, and they influence the level of circulating cholesterol as well.

The isolation and cloning of the LDL receptor gene in 1984 were a critical step in understanding exactly how LDL receptor defects cause FH. This gene, located on chromosome 19, is 45 kb in length and consists of 18 exons and 17 introns. It encodes a 5.3-kb mRNA transcript that ultimately produces a mature protein of 839 amino acids. More than 150 different mutations, including missense and nonsense substitutions as well as insertions and deletions, have been identified in the LDL receptor gene. These can be grouped into five broad classes, according to their effects on the activity of the receptor. Class I mutations result in no detectable protein product. Thus heterozygotes would produce only half the normal number of LDL receptors. Class II mutations in the LDL receptor gene result in production of the LDL receptor, but it is altered such that it cannot leave the endoplasmic reticulum. It is eventually degraded. Class III mutations produce an LDL receptor that is capable of migrating to the cell surface but incapable of normal binding to LDL. Class IV mutations, which are comparatively rare, produce receptors that are normal except that they do not migrate specifically to coated pits and thus cannot carry LDL into the cell. The final group of mutations, class V, produces an LDL receptor that cannot disassociate from the LDL particle after entry into the cell. The receptor cannot return to the cell surface and is degraded. Each class of mutations reduces the number of effective LDL receptors, resulting in decreased LDL uptake and hence elevated levels of circulating cholesterol. The number of effective receptors is reduced by about half in FH heterozygotes, and homozygotes have virtually no functional LDL receptors.

Understanding the defects that lead to FH has helped to develop effective therapies for the disorder. Dietary reduction of cholesterol (primarily through the reduced intake of saturated fats) has only modest effects on cholesterol levels in FH heterozygotes. Because cholesterol is reabsorbed into the gut and then recycled through the liver (where most cholesterol synthesis takes place), serum cholesterol levels can be reduced by the administration of bile acid-absorbing resins, such as cholestyramine. The absorbed cholesterol is then excreted. Interestingly,

Continued.

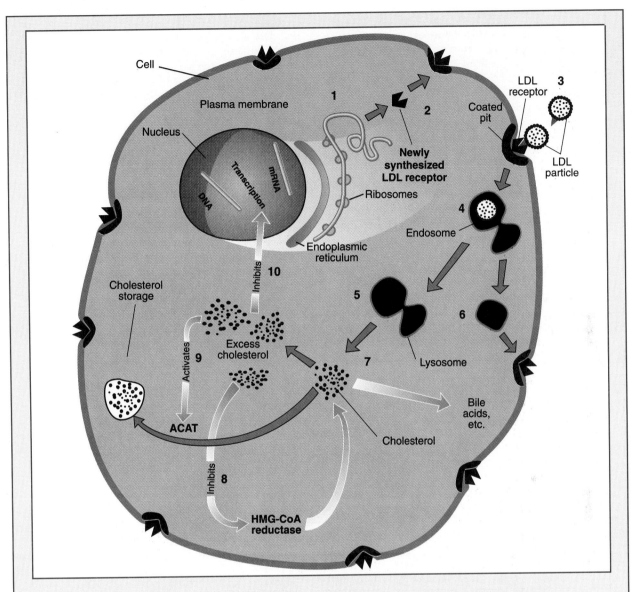

Figure 10-7 ■ The process of receptor-mediated endocytosis. *1,* The LDL receptors, which are glycoproteins, are synthesized in the endoplasmic reticulum of the cell. *2,* From here they pass through the Golgi apparatus to the cell surface, where part of the receptor protrudes outside the cell. *3,* The circulating LDL particle is bound by the LDL receptor and localized in cell-surface depressions called "coated pits" (so named because they are coated with the protein *clathrin*). *4,* The coated pit invaginates, bringing the LDL particle inside the cell. *5,* Once inside the cell, the LDL particle is separated from the receptor, taken into a lysosome, and broken down into its constituents by lysosomal enzymes. *6,* The LDL receptor is recirculated to the cell surface to bind another LDL particle (each LDL receptor goes through this cycle approximately once every 10 minutes even if it is not occupied by an LDL particle). *7,* Free cholesterol is released from the lysosome for incorporation into cell membranes or metabolism into bile acids or steroids. Excess cholesterol can be stored in the cell as a cholesterol ester or removed from the cell by associating with HDL. *8,* As cholesterol levels in the cell rise, cellular cholesterol synthesis is reduced by inhibition of the rate-limiting enzyme, HMG-CoA reductase (3-hydroxy-3-methylglutaryl CoA reductase). *9,* Rising cholesterol levels also increase the activity of acyl-CoA:cholesterol acyltransferase (ACAT), an enzyme that modifies cholesterol for storage as cholesterol esters. *10,* In addition, the number of LDL receptors is decreased by lowering the transcription rate of the LDL receptor gene itself. This decreases cholesterol uptake. (Adapted from Goldstein JL and Brown MS. In Scriver CR, Beaudet AL, Sly WS, and Valle D, editors: The metabolic basis of inherited disease, vol 1, ed 6, New York, 1989, McGraw-Hill.)

Continued.

Clinical Commentary 10-2. Familial Hypercholesterolemia—cont'd

reduced recirculation from the gut causes the liver cells to form additional LDL receptors, lowering circulating cholesterol levels. However, the decrease in intracellular cholesterol also stimulates cholesterol synthesis by liver cells, so the overall reduction in plasma LDL is only about 15% to 20%. This treatment is much more effective when combined with agents such as lovastatin, which reduce cholesterol synthesis by inhibiting HMG-CoA reductase (Fig. 10-7). Decreased synthesis leads to further production of LDL receptors. When these therapies are used in combination, serum cholesterol levels in FH heterozygotes can often be reduced to approximately normal levels.

The picture is less encouraging for FH homozygotes. The therapies mentioned above can enhance cholesterol elimination and reduce its synthesis, but they are largely ineffective in homozygotes because these individuals have few or no LDL receptors. Liver transplants, which provide hepatocytes that have nor-

mal LDL receptors, have been successful in some cases, but this option is often limited by a lack of donors. Plasma exchange, carried out every 1 to 2 weeks, in combination with drug therapy, can reduce cholesterol levels by about 50%. However, this therapy is difficult to continue for long periods of time. Somatic cell gene therapy, in which hepatocytes carrying normal LDL receptor genes are introduced into the portal circulation, is now being tested (see Chapter 11). It may eventually prove to be an effective treatment for FH homozygotes.

The FH story illustrates how medical research has made important contributions both to our understanding of basic cell biology and to advancements in clinical therapy. The process of receptor-mediated endocytosis, elucidated largely by research on the LDL receptor defects, is of fundamental significance for cellular processes throughout the body. Equally, this research, by clarifying how cholesterol synthesis and uptake can be modified, has led to significant improvements in therapy for this important cause of heart disease.

Table 10-6 ■ Single genes known to contribute to coronary heart disease risk*

Gene	Chromosomal location	Function
Apolipoprotein gene		
Apo A-I	11q	HDL formation
Apo A-IV	11q	Unknown
Apo C-III	11q	Unknown
Apo B	2p	Chylomicrons; VLDL, IDL, and LDL formation; ligand for LDL receptor
Apo D	2p	Unknown
Apo C-I	19q	LCAT activation
Apo C-II	19q	Lipoprotein lipase activation
Apo E	19q	Ligand for LDL receptor
Apo A-II	1p	Unknown
Other genes		
Lp(a)	6q	Lp(a) particle formation
LDL receptor	19p	Uptake of LDL particles
Lipoprotein lipase	8p	Hydrolysis of lipoprotein lipids
Hepatic triglyceride lipase	15q	Hydrolysis of lipoprotein lipids
LCAT	16q	Cholesteryl esterification
Cholesterol ester transfer protein	16q	Facilitates transfer of cholesterol esters and phospholipid lipoproteins

*From King RA, Rotter JI, and Motulsky AG, editors: The genetic basis of common diseases, New York, 1992, Oxford University Press.

important causes of CHD. There is abundant epidemiologic evidence that cigarette smoking and obesity increase the risk of CHD, whereas exercise and a diet low in saturated fats decrease the risk. Indeed, the approximate 50% decline in CHD incidence in the United States during the past 40 years is usually attributed to a decrease in the proportion of adults who smoke cigarettes, decreased consumption of saturated fats, and an increased emphasis on exercise and a generally healthier lifestyle.

CHD shows familial aggregation. This aggregation is especially strong if there is early age of onset and if there are multiple affected relatives. Specific genes have been identified for some subsets of CHD families, and lifestyle changes (exercise, diet, avoidance of tobacco) can modify CHD risks appreciably.

Hypertension

Systemic hypertension, which is seen in at least 15% of the populations of most developed countries, is a key risk factor for heart disease, stroke, and kidney disease. Studies of blood pressure correlations within families indicate that the heritability of both systolic and diastolic blood pressure is approximately 20% to 40%. Heritability estimates based upon twin studies tend to be higher (about 60%). This difference may reflect an inflation of the heritability estimate because of greater similarities in the environments of MZ twins. The fact that the heritability estimates are substantially less than 100% indicates that environmental factors must also be important causes of blood pressure variation. The most important environmental risk factors for hypertension are increased sodium intake, decreased physical activity, psychosocial stress, and obesity (but as discussed below, the latter factor is itself influenced both by genes and environment).

Blood pressure regulation is a highly complex process that is influenced by many physiologic systems. These include various aspects of kidney function, cellular ion transport, and heart function. Because of this complexity, it is unlikely that family studies of simple blood pressure will reveal much about genes responsible for hypertension. For this reason most research is now focused on specific components that may influence blood pressure variation, such as angiotensin, angiotensinogen, urinary kallikrein, and sodium–lithium countertransport (Fig. 10-8 and Table 10-7). These factors are more likely to be under the control of smaller numbers of genes. For example, linkage and associ-

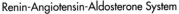

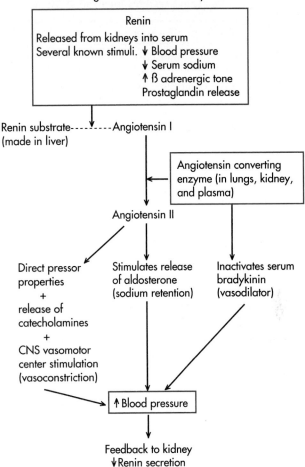

Figure 10-8 ■**The renin-angiotensin-aldosterone system.** (Adapted from King RA, Rotter JI, and Motulsky AG, editors: The genetic basis of common diseases, New York, 1992, Oxford University Press.)

ation studies have recently implicated a gene for angiotensinogen in the causation of both hypertension and preeclampsia (a form of pregnancy-induced hypertension).

The quantitative trait locus method has also been used in attempts to identify hypertension genes. In one application, linkage analysis was undertaken using 181 DNA polymorphisms detected in the offspring of a cross between normal and hypertensive rat strains. Linkage was obtained between hypertension and markers near a gene that is highly similar in DNA sequence to a human gene that encodes the angiotensin-converting enzyme (ACE). This enzyme converts angiotensin I to angiotensin II; the latter functions as a vasoconstrictor (it contracts blood vessels) and is also involved in modulating the excretion of sodium in the kidney. Although it would thus seem a likely candidate as a hypertension gene, most studies indicate no rela-

Table 10-7 ■ Transport systems involved in blood pressure regulation*

Laboratory measurement	Positive findings
Sodium–potassium cotransport (red cells)	Decreased in hypertensives and their children Abnormality found in both white and black subjects
Sodium–lithium countertransport (red cells)	Increased in hypertensives and their first-degree relatives Abnormality rare or absent in black hypertensives No consistent correlation with cotransport abnormalities
Na$^+$, K$^+$–ATPase (white cells)	Decreased sodium excretion in hypertensives and their relatives Humeral inhibitor present in sera from hypertensives

*From King RA, Rotter JI, and Motulsky AG, editors: The genetic basis of common diseases, New York, 1992, Oxford University Press.

tionship between variation in the ACE gene and hypertension in human populations. However, there is evidence that mutations in the ACE gene increase susceptibility to myocardial infarction through mechanisms that are as yet unknown.

Heritability estimates for systolic and diastolic blood pressure range from 20% to 40%. Several genes influencing blood pressure variation have been pinpointed in the human. Other risk factors for hypertension include sodium intake, lack of exercise, psychosocial stress, and obesity.

Cancer

Cancer is the second leading cause of death in the United States, although it is estimated that cancer will surpass heart disease as the leading killer by the year 2000. It is well established that many major types of cancer (e.g., breast, colon, prostate, ovarian) cluster strongly in families. This is due both to shared genes as well as shared environmental factors. While numerous cancer genes are being isolated, environmental factors also play an important role in causing cancer. In particular, tobacco use is estimated to account for one third of all cancer cases in the United States, making it the most important known cause of cancer. Because cancer genetics is the subject of Chapter 9, we confine our attention to several specific examples in which cancer genes have been isolated.

Breast Cancer. Breast cancer is the most common cancer among women, affecting approximately 11% of American women at some time during their lives. It was formerly the leading cause of cancer death among women, but it has recently been surpassed by lung cancer. Breast cancer aggregates strongly in families. If a woman has one affected first-degree relative, her risk of developing breast cancer doubles. This risk increases if the age of onset in the affected relative is early and if the

cancer is bilateral (tumors in both breasts). A recent study indicated that the risk of developing breast cancer climbs to 54% among women who have two first-degree relatives affected with breast cancer before age 55.

It is estimated that an autosomal dominant form of breast cancer accounts for approximately 5% of breast cancer cases in the United States. Genes responsible for this form of breast cancer have been mapped to chromosomes 17 (*BRCA1*) and 13 (*BRCA2*). Each of these genes has now been cloned. *BRCA1* mutations are also associated with an increased risk of ovarian cancer. Cloning of these genes and identification of disease-causing mutations may lead to early diagnosis of breast cancer, and the evaluation of these genes' protein products will yield valuable evidence on the etiology of breast cancer in general.

Colon Cancer. Colorectal cancer is second only to lung cancer in the number of cases occurring annually in the United States, with 155,000 new cases in 1990. Like breast cancer, it clusters in families (familial clustering of this form of cancer was reported in the medical literature as early as 1881). The risk of colorectal cancer in people with one affected first-degree relative is two to three times higher than in the general population.

This familial aggregation is caused in part by subsets of colon cancer cases that are inherited as single-gene traits. Familial adenomatous polyposis occurs in approximately 1 in 8000 whites. The gene responsible for this disorder was mapped to chromosome 5 several years ago, and the gene itself was subsequently cloned. Cloning of this gene and the study of the probable function of its product have provided important new information on the molecular basis of this disorder (see Chapter 9 for further discussion).

Hereditary nonpolyposis colorectal cancer, which may account for up to 5% of colon cancer cases, is caused by autosomal dominant genes mapped to chromosomes 2 and 3. As discussed in Chapter 9, these genes play a role in correcting DNA mismatches.

Other colon cancer cases are likely to be caused by a complex interaction of multiple genes. In addition, environmental factors, such as a high-fat, low-fiber diet, are likely to increase the risk of colorectal cancer.

Other Cancers. We have previously discussed the genetic basis of various other cancers, including Wilms tumor, chronic myelogenous leukemia, and retinoblastoma. Although each of these cancers is relatively rare, the study of the causative genes has provided many important insights on the nature of carcinogenesis in general. This will lead to more effective treatment and prevention of all cancers.

Most common cancers have genetic components. Recurrence risks tend to be higher when the proband has developed cancer at an early age. Specific genes have been discovered that cause colon and breast cancer in some families.

Diabetes Mellitus

A prominent geneticist once described diabetes as "the geneticist's nightmare." Like the other disorders discussed in this chapter, the etiology of diabetes mellitus is complex and not fully understood. Nevertheless, progress is being made in understanding the genetic basis of this disorder, which is a leading cause of blindness, heart disease, and kidney failure (*SOL* 83, 84). An important advance has been the recognition that diabetes is actually a heterogeneous group of disorders, all characterized by elevated blood sugar. We focus here on the two major types of diabetes, type I (insulin dependent diabetes mellitus, IDDM) and type II (non–insulin-dependent diabetes mellitus, NIDDM).

Type I Diabetes. This form of diabetes, which is characterized by T-cell infiltration of the pancreas and destruction of the insulin-producing β cells, usually (though not always) presents before age 40. Patients with type I diabetes must receive exogenous insulin to survive. The pathology of the disorder, together with the common finding of antibodies against pancreatic β cells and a strong association with several HLA class II alleles, suggests that type I diabetes is an autoimmune disorder. Siblings of individuals with type I diabetes face a substantial elevation in risk: approximately 6% as opposed to a risk of about 0.3% to 0.5% in the general population. Although the sexes are affected

in almost equal proportions (there is a slight excess of males), recurrence risks for offspring vary substantially with the sex of the parent. The risk to offspring of diabetic mothers is only 1% to 3%, while it is 4% to 6% for the offspring of diabetic fathers (note that this is inconsistent with the sex-specific threshold model for multifactorial traits). Twin studies show that the empirical risks for identical twins of type I diabetes patients range from 30% to 50%. The fact that type I diabetes is not 100% concordant among identical twins indicates that genetic factors are not solely responsible for the disorder. There is good evidence that viral infections, for example, contribute to the causation of type I diabetes in at least some individuals.

The association of specific HLA class II alleles and type I diabetes has been studied intensively. Approximately 95% of whites with type I diabetes have the HLA-DR3 and/or DR4 alleles, whereas only about 50% of the general white population has either of these alleles. If an affected proband and a sibling are both heterozygous for the DR3 and DR4 alleles, the sibling's risk of developing type I diabetes is nearly 20% (i.e., about 40 times higher than the risk in the general population). One study showed that the presence of aspartic acid at position 57 of the HLA-DQ$_\beta$ chain is strongly associated with resistance to type I diabetes. Those who have this amino acid at position 57 are 100 times less likely to develop the disease than are individuals homozygous for other amino acids (alanine, serine, or valine). It is probable that this particular amino acid is involved in T-cell recognition and that those who lack it are more likely to suffer an autoimmune episode.

The quantitative trait locus approach has been used to isolate candidate genes for type I diabetes. The nonobese diabetic (NOD) mouse strain was crossed with a normal strain to produce unaffected and diabetic progeny. Linkage analysis was performed using a battery of 61 DNA polymorphisms (including 53 VNTR loci). This procedure revealed two susceptibility loci in the NOD mouse. Further studies, using numerous microsatellite repeat polymorphisms, have revealed at least 12 different loci in the NOD mouse that appear to contribute to type I diabetes susceptibility. These are possible candidates for type I diabetes susceptibility in the human, and their further study may aid in understanding this disorder.

The insulin gene itself, which is located on the short arm of chromosome 11, is another logical candidate for type I diabetes susceptibility. Polymorphisms in and around the insulin gene have been studied extensively, and alleles of some of these polymorphisms are associated with susceptibility to type I diabetes. Recall from Chapter 7 that such associations in populations can be due to direct causation or to linkage disequilibrium between a polymorphism and a causal gene. These associations are not strict: not everybody who carries a given allele will develop type I diabetes. This is expected, given the many other factors, both genetic and nongenetic, that appear to be involved in causing this disease.

Type II Diabetes. Type II diabetes accounts for 80% to 90% of all diabetes cases in the United States. A number of features distinguish it from type I diabetes. Unlike type I diabetes, there is nearly always some endogenous insulin production in persons with type II diabetes, and it can often be treated successfully with dietary modification and/or oral drugs. Type II diabetes patients also suffer from insulin resistance (i.e., their bodies have difficulty in using the insulin they produce). This disease typically occurs among people over age 40 and, in contrast to type I diabetes, is seen more commonly among the obese. Neither HLA associations nor autoantibodies are seen commonly in this form of diabetes. Monozygotic twin concordance rates are substantially higher than in type I diabetes, often exceeding 90% (because of age dependence, the concordance rate increases if older subjects are studied). The empirical recurrence risks for first-degree relatives of type II diabetes cases are higher than those for type I, generally ranging from 10% to 15%. The differences between type I and type II diabetes are summarized in Table 10-8.

Despite the apparently high degree of genetic involvement in type II diabetes, specific genes for this disorder have not yet been identified. The insulin and insulin receptor genes have both been studied, but it appears unlikely that defects in either gene are responsible for a substantial portion of disease cases.

The two most important risk factors for type II diabetes are positive family history and obesity; the latter increases insulin resistance. The disease tends to rise in prevalence when populations adopt a diet and exercise pattern typical of United States and European populations. Increases have been seen, for example, among Japanese immigrants to the United States and among some native populations of the South Pacific, Australia, and the Americas. Several studies, conducted on both male and female subjects, have shown that regular exercise can substantially lower one's risk of developing type II diabetes, even among individuals with a family history of the disease. This is partly because exercise reduces obesity. However, even in the absence of weight loss, exercise increases insulin sensitivity and improves glucose tolerance.

A small proportion of type II diabetes cases manifest the disease early in life, typically before 25 years of age. This subset, termed "maturity onset diabetes of the young" (MODY), can be inherited as an autosomal dominant trait. Studies of MODY pedigrees have shown that some cases of the disease are caused by mutations in the glucokinase gene. Glucokinase converts glucose to glucose-6-phosphate in the pancreas. The possible role of glucokinase in late-onset type II diabetes is also being explored.

Type I (insulin-dependent) and type II (non–insulin-dependent) diabetes both cluster in families, with stronger familial clustering observed for type II diabetes. Type I has an earlier average age of onset, is HLA-associated, and is an autoimmune disease. Type II is not an autoimmune disorder and is more likely to be seen in obese individuals. Some cases of MODY, a subset of type II diabetes, are caused by mutations of the glucokinase gene.

Table 10-8 ■ A comparison of the major features of type I and type II diabetes mellitus

Feature	Type I diabetes	Type II diabetes
Age of onset	Usually <40 yr	Usually >40 yr (except MODY)
Insulin production	None	Partial
Insulin resistance	No	Yes
Autoimmunity	Yes	No
Obesity	Not common	Common
MZ twin concordance	0.55	0.90
Sibling recurrence risk	1%–6%	10%–15%

Obesity

Obesity is often defined as a body weight exceeding 20% of the upper limit of the normal range. Using this criterion approximately 20% of American adults are obese. The body mass index [BMI, defined as weight (kg) divided by height (m) squared] is also used as a measure of obesity. Using the criterion that a BMI above 30 kg/m² indicates obesity, 12% of American adults are obese (one of the highest percentages in the world). Although obesity itself is perhaps not a "disease," it is an important risk factor for several common diseases, including heart disease, stroke, and type II diabetes.

As one might expect, there is a strong correlation between obesity in parents and their children. This could easily be ascribed to common environmental effects: parents and children usually share similar dietary and exercise habits. Indeed, it may seem that obesity should be influenced almost exclusively by environmental factors. However, there is good evidence for genetic components as well. Four different adoption studies each showed that the body weights of adopted individuals correlated significantly with their natural parents' body weights but not with those of their adoptive parents. Twin studies also provide evidence for a genetic effect on body weight, with most studies yielding heritability estimates between 0.60 and 0.80. Statistical analyses of family data have shown that there may be major genes, as well as polygenic effects, associated with obesity. A gene that encodes leptin, a protein involved in appetite regulation, has been cloned in mice and humans. A leptin receptor gene has also been cloned.

Adoption and twin studies indicate that at least half of the population variation in obesity may be caused by genes.

Alzheimer Disease

It is estimated that Alzheimer disease (AD) affects approximately 10% of Americans over age 65 and up to half of those over age 85. The annual cost of caring for AD patients is at least $25 billion. This disorder is characterized by progressive dementia and loss of memory and by the formation of amyloid plaques and neurofibrillary tangles in the brain, particularly in the cerebral cortex and hippocampus (*SOL* 54-56). Death usually occurs within 5 to 10 years after the first appearance of symptoms. Individuals with an affected first-degree relative have, on average, a 10% chance of developing the disorder; however, because of the age dependence and heterogeneity of AD, this value is approximate. Whereas most cases of AD do not appear to be

caused by single loci, 5% to 15% follow an autosomal dominant mode of transmission. Early-onset AD (before age 65) accounts for about 25% of AD cases and is much more likely to be inherited in autosomal dominant fashion.

AD is a genetically heterogeneous disorder. Genes for early-onset disease map to chromosomes 1 and 14, and these two genes encode highly similar protein products. Mutations of the amyloid precursor protein gene, on chromosome 21 have also been shown to cause AD in a small minority of patients. In addition, some cases of the more common late-onset form may be linked to the region on chromosome 19 that contains the apolipoprotein E (*APOE*) locus. One study showed that, among individuals who are members of late-onset AD families, those who inherit two copies of the $\epsilon4$ allele of the *APOE* locus had a 90% chance of developing the disease by age 75. Those who inherited one copy of $\epsilon4$ had a 45% chance, and those who inherited no copies of the allele had only a 20% chance of developing AD (note that, because the study population consisted of families with multiple affected members, the risk estimates for these genotypes do not necessarily apply to the general population). This association is especially interesting because the *APOE-$\epsilon4$* protein product binds more rapidly to amyloid than does the product of the more common allele, *APOE-$\epsilon3$*.

AD has several features that make it especially refractory to genetic analysis. Its genetic heterogeneity has already been described. In addition, because a definitive diagnosis can only be obtained by a brain autopsy, it is not possible to diagnose living family members with certainty (although clinical features and brain imaging techniques can provide strong evidence that an individual is affected with AD). Finally, because the age of onset can be very late, individuals carrying a gene for AD could die of another cause before developing the disease. They would then be misdiagnosed as noncarriers. These types of difficulties arise not only in studying AD but in many other common adult diseases as well. In spite of these difficulties, further studies of the genes linked to AD will shed light not only on the most common cause of dementia among the elderly but also on the aging process in general.

Approximately 5% to 15% of AD cases are caused by autosomal dominant genes. Early-onset cases cluster more strongly in families and are more likely to follow an autosomal dominant inheritance pattern. This disease is genetically heterogeneous: linkage studies have mapped AD genes to chromosomes 1, 14, 19, and 21.

Alcoholism

At some point in their lives, alcoholism is diagnosed in approximately 10% of adult males and 3% to 5% of adult females in America. The national cost of alcoholism, in terms of lost productivity and direct medical costs, exceeds $100 billion per year. More than 100 studies have shown that this disease clusters in families. The risk of developing alcoholism among individuals with one affected parent is 3 to 5 times higher than for those with unaffected parents. Most twin studies have yielded concordance rates for DZ twins less than 30% and concordance rates for MZ twins in excess of 60%. Adoption studies have shown that the offspring of an alcoholic parent, even when raised by nonalcoholic parents, have a fourfold increased risk of developing the disorder. To control for possible prenatal effects in an alcoholic mother, some studies have included only the offspring of alcoholic fathers. The results have remained the same. Intriguingly, one study showed that the offspring of nonalcoholic parents, when reared by alcoholics, did *not* have an increased risk of developing alcoholism. These data argue that there may be genes that predispose some people to alcoholism.

Some researchers distinguish two major subtypes of alcoholism. Type I is characterized by a later age of onset (after age 25), occurrence in both males and females, and greater psychologic dependency upon alcohol. Type I alcoholics are more likely to be introverted, solitary drinkers. This form of alcoholism is less likely to cluster in families (one study yielded a heritability estimate of 0.21), has a less severe course, and is more easily treated. Type II alcoholism is seen predominantly in males, typically occurs before age 25, and tends to involve individuals who are extroverted and thrill-seeking. This form is more difficult to treat successfully and tends to cluster much more strongly in families, with one study obtaining a heritability estimate of 0.88.

Published studies have shown an association between alcoholism and a DNA polymorphism linked to the dopamine D2 receptor gene on chromosome 11. Because the dopamine receptors are part of the brain's reward pathway, this association has some intuitive appeal. However, seven additional studies in other populations have failed to replicate the association. The inability to replicate this finding reflects some of the difficulties encountered in population association studies (see Chapter 7). It now appears unlikely that this polymorphism contributes importantly to alcoholism susceptibility. Nevertheless, the twin and adoption studies mentioned above are compelling, and it is possible that further studies may reveal genes that do in fact influence susceptibility to this important disease.

It should be underscored that we refer to genes that may increase one's *susceptibility* to alcoholism. This is obviously a disease that requires an environmental component. Regardless of genetic constitution, someone who never consumes alcohol cannot become an alcoholic.

> **Twin and adoption studies show that alcoholism clusters strongly in families, reflecting a possible genetic contribution to this disease. Familial clustering is particularly strong for type II alcoholism (early onset form primarily affecting males).**

Psychiatric Disorders

The major psychiatric diseases, schizophrenia and affective disorder, have both been the subjects of numerous genetic studies. Twin, adoption, and family studies have shown that both disorders aggregate in families.

Schizophrenia. Schizophrenia is a severe emotional disorder characterized by delusions, hallucinations, retreat from reality, and bizarre, withdrawn, or inappropriate behavior (contrary to popular belief, schizophrenia is not a "split personality" disorder). The lifetime recurrence risk for schizophrenia among the offspring of one affected parent is approximately 8% to 10%, which is about 10 times higher than the risk in the general population. As one might expect, the empirical risks increase when more relatives are affected. For example, an individual with an affected sibling and an affected parent has a risk of about 17%, and an individual with two affected parents has a risk of 40-50%. The risks decrease when the affected family member is a second- or third-degree relative. Details are given in Table 10-9. On inspection of this table, it may seem puzzling that the proportion of schizophrenic probands who have a schizophrenic parent is only about 5%, which is substantially lower than the risk for other first-degree relatives (e.g., siblings, affected parents and their offspring). This can be explained by the fact that schizophrenics are less likely to marry and produce children than are other individuals. There is thus substantial selection against schizophrenia in the population.

Twin and adoption studies indicate that genetic factors are likely to be involved in schizophrenia. Data pooled from five different twin studies show a 47% concordance rate for MZ twins, compared

Table 10-9 ▪ Recurrence risk for relatives of schizophrenic probands*

Relationship to proband	Recurrence risk (%)
Monozygotic twin	44.3
Dizygotic twin	12.1
Offspring	9.4
Sibling	7.3
Niece/nephew	2.7
Grandchild	2.8
First cousin	1.6
Spouse	1.0

*Adapted from McGue et al: Behav Genet 16:75–87, 1986. Data are based on multiple studies of Western European populations.

with a concordance rate of only 12% for DZ twins. When the offspring of a schizophrenic parent are adopted by normal parents, their risk of developing the disease is about 10%, which is approximately the same as the risk when raised by a schizophrenic biologic parent.

A study reported several years ago showed significant linkage between schizophrenia and a marker on chromosome 5. However, despite numerous attempts, this result has not been replicated in other populations. More recently, strong evidence has been obtained for a schizophronia susceptibility locus on chromosome 6.

Bipolar Affective Disorder. Bipolar affective disorder, also known as manic-depressive disorder, is a form of psychosis in which extreme mood swings and emotional instability are seen. The prevalence of the disorder in the general population is approximately 0.5%, but it rises to 5% to 10% among those with an affected first-degree relative. A study based upon the Danish twin registry yielded concordance rates of 79% and 24% for MZ and DZ twins, respectively. The corresponding concordance rates for unipolar disorder (major depression) were 54% and 19%. In general, it appears that bipolar disorder is more strongly influenced by genetic factors than is unipolar disorder.

Considerable excitement was generated by a report linking bipolar affective disorder to a polymorphism on chromosome 11p. This study examined a series of Old Order Amish families in which the disorder is transmitted in autosomal dominant fashion. Linkage analysis initially yielded a LOD score (see Chapter 7) of 4.0. However, the result was later reversed with the addition of another branch of the pedigree and when two initially unaffected family members, who did not carry the

marker allele segregating with the disorder, subsequently developed the disorder. This demonstrates the sensitivity of linkage analysis to changes in disease status. Many additional families have been studied since, and the LOD score is now approximately −9.0 (i.e., the odds are 1 billion to one *against* linkage to the chromosome 11 marker).

Comments on Psychiatric Disorders. Large-scale linkage studies involving hundreds of polymorphisms throughout the genome have now been carried out for both schizophrenia and bipolar affective disorder. Most of these studies have produced negative results, although a few recent large-scale studies have yielded promising findings. A number of candidate genes have been tested for linkage or association with both diseases. Most of these candidates were chosen on the basis of the known involvement of certain neurotransmitters, receptors, or neurotransmitter-related enzymes in each disease (e.g., schizophrenia can be treated by drugs that block dopamine receptors, and bipolar affective disorder is sometimes treated with lithium). None of the candidate genes tested thus far, including those for sodium–lithium countertransport, various components of the dopaminergic system, and several neurotransmitter-related enzymes (such as monoamine oxidase, dopamine-β-hydroxylase, and tyrosine hydroxylase), has been shown unequivocally to be linked or associated with either disease.

These results reflect some of the difficulties encountered in doing genetic studies of psychiatric disorders. These disorders are undoubtedly heterogeneous, reflecting the influence of numerous genetic and environmental factors. Also definition of the phenotype is not always straightforward, and it may change through time. As the bipolar affective disorder linkage story shows, this can be critical.

Marked familial aggregation has been observed for schizophrenia and bipolar affective disorder. Genes for neurotransmitters, receptors, and neurotransmitter-related enzymes have been studied in families, and linkage studies with hundreds of random markers have been carried out.

Some General Principles and Conclusions

Some general principles can be deduced from the results obtained thus far on the genetics of complex disorders. First, the more strongly inherited forms of complex disorders generally have an earlier age of onset (examples include breast cancer, Alzheimer disease, and heart disease). Often these represent subsets of cases in which there is single-gene inheritance. Second, when there is laterality, the bilateral forms are more likely to cluster strongly in families (e.g., breast cancer, cleft lip/palate). Third, while the sex-specific threshold model fits some of the complex disorders (e.g., pyloric stenosis, cleft lip/palate, autism, heart disease), it fails to fit others (e.g., type I diabetes).

There is a tendency, particularly among the lay public, to assume that the presence of a genetic component means that the course of a disease cannot be altered (''if it's genetic, you can't change it''). This is incorrect. Most of the diseases discussed in this chapter have both genetic and environmental components. Thus environmental modification (e.g., diet, exercise, stress reduction) can often reduce risk significantly. Such modification may be especially important for individuals with a family history of a disease because they are likely to develop the disease earlier in life. Those with a family history of heart disease, for example, can often add many years of productive living with relatively minor lifestyle alterations. By targeting those who can benefit most from intervention, genetics helps to serve the goal of preventive medicine.

In addition, it should be stressed that the identification of a specific genetic lesion can lead to more effective prevention and treatment of the disease. Identification of mutations causing autosomal dominant breast cancer may enable early screening and prevention of metastasis. Pinpointing a gene responsible for a neurotransmitter defect in a behavioral disorder, such as schizophrenia, could lead to the development of more effective drug treatments. In some cases, such as familial hypercholesterolemia, gene therapy may be useful. It is important for health care practitioners to make their patients aware of these facts.

Although the genetics of common disorders is complex and often confusing, the public health impact of these diseases and the evidence for hereditary factors in their etiology demand that genetic studies be pursued. Substantial progress is already being made. The next decade will undoubtedly witness many further advancements in our understanding and treatment of these disorders.

■ STUDY QUESTIONS

1. Consider a multifactorial trait that is twice as common in females as in males. Indicate which type of mating is at higher risk for producing affected children (affected father and normal mother vs. normal father and affected mother). Is the recurrence risk higher for their *sons* or their *daughters*?

2. Consider a disease that is known to have a 5% sibling recurrence risk. This recurrence risk could be either the result of multifactorial inheritance or a single autosomal dominant gene with 10% penetrance. How would you test which of these possibilities is correct?

3. One member of a pair of monozygotic twins is affected by an autosomal dominant disease, whereas the other member of the pair is not. List two different ways in which this could happen.

4. Suppose that the heritability of body fat is 0.80 when correlations between siblings are studied, but it is only 0.50 when correlations between parents and offspring are studied. Suppose also that a significant positive correlation is observed in the body fat measurements of spouses. How would you interpret these results?

■ ADDITIONAL READING

Atkinson MA, Maclaren NK: The pathogenesis of insulin-dependent diabetes mellitus, N Eng J Med 331:1428–1436, 1994.

Bishop DT: Multifactorial inheritance. In Emery AEH and Rimoin DL, editors: Principles and practice of medical genetics, vol 1, ed 2, Edinburgh, 1990, Churchill Livingstone.

Bouchard TJ, Lykken DT, McGue M, et al: Sources of human psychological differences: the Minnesota study of twins reared apart, Science 258:223–228, 1990.

Carpenter WT, Buchanan RW: Schizophrenia. N Eng J Med 330:681–690, 1994.

Cavalli-Sforza LL and Bodmer WF: The genetics of human populations, San Francisco, 1971, WH Freeman.

Cordell HJ, Todd JA: Multifactorial inheritance in type 1 diabetes, Trends Genet 11:499–504, 1995.

Czeizel AE and Dudás I: Prevention of the first occurrence of neural-tube defects by periconceptional vitamin supplementation, N Engl J Med 327:1832–1835, 1992.

Daly LE, Kirke PN, Molloy A, Weir DG, Scott JM: Folate levels and neural tube defects: implications for prevention, JAMA 274:1698–1702, 1995.

Devor EJ and Cloninger CR: Genetics of alcoholism, Annu Rev Genet 23:19–36, 1989.

Dewji NN, Singer SJ: Genetic clues to Alzheimer's disease, Science 271:159–160, 1996.

Fraser FC: Evolution of a palatable multifactorial threshold model, Am J Hum Genet 32:796–813, 1980.

Futreal PA, Liu Q, Shattuck-Eidens D, Cochran C, Harshman K, Tavtigian S, Bennett LM, et al.: BRCA1 mutations in primary breast and ovarian carcinomas, Science 266:120–122, 1994.

Gelernter J, Goldman D, and Risch N: The A1 allele at the D_2 dopamine receptor gene and alcoholism: a reappraisal, JAMA 269:1673–1677, 1993.

Goldstein JL and Brown MS: Familial hypercholesterolemia. In Scriver CR, Beaudet AL, Sly WS, and Valle D, editors: The metabolic basis of inherited disease, vol 1, ed 7, New York, 1995, McGraw-Hill.

Groden J, Thliveris A, Samowitz W, et al: Identification and characterization of the familial adenomatous polyposis coli gene, Cell 66:589–600, 1991.

Hall JG, Friedman JM, Kenna BA, et al: Clinical, genetic, and epidemiological factors in neural tube defects, Am J Hum Genet 43:827–837, 1988.

Hobbs HH, Brown MS, and Goldstein JL: Molecular genetics of the LDL receptor gene in familial hypercholesterolemia, Hum Mutation 1:445–466, 1992.

Kelly DP, Strauss AW: Inherited cardiomyopathies. N Eng J Med 330:913–919, 1994.

King RA, Rotter JI, Motulsky AG, editors: The genetic basis of common diseases, New York, 1992, Oxford University Press.

Lander ES, Schork NJ: Genetic dissection of complex traits, Science 265:2037–2048, 1994.

Levy-Lahad E, Wasco W. Poorkaj P, Romano DM, Oshima J, Pettingell WH, Yu C, et al.: Candidate gene for the chromosome 1 familial Alzheimer's disease locus, Science 269:973–977, 1995.

Lifton RP: Genetic determinants of human hypertension, Proc Natl Acad Sci USA 92:8545–8551, 1995.

McInnes LA, Freimer NB: Mapping genes for psychiatric disorders and behavioral traits, Curr Opin Genet Dev 5:376–381, 1995.

Neale MC and Cardon LR: Methodology for genetic studies of twins and families, Dordrecht, The Netherlands, 1992, Kluwer Academic Publishers.

Peltomäki P, Aaltonen LA, Sistonen P, et al: Genetic mapping of a locus predisposing to human colorectal cancer, Science 260:810–812, 1993.

Pericak-Vance MA, Haines JL: Genetic susceptibility to Alzheimer disease, Trends Genet 11:504–508, 1995.

Plomin R: The role of inheritance in behavior, Science 248:183–188, 1990.

Plomin R, Owen MJ, McGuffin P: The genetic basis of complex behaviors. Science 264:1733–1739, 1994.

Rohner-Jeanrenaud F, Jeanrenaud B: Obesity, leptin, and the brain, N Eng J Med 334:324–325, 1996.

Roses AD: Apolipoprotein E and Alzheimer disease, Scientific American Science and Medicine 2:16–25, 1995.

Rubin EM, Smith DJ: Atherosclerosis in mice: getting to the heart of a polygenic disorder, Trends Genet 10:199–203, 1994.

Steel KP, Brown SDM: Genes and deafness, Trends Genet 10:428–435, 1994.

Stratton MR, Wooster R: Hereditary predisposition to breast cancer, Curr Opin Genet Dev 6:93–97, 1996.

Straub RE, MacLean CJ, O'Neill A, Burke J, Murphy B, Duke F, Shinkwin R, et al.: A potential vulnerability locus for schizophrenia on chromosome 6p24–22: evidence for genetic heterogeneity, Nature Genet 11:287–293, 1995.

Szabo CI, King M-C: Inherited breast and ovarian cancer, Hum Molec Genet 4:1811–1817, 1995.

Weissman SM: Genetic bases for common polygenic diseases, Proc Natl Acad Sci USA 92:8543–8544, 1995.

Wooster R, Bignell G, Lancaster J, Swift S, Seal S, Mangion J, Collins N, et al.: Identification of the breast cancer susceptibility gene BRCA2, Nature 378:789–792, 1995.

Zhang Y, Proenca R, Maffei M, Barone M, Leopold L, Friedman JM: Positional cloning of the mouse obese gene and its human homologue, Nature 372:425–432, 1994.

11 Genetic Screening, Genetic Diagnosis, and Gene Therapy

As we have seen in previous chapters, significant advances have occurred in DNA technology, gene mapping, cytogenetics, and many other areas of medical genetics. These developments have paved the way for more accurate and efficient diagnoses of genetic disorders. In particular, population screening and prenatal diagnosis of genetic disorders are becoming increasingly widespread. The principles and application of genetic diagnosis in these contexts are one focus of this chapter.

Another focus is the treatment of genetic disease. Many aspects of disease management involve areas of medicine, such as surgery and drug treatment, that are beyond the scope of this book. However, gene therapy, in which normal genes are placed in the cells of patients to combat specific diseases, falls well within the purview of this text and will be discussed in some detail.

■ POPULATION SCREENING FOR GENETIC DISEASE

Screening tests represent an important component of routine health care. These tests are usually designed to detect treatable human diseases in their presymptomatic stage. Pap tests for the recognition of cervical dysplasia and population screening for hypercholesterolemia are well-known examples of this public health strategy. **Population screening** has been defined as "the presumptive identification of an unrecognized disease or defect by the application of tests, examinations, or other procedures which can be applied rapidly to sort out apparently well persons who *probably* have a disease from those who *probably do not*" (Mausner and Bahn, 1974). Screening tests are not intended to provide definitive diagnoses but rather are aimed at identifying a subset of the population on whom further diagnostic tests should be carried out.

Genetic screening is defined as the "search in a population for persons possessing certain geno-

types that: (1) are already associated with disease or predisposition to disease or (2) may lead to disease in their descendants." (National Academy of Sciences, 1975) Newborn screening for inherited metabolic diseases is a good example of the first type of genetic screening, and heterozygote detection for Tay-Sachs disease (discussed below) exemplifies the second. While these two examples involve screening of populations, genetic screening can also be applied to members of families that have a positive history of a genetic condition. An example would be testing for a balanced reciprocal translocation in families in which one or more members have had a chromosome disorder (see Chapter 6). Box 11-1 lists the various types of genetic screening, including several forms of prenatal diagnosis, that are discussed in this chapter.

> The goal of screening is early recognition of a disorder so that intervention will prevent or reverse the disease process (as in newborn screening for inborn errors of metabolism) or so that informed reproductive decisions can be made (as in the prenatal diagnosis of congenital malformations).

Principles of Screening

The basic principles of screening were developed in the 1960s and are still widely applied. The following points should be considered when deciding whether population screening is appropriate:

1. *Disease characteristics.* The condition should be serious and relatively common. This ensures that sufficient benefits will be derived from the screening program to justify its costs. The natural history of the disease should be clearly understood. There should be an acceptable and effective treatment or, in the case of some genetic conditions, prenatal diagnosis should be available.

Box 11-1. Genetic screening and prenatal diagnosis

I. Population screening of genetic disorders
   A. Newborn screening
      1. Blood
         a. PKU, all 50 states in the United States
         b. Galactosemia, all 50 states in the Unites States
         c. Hypothyroidism, 45 of 50 states in the United States
         d. Other: hemoglobinopathies, cystic fibrosis
      2. Urine: aminoacidopathies
   B. Heterozygote screening
      1. Tay-Sachs disease, Ashkenazi Jewish population
      2. Sickle cell disease, African-American population
      3. Thalassemias, at-risk ethnic groups
      4. Cystic fibrosis, pilot programs only
II. Prenatal diagnosis of genetic disorders
   A. Diagnostic testing (invasive prenatal diagnosis)
      1. Amniocentesis
      2. Chorionic villus sampling
      3. Percutaneous umbilical blood sampling (PUBS)
   B. Fetal visualization techniques
      1. Ultrasonography
      2. Radiography
   C. Population screening
      1. Maternal age > 35 years
      2. Family history of condition diagnosable by prenatal techniques
      3. Abnormal maternal serum α-feto-protein
      4. Triple screen: maternal serum α-feto-protein, estriol, human chorionic gonadotropin
III. Family screening of genetic disorders
   A. Family history of chromosomal rearrangement (e.g., translocation)
   B. Screening female relatives in an X-linked pedigree (e.g., Duchenne muscular dystrophy, fragile X syndrome)
   C. Heterozygote screening within at-risk families (e.g., cystic fibrosis)
   D. Presymptomatic screening (e.g. Huntington disease, breast cancer, colon cancer)

---

2. *Test characteristics.* The screening test should be acceptable to the population, easy to perform, and relatively inexpensive. The screening test should be valid and reliable.
3. *System characteristics.* The resources for diagnosis and treatment of the disorder must be

accessible. A strategy for communicating results efficiently and effectively must be in place.

As summarized in Clinical Commentary 11-1, the phenylketonuria (PKU) screening program meets these criteria quite well.

Screening programs typically use tests that are widely applicable and inexpensive in order to identify an at-risk population. Members of this population are then targeted for subsequent tests that are more accurate but also more expensive and time-consuming. In this context, the **validity** of a screening test deserves emphasis. Validity refers to the ability of a test to separate individuals who have the disease from those who do not. It involves two components: sensitivity and specificity. **Sensitivity** is defined as the ability to correctly identify those with the disease. It is measured as the proportion of affected individuals in whom the test is positive (i.e., **true positives**). **Specificity** is the ability to correctly identify those without the disease. It is measured as the proportion of unaffected individuals in whom the test is negative (i.e., the **true-negative** rate). Sensitivity and specificity are determined by comparing the screening results with those of a definitive diagnostic test (Table 11-1).

Screening tests are seldom, if ever, 100% sensitive and 100% specific. This is because the range of test values in the disease population overlaps that of the unaffected population (Fig. 11-1). Thus, a screening test (as opposed to the definitive follow-up diagnostic test) will diagnose some members of the population incorrectly. Usually a cutoff for separating the diseased and nondiseased portions of the population is designated. A balance exists between the impact of nondetection or low sensitivity (i.e., an increased **false-negative** rate) versus low specificity (an increased **false-positive** rate). If the penalty for missing affected individuals is high (as in untreated PKU), then the cutoff level

---

Table 11-1 ▪ Definitions of sensitivity and specificity*

Screening test	Disease state	
	Affected	Unaffected
Test positive (+)	a (true positive)	b (false positive)
Test negative (−)	c (false negative)	d (true negative)

*Sensitivity = a/(a + c). Specificity = d/(b + d).

Clinical Commentary 11-1. Neonatal screening for phenylketonuria (PKU)

Disease Characteristics

Population screening of newborns for PKU represents the best example of the application of the screening model to genetic disease. As discussed in Chapter 3, the prevalence of this autosomal recessive disorder of phenylalanine metabolism is about 1 in 10,000 to 15,000 white births. The natural history of PKU is well understood. More than 95% of untreated PKU patients become moderately to severely mentally retarded. The condition is not identified clinically in the first year of life, as the physical signs are subtle and PKU usually manifests only as developmental delay. Dietary restriction of phenylalanine, when begun before 4 weeks of age, is highly effective in altering the course of the disease. Virtually all individuals with classical PKU will have normal intelligence when treated (an important exception is those who have a defect in biopterin metabolism and in whom a different therapy is used). The diet, although not particularly palatable, is effective in treating the disease.

Screening Characteristics

PKU is detected by the measurement of blood phenylalanine using a bacterial inhibition assay, the Guthrie test. Blood is collected in the newborn period, usually by heel stick, and placed on filter paper. The dried blood is placed on an agar plate and incubated with a bacterial strain *(Bacillus subtilis)* that requires phenylalanine for growth. Measurement of bacterial growth permits quantification of the amount of phenylalanine in the blood sample. Positive test results are usually repeated and followed by a quantitative assay of plasma phenylalanine and tyrosine.

If the test is performed after 2 days of age and after regular feeding on a protein diet, the detection rate (sensitivity) is about 98%. If performed at less than 24 hours of age, the sensitivity is about 84%. Thus, early discharge from the nursery requires a repeat test a few weeks after birth. Specificity is close to 100%.

System Characteristics

Because of the requirement of normal protein in the diet, many states request rescreening at 2 to 4 weeks of age. Then sensitivity approaches 100%. Because of the impact of a misdiagnosis, a high sensitivity level is desirable.

Phenylalanine levels in children with classical PKU typically exceed 20 mg/dl. For every 20 positive PKU screens, only one infant will have classical PKU. The others will be either false-positives (usually due to a transient reversible tyrosinemia) or will have a form of hyperphenylalaninemia (elevated phenylalanine) not due to classical PKU.

The cost of a Guthrie test is about $1.25. Several studies have shown that the cost of nationwide PKU screening is significantly less than the savings it achieves by avoiding institutionalization costs and lost productivity.

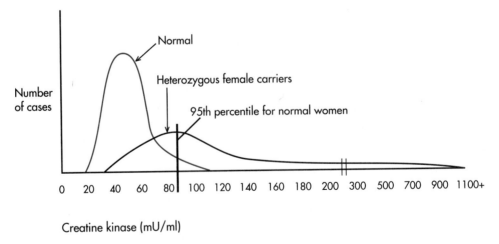

Creatine kinase (mU/ml)

Figure 11-1 ■ **The distribution of creatine kinase (CK) in normal women and in women who are heterozygous carriers for a mutation in the Duchenne muscular dystrophy gene. Note the overlap in distribution between the two groups: about two thirds of carriers have CK levels that exceed the 95th percentile in normal women. If the 95th percentile is used as a cutoff to identify carriers, then the sensitivity of the test is 67% (i.e., two thirds of carriers will be detected), and the specificity is 95% (95% of normal women will be correctly identified).** (From Sibert JR, Harper PS, Thompson RJ et al: Arch Dis Child 54:534–537, 1979.)

is lowered so that nearly all disease cases will be detected (higher sensitivity), while increasing the number of nondisease cases (lower specificity) targeted for subsequent diagnosis. If confirmation of a positive test is expensive and hazardous, then false-positive rates are minimized (i.e., the cutoff level is increased, producing high specificity at the expense of sensitivity).

> **The basic elements of validity include the test's sensitivity (proportion of true positives detected) and specificity (proportion of true negatives detected). When sensitivity is increased, specificity decreases, and vice-versa.**

A primary concern in the clinical setting is the accuracy of a positive screening test. One needs to know the proportion of persons with a positive test who truly have the disease in question [i.e., $a/(a+b)$ in Table 11-1]. This quantity is defined as the **positive predictive value**.

The concepts of sensitivity, specificity, and positive predictive value can be illustrated by an example. Congenital adrenal hyperplasia (CAH) due to a deficiency of 21 hydroxylase is an inborn error of steroid biosynthesis that may produce ambiguous genitalia in females and adrenal crises in males and females. The screening test, a 17-hydroxyprogesterone assay, has a sensitivity of about 95% and a specificity of 99% (Table 11-2). The prevalence of CAH is about 1 in 10,000 in most white populations but rises to about 1 in 400 in the Yupik Eskimo population.

Let us assume that a screening program for CAH has been developed in both of these populations. In a population of 500,000 whites, the false-positive rate (1 − specificity) is 1%. Thus, about 5000 normal individuals will have a positive test. With

95% sensitivity, 47 of the 50 individuals who have CAH will be detected through a positive test. Note that the great majority of people who have a positive test result would *not* have CAH: the positive predictive value is $47/(47 + 5000)$, or less than 1%. Suppose that 10,000 members of the Yupik population are screened for CAH. As Table 11-2 shows, 24 of 25 individuals with CAH will test positive, and 100 without CAH will test positive. Here the positive predictive value is much higher than in whites: $24/(24 + 100) = 19\%$. This example illustrates an important principle: *the positive predictive value of a test increases as the prevalence of the disease increases.*

> **The positive predictive value of a screening test is defined as the proportion of positive tests that are true positives. It increases as the prevalence of the target disorder increases.**

Newborn Screening

Newborn screening programs represent an ideal opportunity for presymptomatic detection and prevention of genetic disease. At present, all states in the United States screen newborns for PKU and galactosemia, an autosomal recessive disorder of carbohydrate metabolism. Most states also screen for hypothyroidism. All of these conditions fulfill the above-stated criteria for population screening. Each is a disorder in which the individual is at significant risk for mental retardation; early detection enables effective intervention and prevention.

In recent years, many parts of the United States and other nations have instituted screening programs to identify neonates with hemoglobin disorders (e.g., sickle cell disease). These programs are justified by the fact that up to 15% of children with sickle cell disease will die of infections before age 5 (see Chapter 3). Effective treatment, in the form of prophylactic antibiotics, is available.

Some communities have begun screening for Duchenne muscular dystrophy (DMD) by measuring creatine kinase levels in newborns. The object is not presymptomatic treatment; rather it is identification of families who should receive genetic counseling to make informed reproductive decisions. Conditions for which newborn screening is commonly performed are summarized in Table 11-3.

> **Newborn screening is an effective public health strategy for treatable disorders such as PKU, hypothyroidism, galactosemia, and sickle cell disease.**

Table 11-2 ■ **Hypothetical results of screening for congenital adrenal hyperplasia (CAH) in a low-prevalence white population and a high-prevalence Yupik population***

Screening test	CAH present	CAH absent
Positive		
White	47	5000
Yupik	24	100
Negative		
White	3	494,950
Yupik	1	9875

*White positive predictive value = $47/(47 + 5000) = 1\%$.
Yupik positive predictive value = $24/(24 + 100) = 19\%$.

Table 11-3 ▪ Characteristics of selected newborn screening programs

Disease	Inheritance	Prevalence	Screening test	Cost	Treatment
Phenylketonuria	Autosomal recessive	1/10–15,000	Guthrie test	$1.25	Dietary restriction of phenylalanine
Galactosemia	Autosomal recessive	1/50–100,000	Transferase assay	1.00	Dietary restriction of galactose
Congenital hypothyroidism	Usually sporadic	1/5000	Measurement of T4 or TSH	1.50	Hormone replacement
Sickle cell disease	Autosomal recessive	1/400–600 African-Americans	Isoelectric focusing or DNA diagnosis	1.50	Prophylactic penicillin

Adapted from American Academy of Pediatrics Committee on Genetics: Newborn screening fact sheets, Pediatrics 83:449–464, 1989.

Heterozygote Screening

The aforementioned principles of population screening can be applied to the detection of unaffected carriers of disease-causing genes. The target population is a group known to be at risk. The "intervention" consists of the presentation of risk figures and the option of prenatal diagnosis. Genetic diseases amenable to heterozygote screening are typically autosomal recessive disorders for which prenatal diagnosis and genetic counseling are available, feasible, and accurate.

An example of a highly successful heterozygote screening effort is the Tay-Sachs screening program in North America. Infantile Tay-Sachs disease is an autosomal recessive disorder in which the lysosomal enzyme β-hexosaminidase A (HEX A) is deficient. This causes a buildup of the substrate, GM_2 ganglioside, in neuronal lysosomes (*SOL* 31).* The accumulation of this substrate damages the neurons and leads to blindness, seizures, hypotonia, and death by about the age of 5.

Tay-Sachs disease is especially common among Ashkenazi Jews, with a heterozygote frequency of about 1 in 30. Thus, this population is a reasonable candidate for heterozygote screening. Accurate carrier testing is available (assays for HEX A or, in some populations, direct testing for mutations). Because the disease is uniformly fatal, options such as pregnancy termination or artificial insemination by noncarrier donors are acceptable to most couples. A well-planned effort was made to educate members of the target population about risks, testing, and available options. As a result of screening, the number of Tay-Sachs disease births in the

United States and Canada has declined by 90%, from 40 to 50 per year before 1970 to 3 to 5 per year in the 1990s.

Cystic fibrosis is another autosomal recessive disorder for which carrier screening is possible. However, the relative costs and benefits of such a screening program are less clear-cut than those of Tay-Sachs disease (Clinical Commentary 11-2). Table 11-4 presents a list of selected conditions in which heterozygote screening programs have been developed in industrial countries.

In addition to the criteria for establishing a population screening program for genetic disorders, guidelines have been developed regarding the ethical and legal aspects of heterozygote screening programs. These are summarized in Box 11-2.

Box 11-2. Public policy guidelines for heterozygote screening

Recommended guidelines:
1. Screening should be voluntary, and confidentiality must be assured.
2. Screening requires informed consent.
3. Providers of screening services have an obligation to assure that adequate education and counseling are included in the program.
4. Quality control of all aspects of the laboratory testing, including systematic proficiency testing, is required and should be implemented as soon as possible.
5. There should be equal access to testing.

From Elias S, Annas GJ, and Simpson JL: Carrier screening for cystic fibrosis: implications for obstetric and gynecologic practice, Am J Obstet Gynecol 164:1077–1083, 1991.

---

*Like Hurler syndrome (see Chapter 4), Tay-Sachs disease is an example of a **lysosomal storage disorder**.

Clinical Commentary 11-2. Population screening for cystic fibrosis

There are now more than 400 known cystic fibrosis (CF)-causing mutations at the CFTR locus. Clearly, it would be technologically impractical to test for all of them in a population carrier screening program. However, among the mutations that can cause CF in whites, about 70% are the 3-base deletion termed ΔF508 (see Chapter 4). Carrier screening using PCR-based detection of this mutation alone would detect approximately 90% of white couples in which one or both members of the couple are heterozygous carriers of this mutation $(1 - 0.30^2$, where 0.30^2 represents the frequency of carrier couples in which *neither* member of the couple carries the ΔF508 mutation). By testing for several additional relatively common mutations, each with a gene frequency of ≥1%, about 75% to 85% of all CF mutations may now be detectable through population screening. Then 94% to 98% of couples would be recognized in which one or both members carry a CF mutation (i.e., $1 - 0.25^2$ to $1 - 0.15^2$). The sensitivity of the screening test would be high.

These carriers would define a population in which prenatal diagnosis for CF might be offered. Given the

CF heterozygote frequency of about 1 in 23 (Chapter 4), only about 1 in every 500 couples would consist of two heterozygotes $(1$ of $23^2)$. Only some of these couples would produce a child affected with CF. Considering the cost of screening tests for couples, it has been estimated that the cost of identifying one homozygous affected fetus through carrier screening would be about $1,000,000.

Moreover, an enormous amount of counseling time would be required to explain the complexities of these results to the at-risk families identified by screening (in this context, it is important that one study of the parents of children with CF showed that only 64% could accurately state the recurrence risk for their future children). It is estimated that *half* of all board-certified geneticists and genetic counselors in the United States would have to devote all of their time to CF screening to meet this need. Obviously this is impractical.

Although carrier screening for individuals with a positive family history of CF is appropriate, it is less certain that general population screening is warranted or feasible. Several centers have initiated pilot programs for CF population screening. The final decision regarding CF screening will await further data from these centers and further technological development.

Heterozygote screening consists of testing (at the phenotype or genotype level) a target population to identify unaffected carriers of a disease gene. The carriers can then be given information about risks and reproductive options.

Presymptomatic Diagnosis

With the development of genetic diagnosis through linkage analysis and direct mutation detection, **presymptomatic diagnosis** has become feasible for some genetic diseases. Individuals known to be at risk for a disorder can be tested to determine whether they have inherited a disease-

causing mutation *before* they develop clinical symptoms of the disorder. Presymptomatic diagnosis is available, for example, for Huntington disease, adult polycystic kidney disease, neurofibromatosis type 1, and autosomal dominant breast cancer. By informing individuals whether they carry a disease-causing gene, presymptomatic diagnosis can aid in making reproductive decisions. It can provide reassurance to those who learn that they do not carry a disease-causing gene. In some cases early diagnosis may improve health supervision. For example, persons who inherit an autosomal dominant breast cancer gene can undergo mammography at an earlier age to detect a tumor while

Table 11-4 ■ Selected examples of heterozygote screening programs in specific ethnic groups

Disease	Ethnic group	Carrier frequency	At-risk couple frequency	Disease incidence in newborns
Sickle cell disease	African-Americans	1/12	1/150	1/600
Tay-Sachs disease	Ashkenazi Jews	1/30	1/900	1/3600
β-thalassemia	Greeks, Italians	1/30	1/900	1/3600
α-thalassemia	Southeast Asians and Chinese	1/25	1/625	1/2500
Cystic fibrosis	Northern Europeans	1/23	1/500	1/2000

Modified from Kaback MM: Heterozygote screening. In Emery AEH and Rimoin DL, editors: Principles and practice of medical genetics, vol 1, ed 2, Edinburgh, 1990, Churchill Livingstone.

it is still small. Those who inherit genes that cause some forms of familial colon cancer (APC and HNPCC, see Chapter 9) can also benefit from early diagnosis and treatment.

> Genetic testing can sometimes be performed to identify individuals who have inherited a disease-causing gene before they develop symptoms. This is termed presymptomatic testing.

Psychosocial Implications of Genetic Screening

Screening for genetic diseases has many social and psychological implications. The burden of anxiety, cost, and potential stigmatization surrounding a positive test must be weighed against the need for detection. Often, screening tests are misperceived as diagnostically definitive. The concept that a positive screening test does not necessarily indicate disease presence must be emphasized to those who undergo screening.

The initial screening programs for sickle cell trait in the 1970s were plagued by misunderstandings about the implications of carrier status. Occasionally, carrier detection led to cancellation of health insurance. Such experiences underscore the need for effective genetic counseling and public education. Other issues include the right to choose *not* to be tested and the potential for invasion of privacy.

The social, psychological, and ethical aspects of genetic screening will become more complicated as newer techniques of DNA diagnosis become more accessible. For example, even though presymptomatic diagnosis of Huntington disease is available, only about 20% of at-risk individuals elect this option. Largely, this reflects the fact that no effective treatment is presently possible for this disorder.

For other genetic diseases, such as some autosomal dominant cancer syndromes, early diagnosis leads to a much better prognosis. However, as screening for such diseases becomes more common, the issues of privacy and confidentiality, and the need for accurate communication of risk information, must also be addressed.

■ MOLECULAR TOOLS FOR SCREENING AND DIAGNOSIS

Until recently, genetic screening usually relied on assays of the disease phenotype, such as a β-hexosaminidase assay for Tay-Sachs disease or a creatine kinase assay for Duchenne muscular dystrophy (DMD). Advances in DNA technology have

led to diagnosis at the level of the genotype. In some cases linkage analysis can determine whether an individual has inherited a disease gene, and in other cases direct assays of disease-causing mutations have been developed. Genetic diagnosis at the DNA level is now supplementing, and in some cases supplanting, screening tests based on phenotypic assays.

Linkage analysis and/or direct mutation diagnosis have been used for diagnostic testing within families, prenatal diagnosis of genetic disorders, and more recently in population screening. Improved technology and an increased demand for testing have led to the establishment of clinical molecular laboratories in many medical centers in North America and Europe. The molecular techniques utilized in these settings will be now be described.

Linkage Analysis

DNA polymorphisms (RFLPs, VNTRs, and microsatellite repeat polymorphisms) can be used as markers in linkage analysis as described in Chapter 7. Once linkage phase is established in a family, the marker locus can be assayed to determine whether an individual has inherited a chromosome containing a disease gene or a chromosome containing a normal gene (Fig. 11-2). Because this approach uses linked markers but does not involve direct examination of the disease-causing mutation(s), it is a form of **indirect diagnosis**.

Linkage analysis has been employed successfully in diagnosing many of the genetic diseases discussed in this text. In principle, it can be used to diagnose any mapped genetic disease. It has the advantages that the disease gene product and its chromosomal location need not be known. The

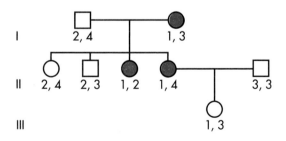

Figure 11-2 ■ In this pedigree for autosomal dominant breast cancer, the analysis of a closely linked marker on chromosome 17 shows that the mutation is on the same chromosome as marker allele 1 in the affected mother in generation II. This indicates that the daughter in generation III has inherited the mutation-bearing chromosome from her mother and is highly likely to develop a breast tumor.

marker simply tells us which chromosome the at-risk individual has inherited. If the location of the marker *is* known, linkage of the disease locus to the marker establishes an approximate physical location for the disease locus.

The disadvantages of this approach are as follows: (1) multiple family members must be tested to establish linkage phase, (2) not all markers are informative (sufficiently heterozygous) in all families, and (3) recombination may occur between the marker and the disease-causing mutation, introducing a source of diagnostic error.

One way to increase the informativeness of markers is to find multiple marker polymorphisms, all of which are closely linked to the disease locus. Particularly useful are markers flanking both sides of the disease locus. This often enables the investigator to determine that a recombination has occurred.

> **Linkage analysis, a form of indirect genetic diagnosis, uses linked markers to determine whether an individual has inherited a chromosome containing a disease gene from his or her parent. The need for typing multiple family members, and the possibilities of recombination and uninformative matings, are disadvantages of this approach.**

Direct Mutation Analysis

Sometimes the mutation causing a disease happens to alter a recognition sequence for a restriction enzyme. In this case the mutation itself creates a restriction site polymorphism that can be detected after digestion with this enzyme. An example is given by the sickle cell disease mutation, which alters an *Mst*II recognition site in the β-globin gene (see Chapter 3, Fig. 3-15). Because the resulting RFLP reflects the disease-causing mutation directly, RFLP analysis provides a **direct diagnosis** of the disease. This approach has the advantages that family information is not needed (the mutation is viewed directly in each individual), lack of informativeness is not a problem, and there is no error due to recombination. The primary disadvantage of this approach is that only about 5% of disease-causing mutations happen to affect known restriction sites.

> **Direct genetic diagnosis is accomplished by typing the disease-causing mutation itself. It is potentially more accurate than indirect diagnosis and does not require family information. RFLP techniques can be used for**

direct diagnosis if the mutation affects a restriction site.

If the DNA sequence surrounding a mutation is known, an oligonucleotide probe can be synthesized that will hybridize (undergo complementary base pairing) only to the mutated sequence (such probes are often termed **allele-specific oligonucleotides**, ASOs). A second probe that will hybridize to the normal DNA sequence is also synthesized. Stringent hybridization conditions are used so that a one-base mismatch will prevent hybridization. DNA from individuals homozygous for the mutation will hybridize only with the ASO containing the mutated sequence, whereas DNA from individuals homozygous for the normal sequence will hybridize with the normal ASO. DNA from heterozygotes will hybridize with both probes (Fig. 11-3). The length of the ASO probes, usually about 18 to 20 nucleotides, is critical. Probes of shorter length would not be unique in the genome and would therefore hybridize to other regions. Longer probes are more difficult to synthesize correctly and could hybridize both to the normal and mutated sequence.

The ASO method of direct diagnosis has the same advantages that were listed for direct diagnosis using RFLPs. It has the additional advantage that it is not limited to mutations that cause alterations in restriction sites. However, it does require that at least part of the disease gene has been cloned and sequenced. In addition, each disease-causing mutation requires a different oligonucleotide probe. For this reason this approach, although powerful, becomes impractical unless a disease is caused by only one or a few relatively common mutations.

> **Direct diagnosis can be performed by hybridization of an individual's DNA with allele-specific oligonucleotide probes. This approach is feasible if the DNA sequence causing a genetic disease is known and if the number of disease-causing mutations is limited.**

Examples of diseases caused by a limited number of mutations include sickle cell disease, α1-antitrypsin deficiency (Clinical Commentary 11-3), and cystic fibrosis (CF). Most cases of CF are caused by one of several mutations, the most common of which is the ΔF508 mutation. Thus, direct diagnosis can be used to identify most CF homozygotes and heterozygous carriers. Prenatal diagnosis is also possible. Direct diagnosis can also be used to detect the deletions or duplications in the dystro-

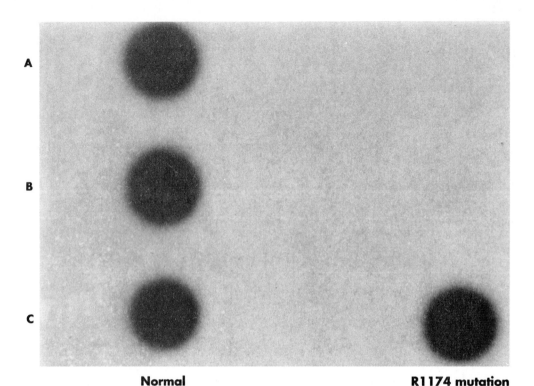

Normal   **R1174 mutation**

Figure 11-3 ▪ Hybridization of allele-specific oligonucleotide (ASO) probes corresponding to normal DNA sequence and a mutation (R1174) that can produce cystic fibrosis. In this "dot blot," the DNA from individuals A and B hybridizes only to the normal sequence; they are normal homozygotes. Individual C's DNA hybridizes to both ASO probes, so he is a heterozygous CF carrier. (Courtesy of Lesa Nelson and Dr. Kenneth Ward, University of Utah Health Sciences Center.)

phin gene that cause most cases of DMD. The most common DNA diagnostic tests performed in a clinical molecular laboratory are presented in Table 11-5.

▪ PRENATAL DIAGNOSIS OF GENETIC DISORDERS AND CONGENITAL DEFECTS

Prenatal diagnosis is a major focus of genetic diagnosis, and several important areas of technology have evolved to provide this service. The principal aim of prenatal diagnosis is to supply at-risk families with information to make informed choices during pregnancy. The potential benefits of prenatal testing include the following: (1) providing reassurance to at-risk families when the result is normal, (2) providing risk information to couples who, in the absence of such information, would not choose to begin a pregnancy, (3) allowing the couple to prepare psychologically for the birth of an affected baby, and (4) helping the physician to plan delivery, management, and care of the infant when the fetus is diagnosed with a disease.

Given the controversy surrounding the issue of pregnancy termination, it should be emphasized that 98% of prenatal diagnoses yield a normal test

Table 11-5 ▪ Selected single-gene disorders for which family screening and prenatal diagnosis by DNA are available

Disease	DNA analysis
Neurofibromatosis type 1	Usually linkage analysis
Myotonic dystrophy	Direct mutation analysis/linkage
Cystic fibrosis	Direct mutation analysis/linkage
Sickle cell disease	Direct mutation analysis/linkage
Fragile X syndrome	Direct mutation analysis/linkage
Hemophilia A	Usually linkage analysis
Huntington disease	Direct mutation analysis/linkage
Duchenne muscular dystrophy	Direct mutation analysis/linkage

result. Thus, the great majority of families receive reassurance, and only a small minority must face the issue of termination.

Prenatal diagnosis includes both screening and diagnostic tests. An example of a population screening test is an assay of maternal serum α-fetoprotein (AFP) at 15 weeks gestation. An abnormal result identifies a subgroup for further testing. **Amniocentesis** (the withdrawal of amniotic fluid during

Clinical Commentary 11-3. The genetic diagnosis of α_1-antitrypsin deficiency

α_1-antitrypsin (α_1-AT) deficiency is one of the most common autosomal recessive disorders among whites, affecting approximately 1 in 2500. α_1-AT, synthesized primarily in the liver, is a serine protease inhibitor. It does bind trypsin, as its name suggests. However, α_1-AT binds much more strongly to neutrophil elastase, a protease that is produced by neutrophils (a type of leukocyte) in response to infections and irritants. It carries out its binding and inhibitory role primarily in the lower respiratory tract, where it prevents elastase from digesting the alveolar septi of the lung.

Individuals with less than 10% to 15% of the normal level of α_1-AT activity will experience significant lung damage and typically develop emphysema during their 30s, 40s, or 50s. In addition, at least 10% develop liver cirrhosis as a result of the accumulation of variant α_1-AT molecules in the liver; α_1-AT deficiency accounts for nearly 20% of all nonalcoholic liver cirrhosis in the United States. An important feature of this disease is that cigarette smokers with α_1-AT deficiency develop emphysema much earlier than do nonsmokers. This is because cigarette smoke irritates lung tissue, increasing secretion of neutrophil elastase. At the same time, it inactivates α_1-AT, so there is also less inhibition of elastase. One study showed that the median age of survival of nonsmokers with α_1-AT deficiency was 62 years, whereas it was only 40 years for smokers with this disease. Because the combination of cigarette smoking (an environmental factor) and the α_1-AT mutation (a genetic factor) produces more severe disease than either factor alone, it is known as an example of a **gene–environment interaction**.

The α_1-AT gene has been localized to chromosome 14q32, and it has been cloned and sequenced. Although there are more than 75 known α_1-AT mutations, the only common mutation with clinically significant effects is a missense mutation in exon 5 that produces an allele known as "Z." The gene frequency of the Z allele is as high as 0.02 in Scandinavia and decreases to less than 0.01 in Southern European populations. It is virtually absent in Japanese and Chinese populations. Because it is the result of a single basepair substitution, the Z mutation can be diagnosed directly by using ASO probes. Typically, PCR is used to amplify the individual's DNA from this region of the gene, and the amplified DNA is blotted onto a membrane. The amplified DNA is hybridized with an ASO probe that has a DNA sequence corresponding to the mutation and a second ASO probe that has the normal DNA sequence. This permits direct determination of the individual's genotype. Thus, rapid, direct diagnosis is possible for this important and common genetic disease.

pregnancy) and **chorionic villus sampling** (CVS) (the biopsy of chorionic villus tissue) represent diagnostic tests. Another example of the distinction between screening and diagnosis is given by amniocentesis for pregnancies in advanced maternal age: the selection of women 35 years of age or older is the screening strategy, and amniocentesis is the diagnostic test. Because of the increased risk of trisomies with advanced maternal age (see Chapter 6), approximately half of North American women older than 35 years currently undergo amniocentesis or CVS during pregnancy.

Prenatal diagnostic methods can be divided into two major types: (1) analysis of fetal tissues (amniocentesis, CVS, cordocentesis, and in vitro fertilization diagnosis) and (2) visualization of the fetus (ultrasonography). In this section, each of these procedures is described, and their accuracy, safety, and feasibility are discussed.

Amniocentesis

Amniocentesis is traditionally performed at 15 to 17 weeks after a pregnant woman's last menstrual period (LMP). A needle is inserted through the abdominal wall into the amniotic sac after real-time ultrasound localizes the placenta and determines the position of the fetus (Fig. 11-4). Twenty to thirty milliliters of amniotic fluid are withdrawn. Amniotic fluid contains living cells (**amniocytes**) that are shed by the fetus. Cytogenetic studies are carried out after culturing the amniocytes to increase their number. Additionally, cells can be grown for biochemical assays or DNA analysis. AFP, which is used to test for the presence of a neural tube defect (see Chapter 10), is also measured in the amniotic fluid. The results of cytogenetic studies are typically completed in 10 to 14 days. Indications for prenatal diagnosis by amniocentesis are listed in Box 11-3.

Box 11-3. Indications for prenatal diagnosis by amniocentesis

Maternal age > 35 years
Previous child with chromosome abnormality
History of structural chromosome abnormality in one of the parents
Family history of genetic defect that is diagnosable by biochemical or DNA analysis
Risk of neural tube defect (NTD)

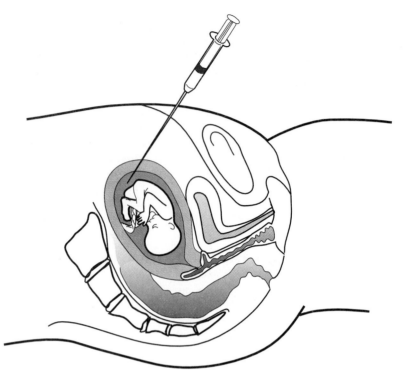

Figure 11-4 ■ A schematic illustration of an amniocentesis, in which 20 to 30 ml of amniotic fluid is withdrawn transabdominally (with ultrasound guidance), usually at 15 to 17 weeks gestation.

The safety and accuracy of amniocentesis have been established by three large collaborative studies performed in the 1970s. The risk of maternal complications is low. Transient fluid leakage occurs in about 1% of mothers, and maternal infections are extremely rare. The risk of primary concern is fetal loss. Amniocentesis increases the risk of fetal loss by an additional 0.5% above the background risk at 15 to 17 weeks post-LMP.

One must weigh the risk of fetal loss against the probability that the fetus is affected with a diagnosable condition. For women younger than 35 years, the former risk usually outweighs the latter. After age 35 the risk of bearing an aneuploid fetus increases considerably, and the latter risk outweighs the former. Thus, amniocentesis is not recommended for women under age 35 unless they have a previous indication of risk for a genetic disease (such as a positive family history) (Clinical Commentary 11-4).

Although amniocentesis provides highly accurate results, chromosomal mosaicism can lead to misdiagnosis. Most apparent mosaicism is caused by the generation of an extra chromosome during in vitro cell culture and is labeled as **pseudomosaicism.**

This can be distinguished easily from true mosaicism if techniques are used in which all cells in a colony are the descendants of a single fetal cell. If only some cells in the colony have the extra chromosome, it is assumed that pseudomosaicism exists. If, however, consistent aneuploidy is visualized in all cells of multiple colonies, then true fetal mosaicism is diagnosed. Further confirmation of fetal mosaicism (which is generally a rare condition) can be obtained by fetal blood sampling, as described below.

Recently, some centers have been evaluating amniocentesis performed earlier in pregnancy, at about 13 to 14 weeks post-LMP. Because less amniotic fluid is present at this time, the risk of fetal loss or injury may be higher. These risks are currently being evaluated in clinical trials.

Amniocentesis, the withdrawal of amniotic fluid during pregnancy, is performed at about 16 weeks post-LMP and is used to diagnose many genetic diseases. The rate of fetal loss attributable to this procedure is approximately 1 in 200.

During the medical care of a pregnant woman older than 35 years, a common discussion with the primary care practitioner involves the decision to undergo amniocentesis. Several factors enter into this decision. First is the age-specific risk for Down syndrome and other chromosomal disorders. A second factor is the risk of fetal loss from the procedure (about 0.5% above the background risk). A third issue is the cost of an amniocentesis with ultrasound and cytogenetic analysis, which is ordinarily about $1,000. These factors must be weighed in terms of their relative costs and benefits for the woman and her family.

As this decision is explored in greater depth, other considerations often arise. If a woman has had previous miscarriages, the 0.5% risk of fetal loss may be weighed more heavily. In addition, the seriousness of bearing a child with disabilities may be perceived differently from family to family. Some couples are uncomfortable with the amount of time that elapses before test results are available (usually 10 to 14 days). Here, the possibility of CVS, which can be performed earlier and which usually yields results more rapidly, may be explored. The possibility of an ambiguous result (e.g., mosaicism) also deserves discussion. Finally, it is important for the clinician to specify that a typical amniocentesis in a woman older than 35 years detects only a specific class of disorders (i.e., chromosome abnormalities and NTDs) and not the entire range of congenital malformations and genetic disorders.

Chorionic Villus Sampling (CVS)

Chorionic villus sampling is performed by aspirating fetal trophoblastic tissue (chorionic villi) by either a transcervical or transabdominal approach (Fig. 11-5). Because it is usually performed at 9 to 12 weeks post-LMP, CVS has the advantage of providing a diagnosis much earlier in pregnancy than amniocentesis. This is beneficial for those couples that consider pregnancy termination an option.

Cell culture (as in amniocentesis) and direct analysis from rapidly growing trophoblasts can provide material for cytogenetic analysis. When chorionic villi are successfully obtained, CVS provides diagnostic results in more than 99% of cases. **Confined placental mosaicism** (mosaicism in the placenta but not in the fetus itself) is seen in about 1% to 2% of cases in which direct analysis of villus material is performed. This confuses the diagnosis, because the mosaicism observed in placental (villus) material is not actually present in the fetus. This confusion can usually be resolved by a follow-up amniocentesis. A disadvantage of CVS is that amniotic fluid AFP cannot be measured. Women who undergo CVS may have their serum AFP level measured at 15 to 16 weeks post-LMP as a screen for neural tube defects.

CVS, like amniocentesis, is generally a safe procedure. Canadian and U.S. collaborative studies revealed a post-CVS fetal loss rate to be 0.5% to 0.8% higher than that of amniocentesis (i.e., a fetal loss rate of approximately 1% to 1.3% above the

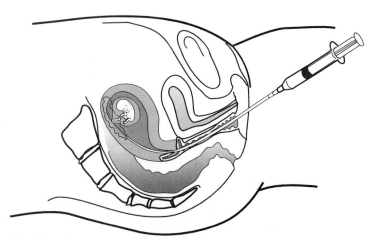

Figure 11-5 ■ A schematic illustration of a transcervical chorionic villus sampling (CVS) procedure. With ultrasound guidance, a catheter is inserted, and several milligrams of villus tissue are aspirated.

background rate, compared with 0.5% for amniocentesis). The most important factors increasing the risk of fetal loss are a lack of experience with the procedure and an increase in the number of transcervical passages to obtain the villus sample. In experienced hands, transcervical and transabdominal procedures appear to entail similar risk levels.

Recently, two studies have indicated that CVS may increase the risk of limb reduction defects. In one study, 5 offspring of 289 women who underwent CVS at 8 to 9 weeks post-LMP were born with shortened limbs or missing parts of a limb. A second study showed that 4 of 394 fetuses had terminal defects of fingers and toes. While other investigations have not indicated an increased risk of limb reduction defects, the apparent association has been of concern because the proposed mechanism (vascular insult leading to hypoperfusion of the limb) is biologically plausible. The increased risk appears to occur primarily when CVS is performed earlier than 10 weeks post-LMP. Accordingly, some professionals now recommend against performing CVS prior to this stage.

> **CVS is performed earlier than amniocentesis (at 10 to 11 weeks post-LMP) using either a transcervical or transabdominal approach. The risk of fetal loss attributable to CVS is approximately 1% to 1.3%. Confined placental mosaicism can confuse the diagnosis. There is some evidence that CVS performed before 10 weeks post-LMP may increase the risk of limb reduction defects.**

Inherited metabolic diseases, which are usually autosomal or X-linked recessive diseases, can be diagnosed prenatally by amniocentesis or CVS if the specific metabolic defect is expressed in amniocytes or trophoblastic tissue. Table 11-6 lists selected metabolic diseases and single gene disorders for which amniocentesis or CVS is available. A comprehensive summary of conditions that may be prenatally diagnosed is provided by Weaver (1992).

Other Methods of Fetal Tissue Sampling

Cordocentesis or **percutaneous umbilical blood sampling** (PUBS) has become the preferred method to access fetal blood, replacing the riskier procedure of fetal blood sampling by **fetoscopy** (direct visualization of the fetus by insertion of an endoscope through the abdominal wall). PUBS is usually carried out after the 16th week of gestation and is accomplished by puncture of the umbilical cord with ultrasound guidance. The fetal loss rate attributable to PUBS is about 1%. The primary applications of PUBS are as follows: (1) Cytogenetic analysis of fetuses with structural anomalies detected by ultrasound when rapid diagnosis is required. Cytogenetic analysis from fetal blood sampling is completed in 2 to 3 days, whereas diagnosis following amniocentesis requires 10 to 14 days because of the necessity of culturing amniocytes. (2) Diagnosis of hemoglobin disorders or other hematologic diseases that are analyzed most effectively in blood samples [e.g., hemophilia A (see Chapter 5) or immunologic disorders such as chronic granulomatous disease (see Chapter 8)].

Table 11-6 ■ **Selected inborn errors of metabolism that are diagnosable through amniocentesis and/or chorionic villus sampling**

Disease	Measurable enzyme
Disorders of amino acid/organic acid metabolism	
Maple syrup urine disease	Branched chain ketoacid decarboxylase
Methylmalonic acidemia	Methylmalonic CoA mutase
Multiple carboxylase deficiency	Biotin responsive carboxylase
Disorders of carbohydrate metabolism	
Glycogen storage disease, type 2	α-glucosidase
Galactosemia	Galactose-1-uridyl transferase
Disorders of lysosomal enzymes	
Gangliosidosis (all types)	β-galactosidase
Mucopolysaccharidosis (all types)	None
Tay-Sachs disease	Hexosaminidase A
Disorders of purine and pyrimidine metabolism	
Lesch-Nyhan syndrome	Hypoxanthine guanine phosophoribosyl transferase
Disorders of peroxisomal metabolism	
Zellweger syndrome	Long-chain fatty acids

Percutaneous umbilical blood sampling (PUBS, or cordocentesis) is a method for the direct sampling of fetal blood and is used to obtain a sample for rapid cytogenetic or hematologic analysis.

Ultrasonography

Technological advances in real-time **ultrasonography** have made this an important tool in prenatal diagnosis. A transducer placed on the mother's abdomen sends pulsed sound waves through the fetus. The fetal tissue reflects the waves in patterns corresponding to tissue density. The reflected waves are displayed on a monitor, allowing real-time visualization of the fetus. Ultrasonography has become the most widely used form of fetal visualization and is useful in the detection of many fetal malformations. It has also assisted in the development and effectiveness of amniocentesis, CVS, and PUBS. Box 11-4 lists some of the congenital malformations diagnosable by fetal ultrasound (a more comprehensive list is provided by Weaver, 1992).

Box 11-4. Selected disorders diagnosed by ultrasound in second trimester*

Symptom complex
  Hydrops
  Oligohydramnios
  Polyhydramnios
  Intrauterine growth retardation
Central nervous system
  Anencephaly
  Encephalocele
  Holoprosencephaly
  Hydrocephalus
Craniofacial
  Cleft lip
Chest
  Congenital heart disease
  Diaphragmatic hernia
Abdomen/pelvis
  Gastrointestinal atresias
  Gastroschisis
  Omphalocele
  Renal agenesis
  Cystic kidneys
  Hydronephrosis
Skeletal system
  Limb reduction defects
  Many chondrodystrophies, including thanatophoric dysplasia and osteogenesis imperfecta

*Detection rate varies by condition.

Ultrasonography is sometimes used to test for a specific condition in an at-risk fetus (e.g., a short-limb skeletal dysplasia). More often, fetal anomalies are detected during the evaluation of obstetric indicators, such as uncertain gestational age, poor fetal growth, or amniotic fluid abnormalities. Several European nations perform routine second-trimester ultrasound screening in all pregnancies. Studies of ultrasound screening suggest that sensitivity for the detection of major congenital malformations is low, ranging from 30% to 50%. Specificity, however, approaches 99%.

While the sensitivity of ultrasonography is rather low for congenital malformations in general, it is high for neural tube defects. Ultrasound can detect virtually all fetuses with anencephaly (Fig. 11-6). Ultrasonography may also sometimes identify a fetus with a chromosome abnormality by detecting a congenital malformation, intrauterine growth retardation, hydrops (abnormal accumulation of fluid in the fetus), or an alteration in the amniotic fluid volume.

Ultrasonography is by far the most common technique now used for fetal visualization, but other techniques are also used. They include radiography and occasionally magnetic resonance imaging (MRI).

Prenatal diagnosis includes invasive techniques designed to analyze fetal tissue (CVS, amniocentesis, or PUBS) and noninvasive procedures that visualize the fetus (ultrasonography).

α-Fetoprotein Measurement in Amniotic Fluid and Maternal Serum

α-Fetoprotein (AFP) is a fetal protein similar to albumin; it is produced initially by the yolk sac and subsequently by the liver. The AFP level normally increases in amniotic fluid until about 10 to 14 weeks of gestation and then decreases steadily. Amniotic fluid AFP is significantly higher in pregnancies in which the fetus has a neural tube defect (NTD). When an amniotic fluid AFP assay is used with ultrasonography in the second trimester, more than 98% of fetuses with an open spina bifida and probably all with anencephaly can be recognized. Currently it is routine for all women having an amniocentesis for cytogenetic analysis to also have their amniotic fluid AFP level measured.

In addition to a fetal NTD, there are several other causes of elevated (or apparently elevated) amniotic fluid AFP. These include underestimation of gestational age, fetal death, presence of twins,

A

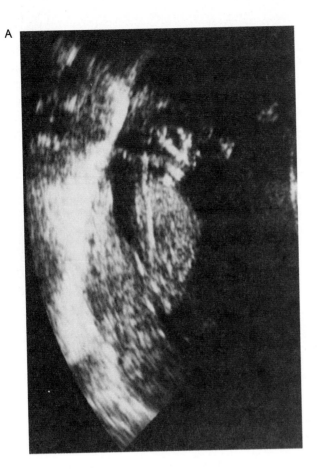

B

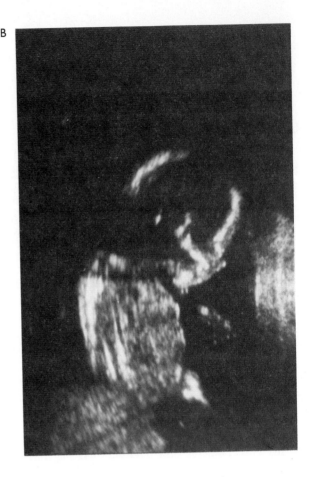

Figure 11-6 ■ *A,* Photograph of an ultrasound result, revealing the presence of a fetus with anencephaly. *B,* Ultrasound result for a normal fetus.

blood contamination, and several specific malformations (e.g., omphalocele or gastroschisis, which are abdominal wall defects). Usually, targeted ultrasonography can distinguish among these alternatives.

> **The amniotic α-fetoprotein level is elevated when the fetus has a neural tube defect and provides a reliable prenatal test for this condition.**

Soon after the link between elevated amniotic fluid AFP and NTDs was recognized, an association between elevated levels of **maternal serum AFP** **(MSAFP)** and NTDs was identified. AFP diffuses across the fetal membranes into the serum of the pregnant female, so MSAFP levels are correlated with amniotic fluid AFP levels. Thus, it possible to measure amniotic fluid AFP noninvasively by obtaining a maternal blood sample.

Because 90% to 95% of NTD births occur in the absence of a previous family history of the condition, a safe, noninvasive population screening procedure for NTDs is highly desirable. However,

there is considerable overlap of MSAFP levels in women carrying NTD and normal fetuses (Fig. 11-7). Thus, the issues of sensitivity and specificity must be considered. Typically, an MSAFP level is

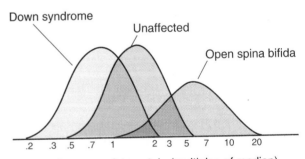

Maternal serum α-fetoprotein (multiples of median)

Figure 11-7 ■ **Maternal serum α-fetoprotein (MSAFP) levels in mothers carrying normal fetuses and in mothers carrying fetuses with Down syndrome and open spina bifida. MSAFP is somewhat lowered when the fetus has Down syndrome, and it is substantially elevated when the fetus has an open spina bifida.** (From Milansky, 1992)

considered to be elevated if it is 2 or 2.5 times higher than the normal median level (adjustments for maternal weight, presence of diabetes mellitus, and race are included in these calculations). Approximately 1% to 2% of pregnant women will exhibit MSAFP levels above this cutoff level. They may then choose to undergo amniocentesis to determine whether they are carrying a fetus with an NTD. After adjustment for advanced gestational age, fetal demise, and presence of twins, about 1 in 15 of these women will have an elevated amniotic fluid AFP. Thus, the positive predictive value of the MSAFP screening test is rather low, approximately 6% (1 of 15). However, the sensitivity of the test is fairly high: MSAFP screening will identify approximately 90% of anencephaly cases and about 80% of open spina bifida cases. Although this sensitivity level is lower than that of amniotic fluid AFP testing, the risk of the MSAFP measurement is also much lower.

An association has also been found between *low* MSAFP and the presence of a fetus with Down syndrome. Previously, population screening for Down syndrome consisted of amniocentesis for women older than 35 years. This screening strategy has a detection rate (sensitivity) of only 20% because only about 20% of all babies with trisomy 21 will be born to mothers older than age 35. MSAFP measurement has expanded the option of population screening for Down syndrome.

As indicated in Figure 11-7, MSAFP levels overlap considerably in normal and Down syndrome pregnancies. The risk for Down syndrome in women younger than age 35 increases by a factor of 3 to 4 when the adjusted MSAFP value is lower than 0.5 multiples of the normal population median. In deriving a risk estimate, complex formulas take into account the mother's weight, age, and MSAFP level. A woman who is 25 years of age ordinarily has a risk of about 1 in 1250 for producing a fetus with Down syndrome, but if she has a weight-adjusted MSAFP of 0.35 multiples of the median, her risk increases to 1 in 171. This risk is higher than that of a 35-year-old woman in the general population. Most screening programs use a risk factor of 1 in 380 (equivalent to the average risk for a 35-year-old woman to produce a newborn with Down syndrome) as an indication for amniocentesis.

It has recently been shown that the accuracy of Down syndrome screening can be increased by measuring the serum levels of unconjugated estriol and human chorionic gonadotropin in addition to MSAFP. The use of these three indicators can identify approximately 60% of Down syndrome pregnancies.

> MSAFP has provided a screening approach that increases the ability to prenatally detect fetuses with various abnormalities, including NTDs and Down syndrome. This noninvasive procedure entails virtually no risk, but its sensitivity for detecting NTDs is lower than that of amniotic AFP diagnosis.

New Diagnostic Techniques: Preimplantation Diagnosis and Circulating Fetal Cell Diagnosis

Several new approaches to prenatal diagnosis are now in the testing or early application stages. These include two preimplantation diagnostic approaches, in vitro fertilization diagnosis and polar body diagnosis, and the diagnosis of fetal cells obtained from the mother's circulation. Because each of these methods involves the analysis of DNA from a single cell or very few cells, each depends critically on the use of the polymerase chain reaction (PCR).

In Vitro Fertilization Diagnosis

In vitro fertilization diagnosis begins with the removal of a single cell from an 8- or 16-cell blastomere that has been generated through in vitro fertilization. The removal of one cell does not adversely affect the development of the blastomere. Using PCR, the DNA from the single cell can be amplified, leading to the diagnosis of single-gene conditions. If the disease-causing mutation is not detected, the blastomere is implanted into the mother's uterus. Several genetic diseases, including chronic granulomatous disease and cystic fibrosis, have been tested using this approach. The subsequent pregnancies have been normal.

Polar Body Diagnosis

Polar body diagnosis involves an examination of the polar body shed at the same time as the ovum. The polar body's DNA is tested to determine whether it contains a disease-causing mutation. If so, it is assumed that the egg does not contain the mutation. This egg is then fertilized and implanted using the usual in vitro techniques. Polar body and blastomere diagnoses both offer the advantage of early detection of genetic disorders. These approaches, however, are costly and technologically challenging, and they are still in the early stages of development.

Diagnosis Using Fetal Cells Isolated from Maternal Blood

During pregnancy a small number of fetal cells find their way into the mother's circulation. One such cell type is the nucleated red blood cell, which is common in the fetus but rare in the adult circulation. These cells can be identified using cell-sorting techniques. Further specificity for fetal cells can be achieved by testing cells for receptors expressed only in early erythrocytes but not mature erythrocytes. Using FISH analysis (see Chapter 6) of fetal cells obtained from maternal circulation, it has been possible to diagnose trisomy 21 and trisomy 18. The major advantage of this approach is that it requires only a blood sample from the mother and thus poses no risk for the fetus. Its accuracy and feasibility are being evaluated.

■ FETAL TREATMENT

A goal of prenatal diagnosis is treatment of the affected fetus. Although this is not currently possible for most conditions, some examples, many of which are still in the experimental stage, can be cited.

Two of the best-established forms of in utero intervention are treatment for rare inborn errors of metabolism and treatment for hormone deficiencies. An important example of a biochemical disorder for which treatment is available is biotin responsive multiple carboxylase deficiency. This autosomal recessive enzyme deficiency can be diagnosed by amniocentesis. In one case report oral administration of biotin to the mother was initiated at 23 weeks of pregnancy. This resulted in the birth of a normal baby.

Congenital adrenal hyperplasia (CAH) is a second example of a condition in which in utero treatment has been successful. Because of excessive androgen secretion by the enlarged adrenal glands, female fetuses with CAH become masculinized. Administration of dexamethasone to the mother beginning at 10 weeks post-LMP diminishes or prevents this masculinization.

Surgical treatment of fetuses, primarily for conditions involving urinary tract obstruction, has met with moderate success. Surgical correction of diaphragmatic hernia at 20 weeks gestation has also been attempted. Preliminary results have been discouraging, but work is continuing. In utero correction of fetal hydrocephalus was halted after initial results showed no beneficial effects.

■ GENE THERAPY

As we have seen, the isolation and cloning of disease genes provide opportunities for improved understanding and diagnosis of genetic diseases. In addition, the possibility of inserting normal copies of genes into individuals with genetic diseases (**gene therapy**) emerges. Although gene therapy is still in its infancy and has only begun to affect the lives of patients, the potential for curing genetic diseases through recombinant DNA techniques has excited a great deal of interest in both professional and lay circles. As of 1995, over 100 gene therapy clinical trials have been initiated (see Table 11-7 for some examples). In this section we review gene therapy techniques and discuss their application to disease therapy.

Somatic Cell Therapy

Somatic cell gene therapy, which has been the focus of gene therapy research in humans, consists of the introduction of normal genes into human somatic cells to treat a specific disorder. The pa-

Table 11-7 ■ A partial list of diseases for which somatic cell gene therapy protocols are being tested

Disease	Target cell	Inserted gene
ADA deficiency	Circulating lymphocytes, bone marrow stem cells	Adenosine deaminase
Hemophilia B	Hepatocytes, skin fibroblasts	Factor IX
Familial hypercholesterolemia	Hepatocytes	Low density lipoprotein receptor
Cystic fibrosis	Airway epithelial cells	CFTR
Malignant melanoma	Tumor-infiltrating lymphocytes	Tumor necrosis factor
Duchenne muscular dystrophy	Myoblasts	Dystrophin
Gaucher disease (lysosomal storage disorder)	Macrophages	Glucocerebrosidase
Lung cancer	Lung cancer cells	Normal p53
Brain tumors	Brain cells	Herpes thymidine kinase
Ovarian cancer	Ovarian cancer cells	Herpes thymidine kinase
AIDS	Cytotoxic T lymphocytes	Herpes thymidine kinase

tient's cells may be extracted and manipulated outside the body (ex vivo therapy), or in some cases the cells may be treated while they are in the body (in vivo therapy). Some types of somatic cells are more amenable to gene therapy than others. Good candidates should be easily accessible and should have a long life span in the body. Proliferating cells are preferred for some gene delivery systems because the vector carrying the gene can then integrate into the cell's DNA. The bone marrow stem cell meets all of these qualifications and thus has been a prime candidate cell for somatic therapy. However, these cells are difficult to manipulate and to isolate from bone marrow (the great majority of bone marrow cells are not stem cells). Consequently, many other cell types have been investigated as potential targets, including skin fibroblasts, muscle cells, vascular endothelial cells, hepatocytes, and lymphocytes. A disadvantage of using cells like lymphocytes is that their life span is relatively short. Thus, therapy using these cells requires repeated treatment and administration of cells.

Not all types of diseases are well suited to gene therapy. Many dominant diseases, in particular those caused by dominant negative mutations, are likely to be difficult to treat because blockage of a gene's effect would be required. Gene therapy is more easily achieved with recessive diseases that involve a defective or missing gene product. Here the insertion of a normal gene will supply the missing product. Many recessive enzyme deficiency disorders can potentially be corrected when only about 10% of the normal enzyme level is produced. Thus, even a partially effective gene therapy strategy may provide significant health benefits.

There are many possible methods for introducing genes into cells, including cell fusion, calcium phosphate coprecipitation (the chemical disturbs the cell membrane, allowing foreign DNA to enter), microinjection, electroporation (electrically shocking the cell so that foreign DNA can pass through the membrane), and liposome fusion. Next, we discuss two of the more commonly used delivery systems, retroviruses and adenoviruses.

Retroviral Vectors

As mentioned in Chapter 9, retroviruses are able to insert copies of their genomes into host cells after reverse-transcribing their viral RNA into DNA. They integrate into the host DNA with a high degree of efficiency, making them a reasonable choice as a gene-delivery vector (Fig. 11-8). The retrovirus must be modified so that it cannot replicate and

infect the host. This is done by using recombinant DNA techniques to delete most of the retroviral genome, replacing it with a normal copy of a human gene, its regulatory elements, and a polyadenylation signal (the human genetic material is termed the "insert"). Retroviruses are capable of accepting inserts as large as 8 kb.

These replication-defective retroviruses are propagated in **packaging cells** (sometimes called helper cells) that compensate for the missing replicative machinery of the retrovirus. This allows the production of multiple copies of retroviruses that contain the human gene but cannot replicate themselves. Retrovirus-containing particles are then incubated with the patient's somatic cells (e.g., human bone marrow stem cells or lymphocytes). The modified retrovirus inserts the normal human gene into the DNA of the host cell. Ideally, the normal gene will then encode a normal gene product in the patient's somatic cells. This type of protocol has been initially successful in treating adenosine deaminase deficiency (Clinical Commentary 11-5).

Although retroviral gene therapy holds considerable promise, there are several important obstacles:
1. *Transient and low-level expression.* The gene product may be expressed at subtherapeutic levels, often less than 1% of the normal amount. In part, this reflects the fact that only some of the target cells successfully incorporate the normal gene. In addition, random insertion of the retrovirus into the host's genome may affect gene regulation. Transcription of the gene often ceases after a few weeks or months.
2. *Difficulties in reaching target tissue.* While some systemic disorders may be relatively easy to target by modifying lymphocytes or possibly bone marrow stem cells, others present formidable challenges. It is often difficult, for example, to target affected neurons responsible for central nervous system disorders.
3. *Potential for oncogenesis.* Because a retrovirus integrates randomly into the host's DNA, it could locate near a proto-oncogene, activating it, and thus causing tumor formation. The retroviral promoters are altered to minimize this possibility, and thus far no cases of oncogenesis directly attributable to retrovirus insertion have been observed.
4. *Necessity for precise regulation of gene activity.* Accurate regulation of gene activity is not a concern for some diseases (e.g., a 50-fold overexpression of adenosine deaminase has no clinically significant effects). However, it is critical

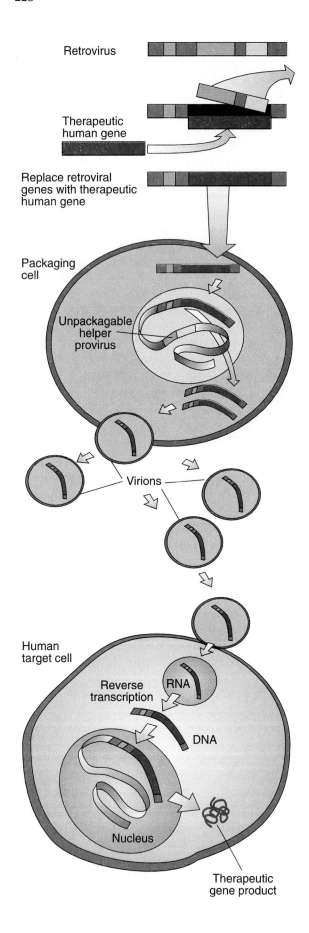

Retrovirus

Therapeutic human gene

Replace retroviral genes with therapeutic human gene

Packaging cell

Unpackagable helper provirus

Virions

Human target cell

Reverse transcription

RNA

DNA

Nucleus

Therapeutic gene product

for diseases such as thalassemia, in which the number of α-globin and β-globin chains must be closely balanced (see Chapter 3). It is difficult to achieve such precision using retroviral gene therapy.

5. *Retroviruses will infect only actively dividing cells.* This property of retroviruses precludes their use in nondividing or slowly dividing cells (e.g., neurons).

Considerable research is being devoted to overcoming these problems. In particular, methods for targeted insertion of genes are being explored, and ways to increase the levels and permanence of gene expression are being developed.

Adenovirus Vectors

Because of the inability of retroviruses to invade nondividing cells, other delivery systems have been explored that are not limited in this way. An important example is the **adenovirus**, a double-stranded DNA virus that is often used in vaccine preparations. Like the retrovirus, the adenovirus can accept an insert of no more than 7 to 8 kb in size. It must be made replication-defective before use in gene therapy. Because of its ability to target nondividing cells, adenoviruses are now being used in trials in which the normal CFTR gene (see Chapter 4) is delivered by an aerosol method to epithelial cells (in vivo gene therapy). It is hoped that this treatment may alter chloride ion channel activity in CF patients. A disadvantage of adenoviruses is that they do not integrate into the host cell's DNA. Thus, they are eventually lost, resulting in transient gene expression and the necessity for reintroduction of the vector. A current difficulty in clinical trials is that adenoviruses induce inflammatory responses in patients. Other vectors, such as liposomes and adeno-associated viruses, may circumvent this problem.

Gene Therapy for Noninherited Diseases

As indicated in Table 11-7, the application of gene therapy techniques is by no means limited to inherited diseases. For example, a gene encoding tumor necrosis factor (TNF) has been inserted ex

Figure 11-8 ■ **Gene therapy using a retroviral vector. The retrovirus is prevented from replicating by removing most of its genome, a normal human gene is inserted into the retrovirus, and the retrovirus is propagated in a packaging cell. Virions from the packaging cell are incubated with human somatic cells, allowing the retrovirus to insert copies of the normal human gene into the cell. Once integrated into the cell's DNA, the inserted gene produces normal gene product.**

Clinical Commentary 11-5. Adenosine deaminase deficiency and gene therapy

Adenosine deaminase (ADA) is produced primarily in lymphoid tissues. It is an important component of the purine salvage pathway, catalyzing the deamination of adenosine into inosine as well as deoxyadenosine (dAdo) into deoxyinosine. ADA deficiency, an autosomal recessive disorder, results in the accumulation of dAdo and its metabolites. This inhibits DNA synthesis in cells and is especially toxic to T lymphocytes. Subsequently, B lymphocytes are also reduced in function and number. The resulting severe combined immune deficiency (SCID, Chapter 8) is usually fatal by the age of 2 if untreated. It is estimated that approximately 25% to 30% of SCID cases are caused by ADA deficiency.

The preferred treatment for ADA deficiency is a bone marrow transplant. However, complications of bone marrow transplants increase patient morbidity and are sometimes fatal. In addition, major histocompatibility complex-compatible sibling donors are available for fewer than 30% of ADA deficiency patients. Patients may be treated with polyethylene glycol (PEG)–conjugated ADA (administered once or twice weekly by intramuscular injection), but the response to this treatment is variable, and some patients develop antibodies against PEG-ADA.

Because it is a systemic, autosomal recessive disorder caused by an enzyme deficiency, ADA deficiency represents a good candidate for gene therapy. Ideally, proliferating bone marrow stem cells would be modified by retroviral vectors containing the normal ADA gene, resulting in a permanent cure for the disorder. Because of difficulties in dealing with bone marrow stem cells, gene therapy for ADA deficiency has been initiated instead by retroviral insertion of ADA genes into lymphocytes that have been extracted from patients and artificially stimulated to replicate. After retroviral insertion, the lymphocytes are injected back into the patient's peripheral circulation.

In two girls in whom this therapy has been applied, the results have been encouraging. Following gene therapy, their ADA levels increased eventually to about 25% of the normal level. Their T lymphocyte counts improved dramatically, and the number of infections they experience is described as "average." Both are now attending public schools. Because of the limited life span of T lymphocytes, these patients must be reinjected with modified T cells once every several months.

There are potential concerns associated with this procedure. For example, there is a possibility of retrovirally induced oncogenesis in a T cell. Also, because only a sample of mature T cells is treated, the immune systems of these patients are likely to be incomplete (i.e., there would be less T cell receptor diversity than in a normal individual). Nonetheless, the initial results are promising, and they provide invaluable information for the development of gene therapy protocols for other genetic diseases.

---

vivo into tumor-infiltrating lymphocytes in the treatment of malignant melanoma. Although TNF is toxic when administered systemically, it is hoped that the patient's tumor-infiltrating lymphocytes, which naturally target the melanomas, will direct TNF specifically to the tumors and destroy them. Gene therapy is even being tested in the treatment of rheumatoid arthritis, where the goal is to block the inflammatory effects of interleukin-1 (IL-1). A gene that encodes IL-1 receptor antagonist protein (IRAP) is inserted into the synovial cells that line the joints, thereby limiting IL-1-caused inflammation.

Germline Therapy

Somatic cell therapy consists of the alteration only of specific somatic cells and thus differs little in principle from many other types of medical intervention (e.g., bone marrow transplants). In contrast, **germline gene therapy** involves the alteration of all cells of the body, including those giving rise to the gametes. Thus, this type of gene therapy would affect not only the patient but all of his or her descendants.

Germline therapy was achieved in the mouse in 1983, when copies of a human growth hormone gene were successfully introduced into mouse embryos by microinjection (the gene is inserted directly into the embryo using a small needle). Among the minority of embryos in which the gene integrated, the gametes were also modified, and the human growth hormone gene was transmitted to future generations (the mice, incidentally, were abnormally large). Although germline therapy is in principle possible in humans, it presents significant problems. First, injected embryos usually die, and some develop tumors and malformations. Second, even in an autosomal dominant disorder, half of the embryos will be genetically normal. If it is possible to distinguish the genetically normal embryos (e.g., through PCR diagnosis of in vitro fertilization products), then it would be simpler to implant the normal embryos than to alter the abnormal ones. Finally, there are numerous ethical questions associated with the permanent alteration of a human's genetic heritage. For these reasons, it appears unlikely that human germline therapy would be useful or desirable.

■ STUDY QUESTIONS

1. A newborn screening program for a metabolic disease has just been initiated. Of 100,000 newborns, 100 were shown by a definitive test to have been affected with the disease. The screening test identified 93 of these individuals as affected and 7 as unaffected. It also identified 1000 individuals as affected who were later shown to be unaffected. Calculate the sensitivity, specificity, and positive predictive value of the screening test, and specify the rate of false-positives and false-negatives.

2. Study the family shown in the accompanying pedigree. Individual 3 has PKU, an autosomal recessive disease. A 2-allele RFLP closely linked to the PKU locus has been assayed for each family member, and the figure shows the genotypes of each individual. The marker alleles are 5 kb and 3 kb in size. Based on the genotypes of the linked marker, is individual 6 affected, a heterozygous carrier, or a normal homozygote?

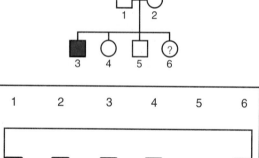

3. Study the family shown in the accompanying pedigree. The affected individuals have Huntington disease, an autosomal dominant condition. A 4-allele VNTR system closely linked to

the Huntington disease locus has been typed for each family member. Based on the genotypes shown in the accompanying figure, will individual 6 develop Huntington disease?

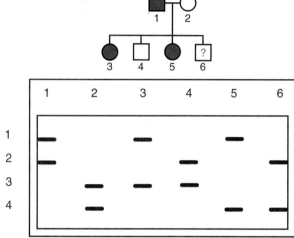

4. In the accompanying pedigree for an autosomal dominant disorder, a tightly linked 2-allele RFLP has been typed in each family member. Based on this information, what can you tell the family about the risk that the offspring in generation III will develop the disorder? How might diagnostic accuracy be improved in this case?

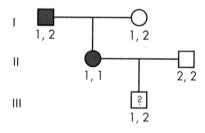

5. Compare the advantages and disadvantages of amniocentesis and chorionic villus sampling (CVS).

6. Why might Huntington disease be a poor candidate for gene therapy?

■ ADDITIONAL READING

American Academy of Pediatrics Committee on Genetics: Newborn screening fact sheets, Pediatrics 83:449–464, 1989.

Blaese RM, Culver KW, Miller AD, Carter CS, Fleisher T, Clerici M, Shearer G, et al. T lymphocyte-directed gene therapy for ADA-SCID: initial trial results after 4 years, Science 270:475–480, 1995.

Boucher RC: Current status of CF therapy, Trends Genet 12:81–84, 1996.

Burton BK: Elevated maternal serum alpha-fetoprotein (MSAFP): interpretation and follow-up, Clin Obstet Gynecol 31:293–305, 1988.

Caskey CT: Presymptomatic diagnosis: a first step toward genetic health care, Science 262:48–49, 1993.

Charrow J, Nadler HL, and Evans MI: Prenatal diagnosis and therapy. In Emery AEH and Rimoin DL, editors: Principles and practice of medical genetics, vol 1, ed 2, Edinburgh, 1990, Churchill Livingstone.

Crystal RG: Transfer of genes to humans: early lessons and obstacles to success, Science 270:404–410, 1995.

D'Alton ME and DeCherney AH: Prenatal diagnosis, N Engl J Med 328:114–119, 1993.

Elias S, Annas GJ, and Simpson JL: Carrier screening for cystic fibrosis: implications for obstetric and gynecologic practice, Am J Obstet Gynecol 164:1077–1083, 1991.

Elias S: Maternal serum screening for fetal genetic disorders. Edinburgh, Churchill Livingstone, 1992.

Friedmann T: Gene therapy for neurological disorders, Trends Genet 10:210–214, 1994.

Fries MH, Golbus MS: Prenatal diagnosis. In Leder P, Clayton DA, Rubenstein E, editors: Introduction to Molecular Medicine, New York, 1994, Scientific American.

Handyside AH, Lesko JG, Tarín JJ, et al: Birth of a normal girl after in vitro fertilization and preimplantation diagnostic testing for cystic fibrosis, N Engl J Med 327:905–909, 1992.

Kaback MM: Heterozygote screening. In Emery AEH and Rimoin DL, editors: Principles and practice of medical genetics, vol 1, ed 2, Edinburgh, 1990, Churchill Livingstone.

Kaback M, Lim-Steele J, Dabholkar D, et al: Tay-Sachs disease—carrier screening, prenatal diagnosis, and the molecular era: an international perspective, 1970 to 1993, JAMA 270:2307–2315, 1993.

Korf B: Molecular diagnosis, N Eng J Med 332:1218–1220, 1995.

Marshall E: Gene therapy's growing pains, Science 269:1050–1055, 1995.

Mausner JS and Bahn AK: Epidemiology: an introductory text, Philadelphia, 1974, WB Saunders.

Milunsky A, editor: Genetic disorders and the fetus: diagnosis, prevention, and treatment, ed 3, Baltimore, 1992, Johns Hopkins University Press.

Motulsky A: Invited editorial: Predictive genetic diagnosis, Am J Hum Genet 55:603–605, 1994.

National Academy of Sciences: Genetic screening: programs, principles and research, Washington, DC, 1975, National Academy of Sciences.

O'Neal WK, Beaudet AL: Somatic gene therapy for cystic fibrosis, Hum Molec Genet 3:1497–1502, 1994.

Pitkin RM: Screening and detection of congenital malformation, Am J Obstet Gynecol 164:1045–1048, 1991.

Simpson JL: Isolating fetal cells from maternal blood: advances in prenatal diagnosis through molecular technology, JAMA 270:2357–2361, 1993.

Trent RJ: Molecular medicine: an introductory text for students, Edinburgh, 1993, Churchill Livingstone.

Wang BT, Peng W, Cheng K-T, Chiu S-F, Ho W, Khan Y, Wittman M, et al.: Chorionic villi sampling: laboratory experience with 4,000 consecutive cases, Am J Med Genet 53:307–316, 1994.

Weaver D: Catalog of prenatally diagnosed conditions, ed 2, Baltimore, 1992, Johns Hopkins University Press.

Wilfond BS and Fost N: The cystic fibrosis gene: medical and social implications for heterozygote detection, JAMA 263:2777–2783, 1990.

Wu Y and Foreman RC: The molecular genetics of α1-antitrypsin deficiency, Bioessays 13:163–169, 1991.

Wulfsberg EA, Hoffman DE, and Cohen MM: α1-Antitrypsin deficiency: impact of genetic discovery on medicine and society, JAMA 271:217–222, 1994.

12 Clinical Genetics and Genetic Counseling

Medical genetics has recently emerged as a true specialty in medicine. In the 1960s the fields of biochemical genetics, clinical cytogenetics, and **dysmorphology** (the study of abnormal physical development) developed. The 1970s witnessed the establishment of the techniques necessary for the prenatal diagnosis of genetic disorders. By the end of the 1970s, discussions about the formation of an American Board of Medical Genetics had occurred, and in 1981 the first certification examination was administered. Ten years later the American Board of Medical Specialties recognized this new field.

Whereas medical genetics is the study of the hereditary nature of human disease, **clinical genetics** deals with the direct clinical care of persons with genetic diseases. The diagnostic, counseling, and management issues surrounding genetic disease are the principal foci of clinical genetics.

In this chapter we summarize the principles of clinical genetics and the process of genetic counseling. In addition, this chapter provides an overview of the field of dysmorphology since the growth of this area has influenced and paralleled the emergence of clinical genetics.

■ THE PRINCIPLES AND PRACTICE OF CLINICAL GENETICS

As mentioned in Chapter 1, genetic conditions as a group are common and are a significant cause of human mortality and morbidity. Typically, genetic disorders are complex, multiorgan, and systemic conditions. The care of persons with these disorders often involves multiple specialties. Thus genetic disorders are part of the differential diagnosis of most symptoms and clinical presentations. For example, when evaluating an infant with a blistering skin disease, the ability to distinguish between one of the many forms of epidermolysis bullosa (an inherited disorder of keratinocytes in which skin blisters develop after mild trauma; *SOL* 67) and

staphylococcal skin disease must be part of the clinician's repertoire.

Because of the complexity and number of human genetic diseases, their clinical diagnosis and treatment can seem overwhelming. To help manage this information, we provide an overview of the most important concepts. These include the importance of accurate diagnosis, the application of the tenets of medical genetics to medical practice, and the role of genetic counseling in the care of persons with genetic disease.

Accurate Diagnosis

The significance of this basic medical principle cannot be overemphasized. The process of genetic counseling, one of the central services of medical genetics, begins with correct diagnosis. All discussions of natural history, prognosis, management, risk determination, options for prenatal diagnosis, and referral to support groups depend on an accurate diagnosis. For example, genetic counseling for a family who has a son with mental retardation usually involves questions of risk for this condition in future offspring. An accurate answer requires the clinician to identify a condition of known etiology. If a specific diagnosis (e.g., fragile X syndrome) is made, then the rest of the genetic counseling process starts: current information can be shared and management initiated (see Clinical Commentary 12-1 for further discussion of this point).

> In clinical genetics, as in all of medicine, accurate diagnosis is the most important first step in patient care.

The process of diagnosing a genetic disorder is a complex sequence of events. It depends upon diagnostic decision-making, biochemistry, dysmorphology, laboratory diagnosis, and the basic principles of medical genetics. For diseases in which the diagnostic criteria are well established, the practi-

Clinical Commentary 12-1. Reasons for Making a Diagnosis of a Syndrome

The long list of syndromes associated with congenital malformations is overwhelming to the clinician. More than 400 conditions are listed in *Smith's Recognizable Patterns of Human Malformations,* and more than 1000 are accessible through the POSSUM computerized data base. This number imparts a sense that the diagnosis of a malformation syndrome lies in the arena of "academic trivia." However, this is not the case.

Consider, for example, the child who is large for gestational age and has a number of physical abnormalities: omphalocele (intestinal protrusion at the umbilicus), large tongue, facial hemangioma, flank mass, and asymmetric limb length (Fig. 12-1). His family has questions such as "what does he have?", "how will he do?", "will he look different?", "will he have mental retardation?", and "what is the chance of his condition occurring again?"

By putting these features together and making the pattern recognition diagnosis of the Wiedemann-Beckwith syndrome, the clinician is able to answer all of the parents' questions fairly precisely. Wiedemann-Beckwith syndrome is an autosomal dominant condition with variable expression and incomplete penetrance. In addition, the gene is thought to exhibit imprinting. When there is no family history, however, the sibling recurrence risk is less than 5%. When there is a family history, the recurrence risk is much higher, and linkage analysis may provide a more precise risk estimate. In future pregnancies prenatal diagnosis using ultrasound can be implemented to look for an omphalocele in the second trimester as well as large size for gestational age, excessive amniotic fluid (polyhydramnios), and large tongue. If a fetus is thought to have Wiedemann-Beckwith syndrome, then the delivery plan would change and the baby should be born in a tertiary care center.

Children with the Wiedemann-Beckwith syndrome do not usually have mental retardation. Although the large tongue can cause orthodontic problems, speech difficulties, and occasionally upper airway problems, these conditions usually improve as one gets older. The facial appearance is not strikingly abnormal in later childhood.

Chromosomes should probably be studied, although most Wiedemann-Beckwith patients do not have the chromosome 11 abnormality which has been reported in a small number of cases. Otherwise the main emphases of the medical care plan include periodic ultrasound to look for intraabdominal malignancies, especially Wilms tumor and hepatoblastoma. Children with Wiedemann-Beckwith syndrome have a 5% to 10% risk of developing these tumors, and both types are treatable if detected early.

In this example it was important to diagnose the Wiedemann-Beckwith syndrome. The correct label led to precise information for genetic counseling, prediction of natural history (including reassurance), organization of appropriate laboratory studies, a health maintenance plan, and referral to a support group. Diagnosis was helpful to the parents, the family physician, and the child.

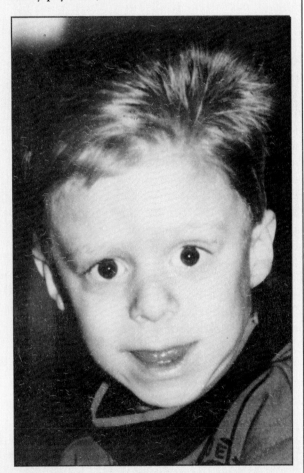

Figure 12-1 ■ A child with Wiedemann-Beckwith syndrome. Note the prominent eyes and large, protruding tongue. (Courtesy of Dr. David Viskochil, University of Utah Health Sciences Center).

tioner has guidelines for making a diagnosis. An example of such criteria would be those recommended by the National Institutes of Health Consensus Development Conference for the diagnosis of neurofibromatosis type 1 (NF1, see Chapter 4). For conditions that are defined by a specific laboratory marker, such as an abnormal karyotype or biochemical assay, the diagnostic procedure is generally straightforward. For many genetic diseases, however, there are no well-established criteria, and the definition and delineation of the disorder are not clear-cut.

Dysmorphic syndromes require knowledge and skills in the recognition of mild malformations, minor anomalies, and phenotypic variations. The diagnosis of other genetic diseases may require expertise from a variety of disciplines. For instance, the diagnosis of any of the forms of retinitis pigmentosa (see Chapter 7) requires input from an ophthalmologist who is familiar with this group of retinal degenerative conditions. The diagnostic process is further complicated by the variable expression, incomplete penetrance, and heterogeneity of many genetic diseases. These concepts were discussed in Chapter 4.

Application of the Principles of Medical Genetics

Developing a genetic approach to human disease in the clinical setting requires the application of all of the basic principles of medical genetics discussed in this book. For example, making or excluding the diagnosis of NF1 requires knowledge of the clinical variability and age of onset of certain features of the condition (see Clinical Commentary 12-2 for further discussion). The recognition of the various forms of neurofibromatosis (i.e, recognition of heterogeneity) is also important.

Knowledge of the other formal principles of medical genetics is also necessary in the care of persons with genetic conditions. The accumulation of family history data and the interpretation of pedigree information are important in answering a family's questions of risk. An understanding of the different modes of inheritance is important in any explanation of recurrence risk. Discussion of the concepts of new mutation and pleiotropy are commonplace in reviewing the cause and pathogenesis of a genetic disease with a family. Even an understanding of meiosis is a requirement for discussions of etiology with the family of a newborn with Down syndrome.

Genetic Counseling
Definition and Principles

Genetic counseling represents one of the central foci of medical genetics. At first glance, use of the term *counseling* implies that this service lies in the domain of mental health, social work, or psychotherapy. In fact, genetic counseling is based on the conventional medical model because it depends significantly on accurate diagnosis and knowledge of medical genetics. As a tradition,

genetic counseling grew out of the field of human genetics rather than from behavioral science, unlike other counseling disciplines.

In 1975 the American Society of Human Genetics adopted a definition of genetic counseling that has stood the test of time:

Genetic counseling is a communication process which deals with the human problems associated with the occurrence or risk of occurrence of a genetic disorder in a family. This process involves an attempt by one or more appropriately trained persons to help the individual or family to: (1) comprehend the medical facts including the diagnosis, probable course of the disorder, and the available management, (2) appreciate the way heredity contributes to the disorder and the risk of recurrence in specified relatives, (3) understand the alternatives for dealing with the risk of recurrence, (4) choose a course of action which seems to them appropriate in their view of their risk, their family goals, and their ethical and religious standards and act in accordance with that decision, and (5) to make the best possible adjustment to the disorder in an affected family member and/or to the risk of recurrence of that disorder.

This definition illustrates the complex tasks that face the practitioner. The first task involves establishing the diagnosis and discussing the natural history and management of the condition. In this regard the treatment of a genetic disease does not differ from that of any other type of disease.

The second task requires an understanding of the basic tenets of medical genetics, especially risk determination. For chromosomal and multifactorial disorders, empirical risks are used to estimate recurrence. Segregation patterns are used to predict the recurrence risk of mendelian disorders. However, the clinical issues are frequently complicated by incomplete penetrance, variable expression, delayed age of onset, and allelic and locus heterogeneity. In some cases, incorporation of additional information using the Bayesian probability approach can significantly alter risk estimates (Clinical Commentary 12-3, page 237).

The third and fourth objectives of the genetic counseling process underlie the primary differences between the genetic model and the traditional biomedical approach. These tasks involve the discussion of reproductive options and the facilitation of decision-making. Implicit in the fourth part of the definition is the notion of respect for the family's autonomy and their perceptions of risk and of the disorder itself. This approach has been called **nondirectiveness**: the counselor leaves all decisions about future reproduction up to the family. This differs somewhat from the more traditional

Clinical Commentary 12-2. Negative Family History

One of the common discussions on ward rounds is the notation that a person's family history is "negative" or "noncontributory." This is often thought to rule out a genetic disorder. However, the *majority* of individuals who have a genetic disease will not have a "positive" family history. A quick review of the mechanisms of mendelian, chromosomal, and multifactorial disease inheritance shows that a lack of other affected persons in the family is common and does not by any means rule out the presence of a genetic disease. For example, the sibling recurrence risk is 25% for diseases with autosomal recessive inheritance. Thus a significant number of families with multiple offspring will only have one affected child and no family history. Even some well-established autosomal dominant disorders may often present a negative family history because of high proportions of new mutations [examples include Marfan syndrome, neurofibromatosis type 1 (NF1), and achondroplasia, in which the proportions of cases caused by new mutations are 30%, 50%, and 80%, respectively]. Chromosomal syndromes usually have a low recurrence risk. Even when a parent carries a balanced chromosome rearrangement, the recurrence risk among the offspring is usually less than 15%. The sibling recurrence risks for multifactorial conditions are usually 5% or less.

Case

A family comes in with a 6-year-old boy who has 10 *café-au-lait* spots exceeding 0.5 cm in diameter and an optic glioma (Fig. 12-2, page 236). The family has questions about the diagnosis and recurrence risk in future pregnancies. On initial telephone contact it is learned that there is no history of a family member with similar features.

There are several possible explanations for this finding. Exploring them underscores the implications of a negative family history:

1. *New mutation of the NF1 gene.* Because of the relatively high proportion of new mutations for this disorder, this is the most likely explanation.
2. *Variable expression.* It is also possible that one of the parents carries the gene with mild expression. Occasionally a parent has multiple *café-au-lait* spots and a few neurofibromas, but a diagnosis of NF1 has never been made.
3. *Incomplete penetrance.* This is a possibility; however, it is unlikely for NF1, in which penetrance is close to 100%. If a family has two children with NF1 and neither parent has the gene, germline mosaicism would be the more likely explanation.
4. *Incorrect diagnosis.* One of the assumptions and basic principles of medical genetics is accurate diagnosis. This patient meets the NIH established criteria for NF1 (see Chapter 4). However, if this individual had only *café-au-lait* spots, then the diagnosis would have been an issue. One would need to know the differential diagnosis of multiple *café-au-lait* spots.
5. *False paternity.* Although relatively unlikely, this possibility must be kept in mind.

We began with an individual having a classical autosomal dominant disorder with no family history. This can be explained in a number of ways. The statement that there is "a negative family history" should not be considered conclusive evidence against the presence of a heritable condition.

Continued.

---

medical approach in which *recommendations* for treatment or intervention are made.

This is an important issue because nondirectiveness sometimes conflicts with the broader view of preventive medicine, which might suggest that the principal goal of genetic counseling should be the reduction of the incidence of genetic diseases. If prevention or reduction of occurrence is the primary goal, then one's approach might be more directive. However, the main goal of genetic counseling is to help families understand and cope with genetic disease, not to reduce the incidence of genetic disease.

Although most geneticists subscribe to the principles of autonomy and nondirectiveness, it may sometimes be impossible to be entirely nondirective simply because of the limited options that the counselor has in a time-restricted session. In addition, information may be presented differently in different contexts. Information about Down syndrome, for example, may be communicated differently depending on whether a diagnosis has been made prenatally or following the birth of an affected newborn (Clinical Commentary 12-4, page 239).

The majority of clinical geneticists subscribe to the principle of nondirectiveness: information about risks, natural history, treatment, and outcome are presented in a balanced and neutral manner, but decisions about reproduction are left to the family.

The facilitation of discussion about reproductive decision-making is central to the task of genetic counseling. Several factors are involved in a family's decision about future pregnancies when there

Clinical Commentary 12-2. Negative Family History—*cont'd*

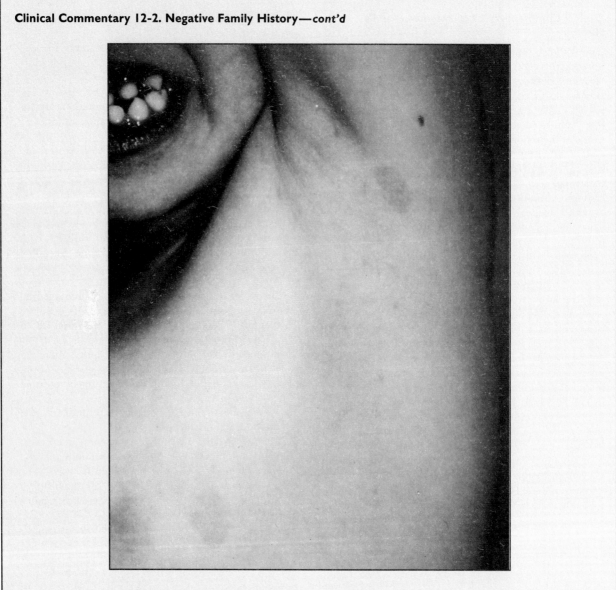

Figure 12-2 ▪ A 6-year-old boy with multiple *café-au-lait* spots and axillary freckling.

is an increased risk. The obvious ones are the magnitude of the risk figure and the burden or impact of the disorder. However, these are not the only significant issues. A family's individual perception of the impact of the condition is probably more important in their decision-making than the professional's perception of the burden. The meaning of children to the individual family, according to their own religious or personal preferences, is weighed heavily in the reproductive decision-making process. In addition, families frequently play out the scenario of coping with a recurrence of the condi-

tion in another child. Identification of these issues for a family often helps to stimulate their own discussions. Some families perceive risk qualitatively rather than quantitatively: they consider themselves to be either "at risk" or not, with the actual risk estimate being a secondary consideration. The fact that there is so much variation in the importance people assign to each of these factors (perception of risk, perception of impact, meaning of children, and the possibility of recurrence) underscores the point that the professional should be a facilitator and not the decision-maker.

Clinical Commentary 12-3. Recurrence Risks and Bayes Theorem

The estimation of recurrence risks was discussed in Chapters 4 and 5. A typical example of recurrence risk estimation would be a case in which a man affected with hemophilia A, an X-linked recessive disorder, produces a daughter (individual II-1 in the pedigree at right). Because the man can transmit only the X chromosome carrying the hemophilia A mutation to his daughter, she must be a carrier. The carrier's daughter, individual III-6, has a 50% chance of receiving the X chromosome carrying the mutation and being herself a carrier. Even though the daughter in generation III has five normal brothers, her risk remains 50% because we know that the mother in generation II is a carrier.

Suppose now that the woman in generation III produces three sons (generation IV), none of whom has hemophilia A. Intuitively, we might begin to suspect that she is not a carrier after all. How can we incorporate this new information into our recurrence risk estimate?

A statistical principle that allows us to make use of such information is called **Bayes theorem** (the application of Bayes theorem is often termed Bayesian analysis or Bayesian inference). The table below summarizes the basic steps involved in Bayesian analysis. We begin with the **prior probability** that the woman in generation III is a carrier. As its name suggests, the prior probability denotes the probability that she is a carrier *before* we account for the fact that she has produced three normal sons. Because we know her mother is a carrier, this prior probability must be 1/2. Then the prior probability that she is not a carrier is also 1/2.

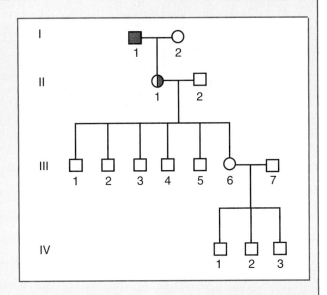

	She is a carrier	She is not a carrier
Prior probability	1/2	1/2
Conditional probability	1/8	1
Joint probability	1/16	1/2
Posterior probability	1/9	8/9

Next we take into account her three normal sons by estimating the probability that all three of them would be normal given that she is a carrier. Because this probability is *conditioned* on her carrier status, it is termed a **conditional probability**. If she is a carrier, the conditional probability that all three of her sons are normal is $(1/2)^3$, or 1/8. We also estimate the probability that all of her sons are normal, given that she is *not* a carrier. This conditional probability is, of course, very close to 1.

Next we want to find the probability that the woman is a carrier *and* that she is a carrier with three

normal sons. To obtain the probability of the co-occurrence of these two events, we multiply the prior probability times the conditional probability to derive a **joint probability** (i.e., the probability of *both* events occurring together, a concept discussed in Chapter 4). The joint probability that she is a carrier is then $1/2 \times 1/8 = 1/16$. Similarly, the joint probability that she is not a carrier is $1/2 \times 1 = 1/2$. These joint probabilities indicate the woman is 8 times more likely *not* to be a carrier than to be a carrier.

The final step is to standardize the joint probabilities so that the two probabilities under consideration (i.e., being a carrier vs. not being a carrier) add to 1. To do this we simply divide the joint probability that the woman is a carrier (1/16) by the sum of the two joint probabilities $(1/16 + 1/2)$. This yields a **posterior probability** of 1/9 that she is a carrier and 8/9 that she is not a carrier. Notice that this standardization process allows us to provide a risk estimate (1/9, or 11%) while preserving the odds of noncarrier versus carrier status indicated by the joint probabilities.

Having worked through the Bayesian analysis, we see that our intuition was confirmed: the fact that the woman in question produced three normal sons reduced her risk of being a carrier substantially, from an initial estimate of 50% to a final probability of only 11%.

Prior to the advent of disease diagnosis through linked markers or mutation detection, Bayesian analysis was often the only way to derive a risk estimate in a situation such as this one. Now, one would attempt to identify the factor VIII mutation that causes hemophilia A in this family directly, or, failing this, linked markers would be used. This is a much more direct and accurate approach for determining carrier status. However, as discussed in Chapter 11, it is not always possible to identify the responsible mutation, particularly when a large number of mutations can cause the

Continued.

Clinical Commentary 12-3. Recurrence Risks and Bayes Theorem—*cont'd*

disorder (as is the case for hemophilia A). In addition, linkage analysis is not always informative. Thus Bayesian analysis is still sometimes a useful tool for refining risk estimates.

The additional information incorporated in Bayesian analysis is not confined to the assessment of health status in relatives, as shown in this example. Another type of information is a biochemical assay, such as factor VIII activity level, that could help to

indicate carrier status. Because there is usually overlap between carriers and normal homozygotes for such tests, the assay cannot determine carrier status with certainty but gives us a *probability* estimate for incorporation into Bayesian analysis. In diseases with delayed age of onset, such as adult polycystic kidney disease, the probability of being affected at a certain age can be used in a Bayesian analysis. Here one considers the fact that the at-risk individual is less and less likely to have the disease gene if he or she remains normal beyond a certain age.

The final task of genetic counseling is to help the family cope with the presence of the disorder and/or its risk of recurrence. This task is similar to the physician's support of a family that deals with any chronic disease and/or disability. What is unique, perhaps, is the family's perception of the *meaning* of a genetic disorder. In many acquired conditions, such as infections or accidents, the ultimate meaning of the condition is externalized. In genetic disorders, the condition is more intrinsic to the individual and the family; it thus often presents a complex personal dilemma. Validation of the plight of families is vital and is probably more effective than simplistic attempts to wipe away guilt. Feelings of guilt and shame are natural to the situation and also need acknowledgment.

The primary care practitioner plays a vital role in the ongoing support of families in which a member has a genetic disease. Additional support strategies include referral of the family to a genetics support group, distribution of written information on the disorder, referral to mental health professionals for ongoing counseling, and frequent follow-up visits that include time for discussions of feelings and thoughts.

Genetic counseling includes five themes: medical management, risk determination, risk options, reproductive decision-making, and support services.

Numerous studies in the last two decades have attempted to evaluate the effectiveness of genetic counseling. The methodology of these studies is complicated, and the evaluation of the results depends on one's interpretation of the goal of genetic counseling. A few general points, however, can be made: Families tend to recall recurrence risks relatively well. A letter sent to them after the visit improves this recall. Families who perceive their

offspring's condition as being serious and one of "burden" recall risk figures better. Most studies suggest that genetic counseling is relatively effective in providing information about the medical aspects and genetic risks of the condition. Issues surrounding decision-making and psychosocial support require additional investigation.

Delivery of Genetic Counseling: Genetic Counselors and Support Groups

As genetic counseling evolved in the 1970s, it became clear that the delivery of this service is complex and time-consuming. Not only did the geneticist need to have skills in most specialties of medicine, but facilitation of decision-making and provision of psychological support were also necessary. As a need for genetics professionals other than the physician became apparent, a number of genetic counseling training programs were initiated. Currently, there are more than a dozen programs in North America that provide master's degree training in genetic counseling. Genetic counselors have become an integral part of the delivery of medical genetic services. From this growth evolved a professional society, the National Society of Genetic Counselors, and more recently the certifying and accrediting board, the American Board of Genetic Counseling. Although the range of skills is wide and job descriptions vary in different medical centers, genetic counselors have established themselves as experts in risk determination, reproductive decision-making, and psychosocial support.

The importance of support groups in assisting families in which a member has a genetic disorder is becoming increasingly obvious. These volunteer groups provide the family with the sense of the "fellow traveler" in a way that the professional is not able to do. The isolation that frequently accom-

Clinical Commentary 12-4. Talking to the Parents of a Newborn with Down Syndrome

The birth of a newborn with Down syndrome presents many challenges. Typically the infant is not acutely ill, and the parents will not be aware of the diagnosis. Thus the practitioner has to approach the parents, often strangers, with disappointing news. The family experiences a series of emotions that are somewhat similar to the reactions after a loss: anger, denial, sadness, and then usually reorganization and adaptation. Families face these situations with markedly different backgrounds: varying attitudes toward crisis, varied demographic and socioeconomic circumstances, and even a wide range of differences in the cultural meaning of a disability or defect. All of these variables, plus the fact that physicians are often not trained in being the bearers of bad news, can make this a difficult situation. Parents remember in detail the way in which the news was presented. The practitioner has both the opportunity and the challenge to help the family through these events.

From studies that have investigated the recommendations of parents who have experienced this event, we can provide a number of practical suggestions:

1. *Talk to both parents together whenever possible.* This is sometimes not practical, but when it can be accomplished it is critical.
2. *Communicate the diagnosis as soon as possible.* All studies of parental interviews show that they prefer early communication of the diagnosis.
3. *Choose a place that is private and quiet where both the parents and the professionals can sit down.* Avoid standing up with the parents seated. Always be sure to introduce yourself. Structure the interview from the beginning.
4. *Humanize the situation as much as possible.* Learn the baby's first name if it has been decided upon, and always know the baby's gender. Refer to the infant as a son or daughter, and be aware of the use of all language. Phrases such as "mental retardation" have great impact. Terms such as "mongolism" are not appropriate because they are stigmatizing, pejorative, and incorrect.
5. *Develop a sense of realistic positivism.* It is important to discuss the developmental limitations in a patient with Down syndrome, but it is also important to have an optimistic and positive attitude. This suggestion comes from the self-help and parents' organizations that have developed in the last two decades.
6. *Answer the parents' questions, but avoid technical overload.* It is important to be accurate and current on the biologic and medical aspects of the disease under discussion. When an answer is not known, mention that it can be reviewed or referred to a consultant.
7. *Listen actively.* Assume that almost all feelings are natural and that parents will be wrestling with their own guilt and shame. Validate all feelings that arise. Most parents will meet this challenge effectively and will not require psychiatric consultation.
8. *Refer the family to the appropriate resources early.* This would include parents' support groups or even individual parents who have a child with Down syndrome. Share any written material that is available, but make certain it is accurate and current.

Above all be aware of the unique plight of families in such a situation, and make an effort to spend time with them. Although it is difficult to present in written form how one can develop attributes such as kindness and empathy, it is important for physicians in training to learn from their mentors and utilize their own personality style as a strength.

---

panies genetic disorders (and rare conditions in general) is often alleviated by meeting someone else in the same situation. Immediate bonds are formed that often assist in the coping process. In the last few decades a clear partnership of professionals and persons with genetic disorders and disabilities has developed. Not only have these groups provided a needed service but they have also promoted the establishment of data bases and research studies. Referral to a support group and distribution of their written information are now a routine part of the care and management of persons with genetic disorders.

Genetic counseling involves a partnership of physicians, genetic counselors, and genetics support groups.

Clinical Genetics Evaluation and Services

With the development of medical genetics as a medical specialty, clinical genetics services have become part of the health care delivery system. Most university medical centers in North America include a genetics clinic whose major objective is the provision of genetic diagnosis and counseling services.

As in all medical visits, evaluation of a person or family for a potential genetic condition requires a thorough history and physical examination. The history includes information about the family's concerns, the prenatal period, labor, delivery, and documentation of family relationships (the pedigree). The physical examination should focus on the physical variations or minor anomalies that provide clues to a diagnosis. Additional family members may need evaluation for the presence or absence of a genetic disorder. Photographs and recording of certain physical measurements are a standard component of the genetic evaluation. Ancillary tests may be required to document specific physical features (e.g., an echocardiogram for aortic dilatation in Marfan syndrome or x-rays to diagnose achondroplasia).

An important type of clinical data gathered in this process is the family history (Box 12-1). The data obtained in a family history are often useful in obtaining an accurate diagnosis of a condition. For example, a strong family history of early-onset coronary disease may indicate the presence of an LDL receptor defect causing familial hypercholesterolemia. A family history of early-onset colon cancer could indicate that a gene for familial adenomatous polyposis or hereditary nonpolyposis colorectal cancer is present in the family. Family history information can also guide the estimation of recurrence risks by helping to determine whether a genetic disease has been transmitted by one's parents or has occurred as a new mutation (this is especially important for diseases with reduced penetrance). The knowledge and skills required to take an accurate and thorough family history are important for all clinicians, not only clinical geneticists.

Routinely the clinician sends the family a letter summarizing the diagnosis, natural history, and risk information regarding the condition. This letter is a valuable resource for the family, as it helps to document the risk information for later review. Information regarding genetics support groups, including pamphlets, booklets, and brochures, is frequently provided. Follow-up visits are recommended depending on the individual situation. Box 12-2 provides a list of clinical genetics services.

Clinical genetic evaluations include physical examination, detailed family history, ancillary tests as needed, and the communication of information to the family through letters and the distribution of published literature.

Box 12-1. Family History

A thorough, accurate family history is an indispensable part of a medical evaluation. At a minimum the following items should be included:

1. The gender of each individual and their relationship to one another should be indicated using standard pedigree symbols (Chapter 4).
2. The family history should include *at least* all first-degree relatives (parents, siblings, and offspring) of the proband. Often it is desirable to include additional relatives. For example, male relatives on the mother's side of the family will be especially important when considering an X-linked recessive disorder.
3. Record the age of each individual. Record whether the individual is affected with the disease in question, and inquire about diseases that may be related to the disease in question (e.g., ovarian cancer in a family being seen for familial breast cancer).
4. Be certain to record all known miscarriages and stillbirths.
5. If possible, record the ethnic origin of the family. This is important because many diseases vary considerably in prevalence among different ethnic groups.
6. Inquire about consanguinity. Although relatively rare in most Western populations, consanguinity is common in many of the world's populations, and immigrant populations will often maintain relatively high rates of consanguinity (see Chapter 4).
7. Family histories change. Family members develop newly diagnosed diseases, and additional children are born. These changes can affect diagnosis and risk estimation, so be certain to keep the family history current.

Box 12-2. Types of Clinical Genetics Services and Programs

Center-based genetics clinic
Outreach clinics
Inpatient consultations
Specialty clinics
    Metabolic clinic
    Spina bifida clinic
    Hemophilia clinic
    Craniofacial clinic
    Other single-disorder clinics (e.g., NF1 clinic)
Prenatal diagnosis program: perinatal genetics
    Amniocentesis/CVS clinics
    Ultrasound program
    Maternal serum AFP program
Genetic screening
    Newborn screening program/follow-up clinic
    Other population screening programs (e.g., Tay-Sachs disease)
Education/training
    Health care professionals
    General public
    School system
    Teratology information services

In recent years the care of persons with genetic disease has included the development of guidelines for follow-up and routine care. Knowledge of the natural history of a condition, coupled with a critical review of screening tests and interventions, can provide a framework for health supervision and anticipatory guidance. The management plan can be subsequently used by the primary care provider. It is primarily for this purpose that many of the specialized clinics, such as NF1 clinics or hemophilia clinics, have been established. An example of this approach is the management checklist for the health maintenance of infants and children with Down syndrome (see Chapter 6).

Traditionally, genetic counseling involves the family who comes in with questions about the diagnosis, management, and recurrence risk of the condition in question. Thus in the majority of situations, genetic counseling is carried out retrospectively. With the increased availability of prenatal, carrier, and presymptomatic testing, "prospective" genetic counseling will become more common. Box 12-3 lists common reasons for referral for genetics evaluation.

DYSMORPHOLOGY AND CLINICAL TERATOLOGY

Dysmorphology was defined at the beginning of this chapter as the study of abnormal physical development (**morphogenesis**). Congenital defects are caused by altered morphogenesis. Although the term *dysmorphology* may seem synonymous with **teratology**, the latter term usually implies the study of the *environmental* causes of congenital anomalies, even though its literal meaning does not refer to etiology. (The term *teratology* is derived from the Greek word for "monster," *teras*. The newer term *dysmorphology* was partly a reaction to the pejorative connotation of teratology).

As mentioned previously, congenital defects represent an important cause of infant mortality and morbidity. Recent studies indicate that the frequency of medically significant malformations diagnosed in the newborn period is 2% to 3%. Investigations that have followed children for a longer period demonstrate that this frequency increases to 3% to 4% by the age of 1 year. In the United States congenital malformations represent the most frequent cause of mortality during the first year of life. Table 12-1 lists some of the most common and important malformation syndromes.

There are several ways in which congenital defects can be classified. The most common classification approach is by organ system or body region (e.g., craniofacial, limb, heart). More clinically useful systems of classification include the following: (1) single defect versus multiple congenital anomaly syndrome, (2) major (medically or surgically significant defects) versus minor anomalies, (3) categorization by the four major types of congenital abnormalities (malformations, deformations, disruptions, and dysplasias) and (4) an etiologic classification.

Box 12-3. Common Indications for Genetics Referral

1. Evaluation of a person with mental retardation or developmental delay
2. Evaluation of a person with single or multiple malformations; question of a dysmorphic syndrome
3. Evaluation of a person with a possible inherited metabolic disease
4. Presence of a possible single gene disorder
5. Presence of a chromosomal disorder, including balanced rearrangements
6. Person at risk for a genetic condition, including questions of presymptomatic diagnosis
7. Person or family with questions about the genetic aspects of any medical condition
8. Couples with a history of recurrent miscarriages
9. Consanguinity in a couple, usually first cousin or closer relationship
10. Teratogen counseling
11. Preconceptional counseling and risk factor counseling, including advanced maternal age and other potential indications for prenatal diagnosis

Table 12-1 ■ Causes of malformations among affected infants

	Number	%
Genetic causes		
Chromosome abnormalities	157 (45)*	10.1
Single mutant genes	48	3.1
Familial	225 (3)	14.5
Multifactorial inheritance	356 (23)	23.0
Teratogens	49	3.2
Uterine factors	39 (5)	2.5
Twinning	6 (2)	0.4
Unknown cause	669 (24)	43.2
TOTAL	1549 (102)	

From Nelson K and Holmes LB: Malformations due to spontaneous mutations in newborn infants, N Engl J Med 320:19–23, 1989.
*Values in parentheses denote therapeutic abortions. Of the 69,277 infants studied, 1549 had malformations, for an incidence of 2.24%

Table 12-2 lists the causes of major defects in a study done by Holmes and associates in Boston. The key messages from these data are the following: (1) the etiology of two thirds of congenital defects is unknown or multifactorial, (2) environmental causes of congenital malformations are infrequent, and (3) a known genetic component is identified in approximately 30% of cases.

Principles of Dysmorphology

In discussing the basic principles of dysmorphology, it is important to define certain key terms. The following definitions are adapted from those suggested by an international working group on dysmorphology (Spranger et al, 1982):

1. **Malformation,** a primary morphologic defect of an organ or body part resulting from an intrinsically abnormal developmental process (e.g., cleft lip or polydactyly).
2. **Dysplasia,** a primary defect involving abnormal organization of cells into tissue (e.g., hemangioma).
3. **Sequence** (formerly **anomalad**), a primary defect with its secondary structural changes (e.g., Pierre Robin sequence, a disorder in which a primary defect in mandibular development produces a small jaw, glossoptosis, and cleft palate).
4. **Syndrome,** a pattern of multiple primary malformations due to a single etiology (e.g., trisomy 13 syndrome).

5. **Deformation,** alteration of the form, shape, or position of a normally formed body part by mechanical forces; usually occurs in the fetal period, not in embryogenesis; a secondary alteration; can be extrinsic as in oligohydramnios (reduced amniotic fluid) or intrinsic as in congenital myotonic dystrophy.
6. **Disruption,** a morphologic defect of an organ, part of an organ, or a larger region of the body resulting from the extrinsic breakdown of, or an interference with, an originally normal developmental process; a secondary malformation (e.g., secondary limb defect resulting from a vascular event).

Note that malformations and dysplasias are primary events in embryogenesis and histogenesis, whereas disruptions and deformations are secondary.

The first question asked in diagnosing a congenital malformation is whether the abnormality represents a single, isolated anomaly or is instead one component of a broader, organized pattern of malformation (i.e., a syndrome). An example is given by the evaluation of a baby with a cleft lip. If a baby has an isolated, nonsyndromic cleft lip and no other malformations, the discussion of natural history, genetics, prognosis, and management is markedly different than if the baby's cleft lip is one feature of the trisomy 13 syndrome (see Chapter 6). The former condition can be repaired surgically and has a relatively low recurrence risk (see Chapter

Table 12-2 ■ The most common multiple congenital anomaly/dysplasia syndromes

Syndrome	Etiology
Down syndrome	Chromosomal
NF1	Single gene (AD)
Oligohydramnios sequence	Heterogeneous
Amnion disruption sequence	Unknown
Osteogenesis imperfecta	Single gene; heterogeneous, defects of type I collagen
Trisomy 18	Chromosomal
VATER associaiton	Unknown
Marfan syndrome	Single gene (AD)
Prader-Willi syndrome	Microdeletion of chromosome 15q
Noonan syndrome	Single gene (AD)
Williams syndrome	Single gene (AD)
Achondroplasia	Single gene (AD)
Trisomy 13	Chromosomal
XO Turner syndrome	Chromosomal
Rubinstein-Taybi syndrome	Microdeletion of chromosome 16p
Klippel-Trenaunay-Weber syndrome	Unknown
Fetal alcohol syndrome	Excessive alcohol
Cornelia de Lange syndrome	Unknown

Adapted from Hall BD: In Kaback M, editor: Genetic issues in pediatrics and obstetrics, Chicago, 1981, Practice Yearbook.

10) and no associated medical problems. Trisomy 13 is a serious chromosomal disorder. In addition to oral-facial clefts, these infants often have congenital heart disease and central nervous system malformations. More importantly, 50% of children with trisomy 13 die in the newborn period and 90% die by 1 year of age.

Another example is a child with cleft lip who also has pits or fistulas of the lower lip. The combination of oral-facial clefts and lip pits signifies an autosomal dominant condition called the *van der Woude syndrome.* Although the natural history of this condition differs little from that of nonsyndromic cleft lip, the discussion of genetic recurrence risks is much different. In the evaluation of a child with van der Woude syndrome, it is important to determine whether one of the parents carries the gene. If so, the sibling recurrence risk is 50%. This is much greater than the 4% sibling recurrence risk usually given for nonsyndromic cleft lip. Because van der Woude syndrome has highly variable expression and frequently manifests itself only by lip fistulas, it is commonly overlooked. Thus a careful physical examination, combined with a knowledge of the genetics of isolated malformations and syndromes, is necessary in determining accurate recurrence risks.

The first question to ask when evaluating a child with a congenital malformation is whether or not the defect is isolated or part of a syndrome pattern.

The increasing knowledge of the pathogenesis of human congenital defects has led to a better understanding of the developmental relationship of the defects in a multiple congenital anomaly pattern. Some well-established conditions that appear to be true syndromes at first glance are really a constellation of defects consisting of a primary malformation with its secondary effects (i.e., a sequence). A sequence represents a condition in which the pattern can be thought of as a developmental unit in which the cascade of secondary pathogenic events is well understood. In contrast, the pathogenic relationship of the primary malformations in a syndrome is poorly understood. It is likely that some conditions now called syndromes will be recognized eventually as sequences.

One of the best examples of a sequence is the so-called Potter phenotype or oligohydramnios sequence (*SOL* 68,69). It is currently believed that any significant and persistent condition leading to oligohydramnios can produce this sequence, whether it be intrauterine renal failure due to kidney malformations or chronic leakage of amniotic fluid. The fetus will develop a pattern of secondary growth deficiency, joint contractures, facial features, and pulmonary hypoplasia. (Fig. 12-3) Before the cause of these features was understood, the phenotype was termed the "Potter syndrome." Now with the understanding that all of the features are secondary to oligohydramnios, the disorder is more properly termed the *oligohydramnios sequence.* As in any malformation, the renal defect can occur *by itself,* or it could be a part of any number of syndromes that have renal malformations as component features (e.g., in autosomal recessive Meckel-Gruber syndrome or the more common nonsyndromic disease, bilateral renal agenesis). Distinguishing between syndromes and sequences can often improve our understanding of the underlying cause of a disorder.

It is important to distinguish between a sequence, which is a primary defect with secondary structural changes, and a syndrome, which is a collection of malformations whose relationship to one another tends to be poorly understood.

Clinical Teratology

A **teratogen** is an agent external to the fetus's genome that induces structural malformations, growth deficiency, and/or functional alterations during prenatal development. Although teratogens cause only a small percentage of all birth defects, the preventive potential alone makes them worthy of study. Box 12-4 provides a classification of the environmental causes of human malformations and lists the well-established human teratogens. Note that there are few well-established teratogens in humans.

It is important to understand the reasoning process that leads to the designation of a substance as a teratogen. This process is based upon an evaluation of epidemiologic, clinical, biochemical, and physiologic evidence. Animal studies may also help to test whether an agent is teratogenic.

Some of the issues involved in determining whether an agent is teratogenic are summarized in Clinical Commentary 12-5. A key clinical point is that it is common for families to ask their doctors questions about the risks of certain exposures during pregnancy. When faced with such a question, the physician has a number of options. One is to review the human literature on a particular

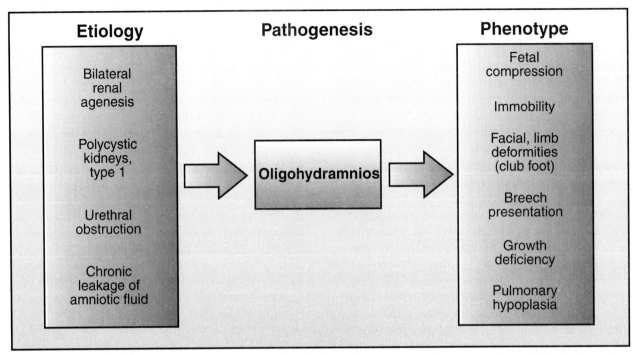

Figure 12-3 ■ The oligohydramnios sequence. Oligohydramnios can arise from a number of distinct causes. It produces a constellation of secondary phenotypic features.

Box 12-4. Well-Established Human Teratogens

Drugs and chemicals
   Thalidomide
   Diethylstilbestrol
   Warfarin
   Hydantoin
   Trimethadione
   Excessive alcohol
   Valproic acid
   Aminopterin/methotrexate
   Tetracycline
   Isotretinoin
   Angiotensin converting enzyme inhibitors
   Penicillamine
   Antithyroid drugs
   Androgen/masculinizing progestogen
   Methylmercury
   Polychlorobiphenyls
Maternal infections
   Rubella
   Cytomegalovirus
   Toxoplasmosis
   Varicella
   Venezuela equine encephalitis
   Syphilis
   Parvovirus
Maternal states
   Diabetes mellitus
   Phenylketonuria
   Systemic lupus erythematosus
   Graves disease
Ionizing radiation

exposure, make a judgment regarding the degree of risk, and then provide counseling. An alternative is to refer the patient or family to a clinical genetics unit or to a teratology information service. Because of the complexity of these issues, teratology information services have sprung up throughout the United States, Canada, and Europe.

Teratogens are external agents that cause a small but important proportion of congenital malformations. It is often difficult to prove conclusively that a substance is teratogenic.

Prevention of Congenital Malformations

Because the majority of structural defects have no obvious cause, their prevention presents a challenge (see Clinical Commentary 12-6, page 246, which discusses fetal alcohol syndrome, one of the more common preventable causes of human malformation). The institution of rubella immunization programs and, recently, the preconceptional administration of folic acid are both examples of successful prevention (Clinical Commentary 12-7, page 246).

Preconceptional counseling is a model for primary prevention. Women who have diabetes mellitus, phenylketonuria, or systemic lupus erythematosus (an autoimmune disorder involving production of autoantibodies that affect multiple organs; *SOL* 72,73) can decrease their risk of pro-

Clinical Commentary 12-5. The Bendectin Saga

Bendectin, or doxyclamine, was an agent introduced in the 1960s for "morning sickness" (nausea and vomiting during pregnancy). The agent was particularly efficacious, and during the 1970s about one third of American women took Bendectin at some time during their first trimester of pregnancy.

Bendectin has probably been studied more than any other individual pregnancy medication. Several epidemiologic studies indicate that there is no conclusive evidence of an increased risk of congenital malformations with usage of Bendectin during pregnancy. The few studies that demonstrated weak associations between Bendectin and birth defects have not shown any consistent patterns. Animal studies also indicate no association. Despite these data, a number of lawsuits were filed in the 1980s against the company that marketed Bendectin. As a result the company removed the drug from the market.

The reasoning process that is used in determining causation in such cases is complex. Before judgments about etiology are made, a critical review of the literature is required. The available epidemiologic studies must be evaluated in terms of their methodology, design, and presence of systematic biases. Up-to-date knowledge of the etiology and pathogenesis of congenital malformations must be included in the design of the study. The basic principles of teratology need application. This includes an evaluation of the **critical period** (i.e., did exposure occur during the period of pregnancy in which the malformed fetal structures were developing?). Clinical evidence includes the search for a pattern of defects (i.e., a specific syndrome) because all well-established ter-

atogens produce consistent patterns (see Box 12-4). Animal models never prove causation in human beings but can provide supportive evidence. In addition, the proposed effect of the agent should be biologically plausible.

A review of the evidence regarding Bendectin shows that it meets none of these criteria. Indeed, because of its extensive testing, Bendectin satisfies standard criteria for "safety" as well as any known medication. What, then, could have produced this litigation? An important part of the answer to this question involves the *coincidental* occurrence of congenital malformations and Bendectin exposure. Considering that 3% of infants will be diagnosed with a major congenital malformation by 1 year of age *and* that about one third of women were taking Bendectin in the first trimester of pregnancy, then about 1% (1/3 × 3%) of all pregnancies in the 1970s would have experienced the co-occurrence of these two events by chance alone. Because about two thirds of congenital malformations have no known cause, it is not surprising that many families of children with these disorders would attribute them to Bendectin use.

It is difficult to prove epidemiologically that any exposure is "safe." The power of such studies does not permit an absolute statement that there is no effect. All that can be demonstrated is that there is no definitive evidence that a particular agent (in this case, Bendectin) causes an adverse outcome. Blanket reassurance or absolute statements of complete safety are not appropriate. However, when the evidence is relatively conclusive, as in the case of Bendectin, it is clinically appropriate to have a reassuring tone in discussing exposure in the pregnancy setting.

ducing an infant with a structural defect with appropriate preconceptional management. Secondary and tertiary levels of prevention occur, respectively, with newborn screening and with the provision of quality medical care for infants and children with congenital malformations. The institution of appropriate guidelines for health maintenance and anticipatory guidance can decrease some of the

complications of these disorders. Public education regarding the limitations of scientific knowledge and the emotional difficulties of families in which a child has a congenital defect are also important. They have the potential to diminish anxiety, improve the family's coping process, and reduce the stigma that surrounds congenital malformations and genetic disorders.

Clinical Commentary 12-6. Fetal Alcohol Syndrome

Among the human teratogens, one of the most common and potentially preventable exposures is excessive alcohol consumption. Women who are chronic alcoholics are at significant risk to bear a child with the fetal alcohol syndrome (FAS). This condition consists of prenatal and postnatal growth deficiency, microcephaly (small head), a wide range of developmental disabilities, and a constel-

lation of facial alterations (Fig. 12-4). The more distinctive and consistent facial features include short palpebral fissures, low nasal root, upturned nose, simple/flat philtral folds, and a thin upper lip. Although most of these signs are not specific for FAS, their mutual occurrence in the context of maternal alcohol abuse allows the clinician to make the diagnosis.

In addition to these findings, infants and children with FAS are at risk for a number of structural

Continued.

Clinical Commentary 12-6. Fetal Alcohol Syndrome—*cont.*

defects, including congenital heart defects, neural tube defects, and renal malformations. Most children with FAS have a mild degree of developmental delay, ranging from mild mental retardation to learning disabilities.

There are still many unanswered questions regarding alcohol use in pregnancy. These include the extent of genetic predisposition to FAS, the risk of binge drinking, the role of moderate and social drinking, and the safe level of alcohol in pregnancy. Suffice it to say that, given our present state of knowledge, the safest amount of alcohol during pregnancy is none at all.

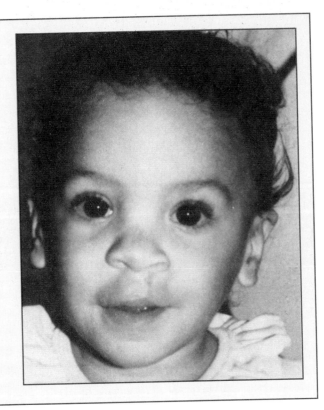

Figure 12-4 ■ A two-year-old child with fetal alcohol syndrome. Note the low nasal root, shortened eyelids, and repaired cleft lip.

Clinical Commentary 12-7. Folate and the Prevention of Neural Tube Defects

The primary prevention of congenital malformations is an important goal of clinical genetics. Because the ultimate cause of most congenital malformations is currently unknown, there are relatively few opportunities for primary prevention. A recent approach to the prevention of congenital defects is the periconceptional use of folate and multivitamin regimens to prevent the occurrence and recurrence of neural tube defects (NTDs).

NTDs consist of malformations of the developing neural tube and express themselves as anencephaly, encephalocele, and meningomyelocele (see Chapter 10). Their impact is serious: Anencephaly is invariably fatal, and the medical complications of spina bifida (lower limb paralysis, hydrocephalus, urinary obstruction) are significant. Because of the potential influence of nutritional elements on embryogenesis, a series of epidemiologic studies were performed in the 1970s and 1980s. With one exception, they demonstrated that the use of vitamins and folate in the periconceptional period reduced the recurrence risk of spina bifida and anencephaly in families that had previously had a child with one of these conditions. In 1991 the Medical Research Council of the United Kingdom published a double-blind study* in which 4 mg folate with or without vitamins was administered to women who had had a child with an NTD. The group receiving folate alone experienced a 70% reduction in the frequency of these malformations in their offspring. In 1992 a Hungarian group demonstrated the usefulness of vitamins and folic acid in preventing the initial occurrence of NTDs. In this study two groups of women, one on vitamins/folic acid and the others not, were followed for the duration of their pregnancies. The vitamin regimen significantly decreased the occurrence of NTDs.

Although it is still not clear whether the purported protective effect is due to folic acid or a combination of folic acid and other vitamins, these data suggest that periconceptional vitamin use is an effective prevention strategy. The mechanism for the apparent effect remains unknown. Nonetheless, the encouraging results of these studies have prompted the Centers for Disease Control to publish two recommendations regarding the use of folate in pregnancy. The first is that all women who have had a previous child with an NTD should take 4 mg/day of folic acid if they are planning to become pregnant. The second recommendation is that all women of reproductive age take 0.4 mg/day of folic acid throughout their reproductive years.

*A **double-blind** study is one in which during the treatment phase of the study neither the subjects nor the investigator knows which subjects are receiving an active ingredient and which are receiving placebos.

■ STUDY QUESTIONS

1. Allen, a 40-year-old man, comes to your office because he is concerned about his family history of heart disease. His father had a fatal myocardial infarction (MI) at the age of 45, and his grandfather (father's father) had a fatal MI at the age of 47. Allen's father had two brothers and two sisters. One of the brothers had an MI at the age of 44, and one of the sisters had an MI at the age of 49. Allen's mother had a brother and sister, both of whom are still alive. Allen's mother's parents both survived into their 80s and died of "natural causes." Draw a pedigree summarizing the information you have taken about Allen's family, and make a recommendation for further study and/or treatment.

2. Mary's two brothers and her mother's brother all had Duchenne muscular dystrophy (DMD) and are now dead. Based only on this information, what is the probability that Mary is a heterozygous carrier for this disorder? What is the probability that she will produce affected offspring? She then has a serum creatine kinase test and is told that her level is above the 95th percentile for homozygous normal individuals. Approximately two thirds of DMD carriers have CK levels above the 95th percentile. Given this information, use Bayes theorem to calculate the probability that she is a carrier and the probability that she will produce affected offspring.

3. Bob's father had Huntington disease and is now deceased. Bob is now 51 years old and has no symptoms of Huntington disease. Age-of-onset curves show that approximately 85% of individuals with an affected father show symptoms by this age (this percentage is slightly lower, about 80%, if the mother is affected). Based on this information, use Bayes theorem to estimate the probability that Bob inherited the Huntington disease mutation from his father.

■ ADDITIONAL READING

Aase JM: Dysmorphologic diagnosis for the pediatric practitioner, Pediatr Clin North Am 39:135–156, 1992.

Brent RL: The Bendectin saga: an American tragedy, Teratology 27: 283-286, 1983.

Carey JC: Health supervision and anticipatory guidance for children with genetic disorders (including specific recommendations for trisomy 21, trisomy 18, and neurofibromatosis I), Pediatr Clin North Am 39:25–53, 1992.

Carey JC, Viskochil DH: Current status of the human malformation map, Birth Defects Original Series 32:13–33, 1996.

Emery AEH and Pullen I: Psychological aspects of genetic counseling, London, 1984, Academic Press.

Friedman JM, Polifka JE: Teratogenic effects of drugs: a resource for clinicians (TERIS), Baltimore, 1994, Johns Hopkins University.

Hall BD: The 25 most common multiple congenital anomaly syndromes. In Kaback M, editor: Genetic issues in pediatrics and obstetrics, Chicago, 1981, Practice Yearbook.

Harper PS: Practical genetic counseling, ed 4, Oxford, 1993, Butterworth Heineman N.

Hoyme HE: Teratogenically induced fetal anomalies, Clin Perinatol 17:547–567, 1990.

Jones KL: Smith's recognizable patterns of human malformations, ed 5, Philadelphia, 1996, WB Saunders.

Kessler S: Genetic counseling: psychological dimensions, New York, 1979, Academic Press.

Marks JH, Heimler A, Reich E, Wexler NS, and Ince SE: Genetic counseling principles in action: a casebook, New York, 1989, March of Dimes Birth Defects Foundation.

Murphy EA and Chase GA: Principles of genetic counseling, St. Louis, 1975, Mosby.

Nelson K and Holmes LB: Malformations due to spontaneous mutations in newborn infants, N Engl J Med 320:19–23, 1989.

Robinson A and Linden MG: Clinical genetics handbook, ed 2, Boston, 1993, Blackwell Scientific Publications.

Schneider KA: Counseling about cancer: strategies for genetic counselors, Dennisport, MA, 1994, Graphic Illusions.

Somer M, Mustonen H and Norio R: Evaluation of genetic counselling: recall of information, post-counselling reproduction, and attitude of the counsellees, Clin Genet 34:352–365, 1988.

Sorenson JR et al: Reproductive plans for genetic counseling clients not eligible for prenatal diagnosis, Am J Med Genet 28:345, 1987.

Sorenson JR and Wertz DC: Couple agreement before and after genetic counseling, Am J Med Genet 25:549, 1986.

Spranger J, Benirschke K, Hall JG, et al: Errors of morphogenesis: concepts and terms, Pediatrics 100:160–165, 1982.

Tingey C: Down syndrome: a resource handbook, Boston, 1988, Little, Brown.

Weiss JO: Support groups for patients with genetic disorders and their families, Pediatr Clin North Am 39:13–23, 1992.

Winter RM: Recent molecular advances in dysmorphology, Hum Molec Genet 4:1699–1704, 1995.

Answers to Study Questions

■CHAPTER 2

1. The mRNA sequence is: 5′–CAG AAG AAA AUU AAC AUG UAA–3′ (remember that transcription moves along the 3′–5′ DNA strand, allowing the mRNA to be synthesized in the 5′ to 3′ direction). This mRNA sequence is translated in the 5′ to 3′ direction to yield the amino acid sequence: Gln-Lys-Lys-Ile-Asn-Met-STOP.

2. The *genome* is the sum total of our genetic material. It is composed of 23 pairs of nuclear *chromosomes* and the mitochondrial chromosome. Each chromosome contains a number of *genes,* the basic unit of heredity. Genes are composed of one or more *exons;* exons alternate with introns. Exons encode mRNA *codons,* which consist of three *nucleotides* each. It is important to remember that DNA coiling patterns also produce a hierarchy: chromosomes are composed of 100-kb chromatin loops, which are in turn composed of solenoids. Each solenoid contains approximately six nucleosomes. Each nucleosome contains about 150 DNA base pairs and may or may not include coding material.

3. Approximately 25% of our DNA consists of repetitive sequences whose function is unknown. Single-copy DNA includes protein-coding genes, but it consists mostly of extragenic sequences and introns that do not encode proteins. Because individual cells have specialized functions, most make only a limited number of protein products. Thus, only a small percentage of the cell's coding DNA is transcriptionally active. This activation is controlled by elements such as enhancers and promoters.

4. Mitosis is the cell division process in which one diploid cell produces two diploid daughter cells. In meiosis a diploid cell produces haploid cells (gametes). Meiosis produces haploid cells because the centromeres are not duplicated in meiosis I and because there is no replication of DNA in the interphase stage between meiosis I and meiosis II. Another difference between mitosis and meiosis is that the homologous chromosomes form pairs and exchange material (crossing over) during meiosis I. Homologs do not pair during mitosis, and mitotic crossing over is rare.

5. Each mitotic division doubles the number of cells in the developing embryo. Thus, the embryo proceeds from 1 to 2 to 4 to 8 cells, and so on. After n cell divisions, there are 2^n cells. For example, after 10 divisions, there are 2^{10}, or 1024 cells. We want a value of n that satisfies the simple relationship $2^n = 10^{14}$. One way to our answer is simply to "plug in" values of n until we get 10^{14}. A more elegant approach is to take the common logarithms of both sides of this equation, yielding $n\log(2) = 14\log(10)$. Since the common logarithm of 10 is 1, we obtain the relationship $n = 14/\log(2)$. Thus $n = 46.5$. It should be emphasized that this result, approximately 46 to 47 cell divisions, is only an average value. Some cell lineages divide more times than others, and many cells are replaced as they die.

6. A total of 400 mature sperm and 100 mature egg cells will be produced. Each primary spermatocyte will produce four mature sperm cells, and each primary oocyte will produce only one

mature egg cell (the other products of meiosis are polar bodies, which degenerate).

■CHAPTER 3

1. Mutation 1 is a nonsense mutation in the fourth codon, producing premature termination of translation. Mutation 2 is a frameshift mutation in the third codon, and mutation 3 is a missense mutation in the second codon.

2. Transcription mutations generally lower the production of a gene product, but often they do not eliminate it completely. Transcription mutations in the β-globin gene usually produce β^+-thalassemia, a condition in which there is some production of β-globin chains. β^+-thalassemia tends to be less severe than β^0-thalassemia. Missense mutations alter only a single amino acid in a polypeptide chain and, when they occur in the β-globin chain, can produce β^+-thalassemia (however, keep in mind that sickle cell disease, which is relatively severe, is also caused by a missense mutation). In contrast, frameshift mutations alter many or all codons downstream from the site of the mutation, so a large number of amino acids may be changed. Frameshifts can also produce a stop codon. Nonsense mutations produce truncated polypeptides, which are often useless (especially if the nonsense mutation occurs near the 5′ end of the gene, eliminating most of the polypeptide chain). Donor–acceptor mutations can delete whole exons or large portions of them. This can substantially alter the amino acid composition of the polypeptide. Nonsense, frameshift, and donor–acceptor mutations all tend to produce the more severe β^0-thalassemia, in which no β-globin chains are present.

3. In thalassemia conditions, one of the chains, α- or β-globin, is reduced in quantity. Most of the harmful consequences are caused by the relative *excess* of the chain that is produced in normal quantity. If both chains are reduced in quantity, there may be a rough balance between the two, resulting in less accumulation of excess chains.

4. Restriction site polymorphisms (RSP) reflect the presence or absence of a restriction site. They thus can have only two alleles. They are detected using RFLP technology. VNTRs are also a type of RFLP, but here the polymorphism is in the number of tandem repeats that lie between two restriction sites, rather than in the presence or absence of a restriction site. Because the number of tandem repeats can vary considerably, VNTRs can have many different alleles in populations. VNTRs are found in minisatellite regions. Microsatellite repeat polymorphisms consist of variations in the number of shorter microsatellite repeats (usually di-, tri-, and tetranucleotides). They are usually detected using polymerase chain reaction (PCR). However, it should be noted that RSPs and VNTRs can also be detected using PCR (instead of RFLP technology), provided that the DNA sequences flanking the polymorphism are known. The autoradiogram represents a microsatellite repeat polymorphism. This is indicated by the fact that there are multiple alleles (distinguishing it from an RSP) and by the fact that the various alleles differ in size by only 4 base pairs (recall from Chapter 2 that the tandem repeat units in minisatellite regions are generally 20 to 70 base pairs long).

5. Because the disease mutation destroys a recognition site, those who have the disease allele will have a longer restriction fragment. This fragment will migrate more slowly on the gel and will be seen higher on the autoradiogram. Individual A has only the longer fragment and thus has two copies of the disease mutation. This individual will have α_1-antitrypsin deficiency. Individual B has only the short fragment and will be genetically and physically normal. Individual C has both fragments and is thus a clinically normal heterozygote.

■CHAPTER 4

1. In this sample of 100 individuals, there are 88 × 2 HbA alleles in the HbA homozygotes and 10 HbA alleles in the heterozygotes. There are thus 186 HbA alleles in the population. The frequency of HbA, p, is 186/200 = 0.93. Then the frequency of HbS, q, is 1 − 0.93 = 0.07. The genotype frequencies in the population are 88/100 = 0.88, 10/100 = 0.10, and 2/100 = 0.02. Assuming Hardy-Weinberg proportions, the expected genotype frequencies are given by p^2, $2pq$, and q^2. This yields expected genotype frequencies of $(0.93)^2$ = 0.865, 2 × 0.93 × 0.07 = 0.130, $(0.07)^2$ = 0.005. In this population the observed and expected genotype frequencies are fairly similar to one another.

2. For an autosomal recessive disease, the prevalence (1 in 10,000) equals the recessive genotype frequency, q^2. Then the PKU gene frequency, q, is given by $\sqrt{q^2} = \sqrt{1/10,000} = 1/100 =$

0.01. The carrier frequency is given by $2pq$, which is approximately $2q$, or 0.02 (1/50).

3. Because this is an autosomal dominant disorder and affected homozygotes die early in life, the man is a heterozygote and has a 50% chance of passing the disease gene to each of his offspring. The probability that all four will be affected is given by the product of each probability: $1/2^4 = 1/16$. The probability that none will be affected is obtained in exactly the same way.

4. The probability that the offspring will inherit the retinoblastoma susceptibility gene is 0.50 because familial retinoblastoma is an autosomal dominant disease. However, we must also consider the penetrance of the disorder. The probability of inheriting the disease gene (0.50) and expressing the disease phenotype (0.90) is given by multiplying the two probabilities together: $0.90 \times 0.50 = 0.45$.

5. Because the woman's sister had Tay-Sachs disease, both parents must be heterozygous carriers. This means that, at birth, one fourth of their offspring will be affected, one half will be carriers, and one fourth will be genetically normal. However, note that the woman in question is 30 years old. She cannot possibly be an affected homozygote. There are thus three equally likely possibilities: (1) the disease allele was inherited from the mother and a normal allele was inherited from the father; (2) the disease allele was inherited from the father and a normal allele was inherited from the mother; and (3) normal alleles were inherited from both parents. Because two of these three possibilities lead to the carrier state, the woman's probability of being a heterozygous carrier is 2/3.

6. This is explained by genomic imprinting. For normal development, differential expression of genes inherited from the father and mother is necessary. If only the expression pattern from one parent is inherited, the embryo cannot develop normally and dies. The experiment works in amphibians because genomic imprinting does not occur in these animals.

7. The coefficient of relationship is $1/2^6 = 1/64$. This gives the probability that the woman also carries the PKU gene. Then, the probability that two carriers produce an affected offspring is 1/4. The overall probability that this couple will produce a PKU baby is given by multiplying the probability that the woman carries the gene

(1/64) by the probability that they both transmit the gene to their offspring (1/4): $1/64 \times 1/4 = 1/256$. This demonstrates that, in this consanguineous mating, the probability of producing an affected offspring is actually small.

■ CHAPTER 5

1. There are four Barr bodies, always one less than the number of X chromosomes.

2. This is most likely a result of X inactivation. The heterozygotes with muscle weakness are the ones with relatively large proportions of active X chromosomes containing the mutant allele.

3. The disease frequency in males is q, while in females it is q^2. The male/female ratio is thus q/q^2 or $1/q$. As q decreases, the male/female ratio thus increases.

4. Because the male's grandfather is affected with the disorder, his mother must be a carrier. His father is phenotypically normal, so he does not have the disease gene. Thus the male in question has a 50% risk of developing hemophilia A. His sister's risk of being a heterozygous carrier is 50%. Her risk of being affected with the disorder is close to zero (barring a new mutation on the X chromosome transmitted by her father).

5. Male–male transmission can be observed in autosomal dominant inheritance, but it will not be observed in X-linked dominant inheritance. Thus males affected with X-linked dominant disorders must always have affected mothers (unless a new mutation has occurred). Males and females are affected in approximately equal proportions in autosomal dominant inheritance, but there are twice as many affected females as males in X-linked dominant inheritance (unless the disorder is lethal prenatally in males, in which case *only* affected females are seen). In X-linked dominant inheritance, *all* of the sons of an affected male are normal, whereas *all* of the daughters are affected. In X-linked dominant diseases, heterozygous females tend to be more mildly affected than are hemizygous males. In autosomal dominant inheritance, there is usually no difference in severity of expression in male and female heterozygotes.

6. In mitochondrial inheritance the disease can be inherited *only* from an affected mother. In contrast to all other types of inheritance, *no* descendants of affected fathers can be affected. Note that males affected with an X-linked recessive

disease who mate with normal females cannot transmit the disease to their offspring, but their grandsons can be affected with the disease.

■ CHAPTER 6

1. Euploid cells have a multiple of 23 chromosomes. Haploid (n = 23), diploid (n = 46), and polyploid (triploid and tetraploid) cells are all euploid. Aneuploid cells do not have a multiple of 23 chromosomes and would include trisomies (47 chromosomes in a somatic cell) and monosomies (45 chromosomes in a somatic cell).

2. A normal egg can be fertilized by two sperm cells (dispermy, the most common cause of triploidy). An egg and polar body can fuse, creating a diploid egg, which is then fertilized by a normal sperm cell. Diploid sperm or egg cells can be created by meiotic failure; subsequent union with a haploid gamete would produce a triploid zygote.

3. The difference in incidence of various chromosome abnormalities reflects the fact that embryos and fetuses with chromosome abnormalities are spontaneously lost during pregnancy. The rate and timing of loss vary among different types of chromosome abnormalities.

4. A karyotype establishes whether the condition is the result of a true trisomy or a translocation. If the latter is the case, the recurrence risk in future pregnancies is elevated. A karyotype also helps to establish whether the patient is a mosaic. This may help to predict and explain the severity of expression of the disorder.

5. Nondisjunction of the X chromosome can occur in both meiosis I and meiosis II. If these two nondisjunctions occur in the same cell, an ovum with four X chromosomes can be produced. If fertilized by an X-bearing sperm cell, the zygote will have the 49,XXXXX karyotype.

6. The meiotic error must have occured in the father because his X chromosome carries the gene for hemophilia A. Because the daughter has normal factor VIII activity, she must have inherited her single X chromosome from her mother.

7. Because a loss of genetic material usually produces more severe consequences than does a gain of material, one would expect the deletion (46,XY,del(8p)) patient to be more severely affected than the duplication patient.

■ CHAPTER 7

1. The affected male in generation 2 inherited the disease allele and marker allele 1 from his affected father, and he inherited a normal allele and marker allele 2 from his mother. Therefore the disease allele must be on the chromosome that contains marker allele 1 in this male (linkage phase). Because he married a female who is homozygous for marker allele 2, we expect to observe allele 1 in the affected offspring under the hypothesis of linkage. Individual III-5 has the 2,2 marker genotype but is affected, and individual 7 has the 1,2 genotype but is normal. They both represent recombinants. Thus there are 2 recombinations observed in 8 meioses, giving a recombination frequency of $2/8 = 25\%$.

2. For marker A, the affected mother in generation 2 must carry allele 2 on the same chromosome as the Huntington disease allele. Under the hypothesis that $\theta = 0.0$, all of her children must also inherit allele 2 if they are affected. Marker A shows a recombinant with the disease allele in individual III-5 and thus produces a likelihood of zero for a recombination frequency of 0.0. The LOD score is $-\infty$ (the logarithm of 0). For marker B, the disease allele is on the chromosome bearing marker allele 1 in the affected mother in generation 2. All offspring inheriting allele 1 also inherit the disease allele, so there are no recombinants. Under the hypothesis that $\theta = 0.0$, the affected mother can transmit only two possible haplotypes: the disease allele with marker allele 1 and the normal allele with marker allele 2. The probability of each of these events is 1/2. Thus the probability of observing six offspring with the marker genotypes shown is $(1/2)^6 = 1/64$. This is the numerator of the likelihood ratio. Under the hypothesis that $\theta = 0.5$ (no linkage), four possible haplotypes can be transmitted, each with probability 1/4. The probability of observing six children with these haplotypes under the hypothesis of no linkage is then $(1/4)^6 = 1/4096$. This is the denominator of the likelihood ratio. The ratio is then $(1/64)/(1/4096) = 64$. The LOD score is given by the common logarithm of 64, 1.8.

3. The table shows a maximum LOD score, 3.5, at a recombination frequency of 10%. Thus the two loci are most likely to be linked at a distance of approximately 10 cM. The odds in favor of linkage at this θ value versus nonlinkage are 3162 $(10^{3.5})$ to 1.

4. The mating in generation 2 is uninformative because the father is a homozygote for the marker allele. It will be necessary to type the family for another closely linked marker (preferably one with more alleles) before any risk information can be given. At this point the only risk information that can be given is that each child has a 50% risk of inheriting the disease gene from the affected father.

5. Synteny refers to loci that are on the same chromosome. Linkage refers to loci that are less than 50 cM apart on a chromosome; alleles at these loci tend to be transmitted together within families. Linked loci are thus syntenic, but syntenic loci are not necessarily linked. Linkage disequilibrium is the nonrandom association of alleles at linked loci, observable when chromosome haplotypes are examined in populations. Association indicates that two traits are observed together in a population more often than expected by chance; the traits may or may not be genetic. Association thus does not necessarily have anything to do with linkage, *unless* we are referring to linkage disequilibrium.

6. Linkage disequilibrium can arise when a disease mutation occurs on a specific chromosome. If there are multiple disease mutations, they are likely to occur on chromosomes with different marker alleles, and little association will be observed between the disease genotype (which actually consists of a *collection* of different mutations at the disease locus) and a specific marker allele.

7. A hybridization signal is seen consistently in clones that include chromosome 5. This indicates that this is the chromosome most likely to contain the cDNA segment.

■ CHAPTER 8

1. The class I molecules present peptides at the surfaces of nearly all of the body's cells. The peptide-class I molecule complex is recognized by cytotoxic T cells, which kill the cell if the class I MHC molecule presents foreign peptide. The class II MHC molecules also present peptides at the cell surface, but only in antigen-presenting cells of the immune system (e.g., dendritic cells, macrophages, and B cells). If the class II molecules present foreign peptide derived from an invading microbe, they are bound by the receptors of helper T cells, which in turn stimulate appropriate B cells to proliferate and produce antibodies that will help to kill the microbes.

2. Immunoglobulins differ among B cells within individuals so that a large variety of infections can be combatted. MHC molecules are identical on each cell surface within an individual, but they vary a great deal between individuals. This interindividual variability may have evolved to prevent infectious agents from spreading easily through a population.

3. T-cell receptors and immunoglobulins are similar in that they are both cell surface receptors that bind to foreign peptides as part of the immune response. Diversity in both types of molecules is generated by multiple germline genes, VDJ recombination, and junctional diversity. They differ in that immunoglobulins are secreted into the circulation (as antibodies) and can bind directly to foreign peptide, whereas T-cell receptors are not secreted and must "see" foreign peptide in conjunction with MHC molecules to recognize them. Also, somatic hypermutation generates diversity in immunoglobulins but not in T-cell receptors.

4. Somatic recombination alone could produce $30 \times 6 \times 200 = 36,000$ different heavy chains of this class.

5. The probability that a sibling will be HLA-identical is 0.25. This is because the probability that two siblings share one gene or haplotype is 0.50 (this is the coefficient of relationship for siblings; see Chapter 4). Then the probability that they share two haplotypes and are HLA-identical is $0.50 \times 0.50 = 0.25$.

6. If a homozygous Rh-positive (DD) man marries an Rh-negative woman, all of the offspring will be Rh-positive heterozygotes (Dd) and incompatible with the mother. If the man is an Rh-positive heterozygote (Dd), half of the children, on average, will be incompatible Rh-positive heterozygotes. However, if the couple is ABO-incompatible, this will largely protect against Rh incompatibility.

■ CHAPTER 9

1. G6PD is on a portion of the X chromosome that is inactivated in one copy in normal females. Thus any single cell will express only one G6PD allele. If *all* tumor cells express the same G6PD allele, this indicates that they all arose from a single ancestral cell. This evidence was used to

support the theory that most tumors are mono-clonal.

2. The probability that a single cell will experience two mutations is given by the square of the mutation rate per cell (i.e., the probability of one mutation *and* a second mutation in the same cell): $(3 \times 10^{-6})^2 \simeq 10^{-11}$. We then multiply this probability times the number of retinoblasts to obtain the probability that an individual will develop sporadic retinoblastoma: $10^{-11} \times 2 \times 10^6 = 2 \times 10^{-5}$. We would thus expect 2 in 100,000 individuals to develop sporadic retinoblastoma, which is consistent with observed prevalence data (i.e., retinoblastoma is seen in about 1 in 20,000 children, and about half of these cases are sporadic). If an individual has inherited one copy of a mutant retinoblastoma gene, then the number of tumors is given by the somatic mutation (second hit) rate per cell times the number of target cells: $3 \times 10^{-6} \times 2 \times 10^6 = 6$ tumors per individual.

3. Oncogenes are produced when proto-oncogenes, which encode substances that affect cell growth, are altered. Oncogenes usually act as dominant genes at the level of the cell and help to produce transformation of a normal cell into one that can give rise to a tumor. Tumor suppressor genes are also involved in growth regulation, but they usually act as recessive genes at the level of the cell (i.e., both copies of the gene must be altered before progression to a tumor can proceed). Because only a single oncogene need be altered to initiate the transformation process, oncogenes have been detected by using transfection and retroviral assays and by observing the effects of chromosome translocations. Such methods are less effective for uncovering tumor suppressors because two altered copies of these genes must be present before their effects can be observed in a cell. Consequently, most tumor suppressor genes have been detected by studying relatively rare cancer syndromes in which one mutant copy of the tumor suppressor is inherited and the second alteration occurs during somatic development.

4. Li-Fraumeni syndrome is caused by the inheritance of a mutation in the *p53* gene. The inherited mutation is present in all cells and greatly increases one's predisposition to tumor formation. However, because of the multistep nature of carcinogenesis, this inherited event is not sufficient to produce a tumor. Other events, occuring in somatic cells, must also take place. These somatic events are rare, so the probability of their occurrence in any given cell is small, explaining the low frequency of any specific tumor type. The involvement of many different tumor types in Li-Fraumeni syndrome is explained by the fact that normal *p53* activity is required for growth regulation in many different tissues. Thus the likelihood that an individual will develop at least one primary tumor, in one of many tissues, is high.

■ CHAPTER 10

1. Because the trait is more common in females than in males, we infer that the threshold is lower in females than in males. Thus an affected father is at greater risk for producing affected offspring than is an affected mother. The recurrence risk is higher in daughters than in sons.

2. For a multifactorial trait, the recurrence risk will decrease rapidly in more remote relatives of a proband. For an autosomal dominant gene with reduced penetrance, the recurrence risk will decrease by 50% with each degree of relationship. Thus it would be 2.5% for second-degree relatives, 1.25% for third-degree relatives, and so on, with the penetrance fraction remaining constant. In addition, if the disease is multifactorial, the recurrence risk should increase in populations in which the disease is more common. There will be no relationship between disease frequency and recurrence risk for an autosomal dominant disease.

3. (1) The disease gene may have reduced penetrance. (2) A somatic mutation may have occurred following cleavage of the embryo, such that one twin is affected by the disorder while the other is not.

4. These results imply that shared environmental factors are increasing the correlations among siblings because siblings tend to share a more common environment than do parents and off-spring. The spouse correlation reinforces the interpretation of a shared environment effect, although it is also possible that individuals with similar body fat levels may marry preferentially.

■ CHAPTER 11

1. The sensitivity of the test is 93% (93 of the 100 true disease cases were detected). The specificity is 99% (98,900 of 99,900 unaffected individuals were correctly identified). The positive

predictive value is 8.5% (93 of the 1093 positive tests actually had the disease). The false-positive rate is 1% (1 − specificity, or 1000 of 99,900), and the false-negative rate is 7% (1 − sensitivity, or 7 of 100).

2. Based on the fact that individual 3 is homozygous for the 5 kb allele, we infer that the disease gene is on the same chromosome as the 5 kb allele in both parents. Thus individual 6, who inherited both copies of the 5 kb allele, also inherited both copies of the PKU disease gene and is affected.

3. The Huntington disease gene is on the same chromosome as allele 1 in the affected father. Thus individual 6, who inherited allele 2 from his father, should be unaffected. Note that our degree of confidence in both answers 1 and 2 depends upon how closely linked the marker and disease loci are.

4. The mating in generation I is uninformative, so we cannot establish linkage phase in the female in generation II. Thus the risk estimate for her daughter cannot be improved from the usual 50% figure used for autosomal dominant genes. Diagnostic accuracy could be improved by assaying another, more polymorphic marker; e.g., a microsatellite repeat polymorphism or a VNTR, both of which would be more likely to permit linkage phase to be assigned.

5. The primary advantages of amniocentesis are a lower rate of fetal loss (approximately 0.5% versus 1% to 1.3% for CVS) and the ability to do an AFP assay for the detection of NTDs. CVS offers the advantages of diagnosis earlier in the pregnancy and a more rapid laboratory diagnosis. The CVS diagnosis may be complicated by confined placental mosaicism, and there is limited evidence for an association between early (prior to 10 weeks post-LMP) CVS and limb reduction defects.

6. One reason why Huntington disease (HD) is likely to be a poor candidate for gene therapy is that it is a dominant disorder and may be caused by a dominant negative effect (this is made likely by the fact that heterozygotes and affected homozygotes have the same phenotype). Thus simple gene insertion is unlikely to correct the disorder. Furthermore this disorder primarily affects neurons, which are relatively difficult to manipulate or target. The fact that HD has a delayed age of onset, however, is encouraging in that identification of the action of the HD gene

may lead to drug therapy to block the gene product's effects before neuronal damage occurs.

■CHAPTER 12

1. Allen's family includes several members who have had MIs at a relatively young age. The pedigree suggests that an autosomal dominant gene predisposing family members to heart disease may be segregating in this family. This could be caused by autosomal dominant familial hypercholesterolemia, or possibly another disorder of lipid metabolism. Allen should be encouraged to have his serum lipid levels tested (total cholesterol, LDL, HDL, and triglyceride). If his LDL level is abnormally high, intervention may be necessary (e.g., dietary modification and/or cholesterol-lowering drugs).

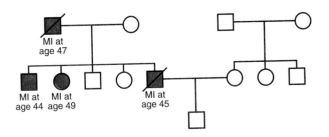

2. Based on the fact that Mary's brothers and uncle are all affected, we can be certain that her mother is a carrier of the Duchenne muscular dystrophy (DMD) gene (if only one of Mary's brothers were affected, we would have to consider the possibility that he was the product of a new mutation). If Mary's mother is a carrier, then there is a probability of 1/2 that Mary is a carrier. As we saw in Chapter 5, a female carrier will transmit the disease gene to half of her sons, on average. Thus the probability that one of her sons will be affected with DMD is 1/2 × 1/2 = 1/4. The creatine kinase test contributes additional information. We can set up the Bayesian calculation as follows:

	Mary is a carrier	Mary is not a carrier
Prior probability	1/2	1/2
Conditional probability that her CK is in the 95th percentile	2/3	0.05
Joint probability	1/3	0.025
Posterior probability	0.93	0.07

It should be clear that the conditional probability of being a carrier given a CK level above the 95th percentile is 2/3. The conditional probability of *not* being a carrier with this CK level must be 0.05 because only 5% of normals will lie above the 95th percentile. Thus the information derived from the CK test has increased Mary's probability of being a carrier from 1/2 to 0.93. Because the probability that she would transmit the DMD gene to her male offspring is 1/2, the probability of producing an affected male increases from 0.25 to 0.47. Currently, it is likely that additional tests, such as screening for DMD mutations and a dystrophin assay, would yield even more precise information.

3. The prior probability that Bob has inherited the gene from his father is 1/2. Because 85% of gene carriers manifest symptoms by age 51 if they inherited the gene from an affected father, the conditional probability that Bob is 51 years old and unaffected, *given* that he inherited the

gene, is 0.15. The probabilities can be set up in the table below. In this example the incorporation of age-of-onset information decreased Bob's chance of inheriting the disease gene from 50% to only 13%. With the cloning of the Huntington disease gene, Bob would likely be offered a DNA diagnostic test to determine with certainty whether he inherited an expanded repeat mutation from his father.

	Bob carries the Huntington disease gene	Bob does not carry the Huntington disease gene
Prior probability	1/2	1/2
Conditional probability that Bob is normal at age 51	0.15	1
Joint probability	0.075	1/2
Posterior probability	0.13	0.87

Glossary

NOTE: When boldface type is used to highlight a word or phrase within a definition, it signifies that the highlighted word or phrase is defined elsewhere in this glossary.

5' cap A chemically modified guanine nucleotide added to the 5' end of a growing mRNA molecule.

acceptor site AG sequence that defines the splice site at the 3' end of an intron.

acrocentric A chromosome whose centromere is close to the end of one arm.

adaptive immune system The portion of the immune system that is capable of changing its DNA sequence to bind foreign particles more effectively. Includes the humoral and cellular components. Compare with **innate immune system.**

addition rule A law of probability which states that the probability of one event *or* another event occurring is derived by adding the probabilities of the two events together, assuming the events occur independently of one another.

adenine One of the four DNA bases. (abbrev.: A)

adenovirus A double-stranded RNA virus that is sometimes used in gene therapy.

adjacent segregation A meiotic segregation pattern in which the pairing of translocated chromosomes leads to unbalanced gametes. Compare with **alternate segregation.**

affinity The binding power of an antibody with an antigen. Low affinity indicates poor binding; high affinity indicates precise binding.

allele Conventional abbreviation for "allelomorph." Refers to the different forms, or DNA sequences, that a gene may have in a population.

allele-specific oligonucleotide A short DNA sequence, usually 18-20 nucleotides, that can hybridize with either disease-causing or normal DNA sequences. Used in DNA diagnosis of mutations.

alpha-fetoprotein An albumin-like protein produced by the fetus. The level of alpha-fetoprotein is increased in pregnancies with neural tube defects and may be decreased in pregnancies with Down syndrome.

alpha-satellite DNA A type of repetitive DNA sequence found near centromeres.

alternate segregation A meiotic segregation pattern in which the pairing of translocated chromosomes leads to balanced gametes. Compare with **adjacent segregation.**

Alu *family* A major group of dispersed repetitive DNA sequences.

amino acid The major building blocks of polypeptides. Each of the 20 amino acids is encoded by one or more mRNA codons.

amniocentesis Prenatal diagnostic technique in which a small amount of amniotic fluid is withdrawn transabdominally at about 16 weeks gestation. Fetal cells can then be tested for some genetic diseases.

amniocyte Fetal cells found in the amniotic fluid.

anaphase One of the stages of cell division in which sister chromatids separate and move toward opposite sides of the cell.

aneuploid Condition in which the number of chromosomes is not a multiple of 23, as in trisomy and monosomy. Compare with **euploid.**

antibody Molecules produced by plasma cells; antibodies bind to invading antigens.

anticipation A feature of pedigrees in which a disease is seen at earlier ages or with increased severity in more recent generations.

anticodon A 3-nucleotide DNA sequence in a tRNA molecule that undergoes complementary base pairing with an mRNA codon.

antigen Molecules that provoke antibody formation (derived from *anti*body *gen*erator).

antigen presenting cell A cell that engulfs foreign bodies, digests them, and then displays the foreign antigens on its cell surface for recognition by T lymphocytes.

apoptosis Programmed cell death.

association The simultaneous occurrence of two traits or events, more often than expected by chance.

autoimmunity Condition in which one's immune system attacks one's own cells.

autoradiogram The image produced by exposing a radioactively labelled substance, such as a probe, to X-ray film. Used, for example, in detecting RFLPs and in performing in situ hybridization.

autosome The 22 pairs of chromosomes excluding the sex chromosomes (X and Y).

B lymphocyte A component of the adaptive immune system that produces antibodies. (also known as B cell)

bacteriophage Viruses that infect bacteria. In recombinant DNA technology, they are used as vectors to carry inserted DNA sequences.

bands 1. Visibly darkened areas on **autoradiograms** that represent the location of alleles on a gel. 2. Alternating dark and light areas visible on chromosomes after certain types of stains are used.

Barr body The inactive X chromosome, visible as a densely stained chromatin mass in the somatic cells of normal females. Also known as **sex chromatin.**

base analog A substance that can mimic the chemical behavior of one of the four DNA bases. Base analogs are a type of **mutagen.**

base One of the four nitrogenous substances (adenine, cytosine, guanine, or thymine) that make up part of the DNA molecule. Combinations of bases specify amino acid sequences.

base pair A unit of complementary DNA bases in a double-stranded DNA molecule (A-T, C-G).

base pair substitution The replacement of one base pair by another. A type of mutation.

Bayes theorem A statistical procedure in which prior and conditional probabilities are used to derive an improved estimate of probability or risk.

benign Describes a neoplasm (tumor) that does not invade surrounding tissue or **metastasize** to other parts of the body. Compare with **malignant.**

bivalent A pair of intertwined homologous chromosomes seen in prophase I of meiosis. Synonymous with **tetrad.**

blood group Molecules found on the surfaces of erythrocytes, some of which (ABO and Rh) determine blood transfusion compatibility.

bp Abbreviation for **base pair.**

breakpoint The location on a chromosome at which a translocation has occurred.

C-banding A type of chromosome staining that highlights the constitutive heterochromatin which lies at and near centromeres.

candidate gene A gene that, on the basis of known properties or protein product, is thought to be the gene causing a specific genetic disease.

carcinogenesis The process of cancer development.

carcinogen Substance that can produce cancer. (adj.: carcinogenic)

carrier An individual who has a copy of a disease-causing gene but does not express the disease. The term is usually used to denote heterozygotes for a recessive disease gene.

cDNA Complementary DNA, formed by reverse transcribing mRNA purified from a collection of cells. This type of DNA corresponds only to coding sequence (exons).

cDNA library A collection of segments of complementary DNA (cDNA) cloned into vehicles such as phage or plasmid. Compare with **genomic library.**

cell adhesion molecule Cell surface molecule that participates in the interaction of T cells and their targets.

cell cycle The alternating sequence of mitosis and interphase.

cellular immune system The T-cell component of the adaptive immune system.

centiMorgan (cM) A unit of measure of the frequency of recombination between two loci, also known as a map unit. One cM corresponds to a recombination frequency of 1%.

centriole Structures in cells that help pull chromosomes apart during meiosis and mitosis.

centromere The region of a chromosome that separates the two arms. Centromeres are the sites of attachment of spindle fibers during cell division.

CG island Unmethylated CG sequences that are often found near the 5' ends of some genes.

chiasma The location of a **crossover** between two homologous chromosomes during meiosis. (pl.: chiasmata)

chorionic villus sampling A prenatal diagnostic technique in which a small sample of chorionic villi is aspirated. Usually performed at 10-12 weeks gestation.

chromatin The combination of proteins (e.g., **histones**) and nucleic acids that makes up chromosomes.

chromatin loop A unit of DNA coiling consisting of a group of **solenoids.** Each loop is approximately 100 kb in size.

chromatin opener Regulatory element that is capable of decondensing or "opening" regions of chromatin.

chromosome Threadlike structure (literally "colored body") consisting of **chromatin.** Genes are arranged along chromosomes.

chromosome abnormalities A major group of genetic diseases, consisting of microscopically observable alterations of chromosome number or structure.

chromosome banding The process of applying specific stains to chromosomes in order to produce characteristic patterns of **bands.** Example: G-banding.

chromosome breakage The fracture of chromosomes. Breakage is increased in the presence of **clastogens.**

chromosome instability syndrome Diseases characterized by the presence of large numbers of chromosome breaks or exchanges, such as **sister chromatid exchange.** Example: Bloom syndrome.

chromosome walking A process in which overlapping clones are used to progress along a chromosome toward a gene of interest.

chromosome-specific library A collection of DNA fragments from a single chromosome.

class switching The process in which heavy chains of B lymphocytes change from one class, or **isotype,** to another; e.g., IgM to IgG.

clastogen A substance that can induce **chromosome breakage.** Example: radiation.

clone A series of identical DNA fragments created by recombinant DNA techniques. Clones also refer to identical cells that are descended from a single common ancestor.

codominant Alleles that are both expressed when they occur together in the heterozygous state. Example: A and B alleles of the ABO blood group system.

codon A group of three mRNA bases, each of which specifies an amino acid when translated.

coefficient of relationship A statistic that measures the proportion of genes shared by two individuals as a result of descent from a common ancestor.

colcemid or colchicine A spindle poison that arrests cells in metaphase, making them easily discernible microscopically.

complement system A component of the immune system, encoded by genes in the Class III MHC region, which can destroy invading organisms. The complement system also interacts with other components of the immune system, such as antibodies and phagocytes.

complementary base pairing A fundamental process in which adenosine pairs only with thymine, and guanine pairs only with cytosine. Also sometimes known as "Watson-Crick pairing".

compound heterozygote An individual who is heterozygous for two different disease-causing mutations at a locus. Compare with **homozygote.** Compound heterozygotes for recessive disease mutations are usually affected with the disorder.

concordant When two individuals have the same trait (e.g., monozygotic twins may be concordant for a disease such as diabetes). Compare with **discordant.** (n.: concordance)

conditional probability The probability that an event will occur, *given* that another event has already occurred. Conditional probabilities are used, for example, in **Bayes theorem.**

confined placental mosaicism A form of **mosaicism** that is observed in the placenta, but not in the fetus.

congenital Present at birth.

consanguinity The mating of related individuals.

consensus sequence A sequence that denotes the DNA bases most often seen in a region of interest. The sequences that are found near **donor** and **acceptor splice sites** are a type of consensus sequence.

conservation The preservation of highly similar DNA sequences among different organisms; conserved sequences are usually found in functional genes.

conserved see **conservation.**

constitutional or constitutive Pertaining to DNA in normal cells of the body, usually used in contrast to tumor DNA.

constitutive heterochromatin See **heterochromatin, constitutive.**

contiguous gene syndrome A disease caused by the deletion or duplication of multiple consecutive genes. *See also* **microdeletion.**

cordocentesis See **percutaneous umbilical blood sampling (PUBS).**

cosmid A phage-plasmid hybrid, capable of accepting larger DNA inserts (up to 40-50 kb) than either phage or plasmids.

costimulatory molecule Cell surface molecule that participates in the binding of T-cell receptors to MHC-antigen complexes.

cross Mating between organisms in genetic studies.

cross-reaction The binding of an antibody to an antigen *other* than the one that originally stimulated antibody formation. Such antigens are usually very similar to the original antibody-generating antigen.

crossing over or **crossover** The exchange of genetic material between homologous chromosomes during meiosis (also occurs rarely during mitosis); produces **recombination.**

cryptic splice site Site at which intron-exon splicing may occur when the usual splice site is altered.

cytogenetics The study of chromosomes and their abnormalities. Combines cytology, the study of cells, and genetics.

cytokine Growth factor that causes cells to proliferate. Example: interleukins.

cytokinesis Cytoplasmic division that occurs during mitosis and meiosis.

cytosine One of the four DNA bases. (abbrev.: C)

cytotoxic T lymphocyte A type of T lymphocyte that destroys a cell when the cell presents a complex of MHC Class I molecule and foreign peptide. Part of the cellular immune system.

daughter cells Cells that result from the division of a parent cell.

deformation Alteration of the form, shape, or position of a normally formed body part by mechanical forces. Example: oligohydramnios sequence.

delayed age of onset Describes phenotypes that are not seen at birth, but later in life. Examples: Huntington disease, familial breast cancer.

deletion The loss of chromosome material. May be terminal or interstitial. Compare with **duplication.**

deletion, interstitial Deletion that removes part of the interior of the chromosome.

deletion, terminal Deletion that removes part of a chromosome, including one telomere.

denaturing gradient gel electrophoresis (DGGE) See **electrophoresis, denaturing gradient gel.**

derivative chromosome A chromosome that has been altered as a result of a translocation. Example: derivative 9, or der(9).

dideoxy method A technique for sequencing DNA in which dideoxynucleotides, which terminate replication, are incorporated into replicating DNA strands.

diploid Having two copies of each chromosome. In humans, the diploid number is 46. Compare with **haploid, polyploid.**

direct diagnosis A form of DNA-based disease diagnosis in which the mutation itself is examined directly. Compare with **indirect diagnosis.**

discordant When two individuals do not share the same trait. Compare with **concordant.** (n.: discordance)

dispermy Fertilization of a single ovum by two sperm cells.

dispersed repetitive DNA A class of repeated DNA sequences in which single repeats are scattered throughout the genome. Compare with **tandem repeats.**

disruption Morphologic defect that results from a breakdown of an otherwise normal developmental process. Example: limb reduction defect resulting from poor vascularization.

dizygotic A type of twinning in which each twin is produced by the fertilization of a different ovum. Synonymous with "fraternal" twin. Compare with **monozygotic.**

DNA (deoxyribonucleic acid) A double-helix molecule that consists of a sugar-phosphate backbone and four nitrogenous bases (A, C, G, and T). DNA bases encode messenger RNA (mRNA) which in turn encodes amino acid sequences.

DNA fingerprint A series of DNA polymorphisms, usually VNTRs, typed in an individual. Because these polymorphisms are highly polymorphic, the combined genotypes are useful in identifying individuals for forensic purposes.

DNA looping The formation of looped structures in DNA; sometimes permits the interaction of various regulatory elements.

DNA polymerase An enzyme involved in DNA replication and repair.

DNA repair A process in which mistakes in the DNA sequence are altered to represent the original sequence.

DNA sequence The order of DNA bases along a chromosome.

dominant Allele that is expressed in the same way in single copy (heterozygotes) as in double copy (homozygotes). Compare with **recessive.**

dominant negative A type of mutation in which the altered protein product in a heterozygote forms a complex with the normal protein product produced by the homologous normal gene, thus disabling it.

donor site GT sequence that defines the splice site at the 5' end of an intron.

dosage compensation As a consequence of X inactivation, the amount of X chromosome-encoded gene product in females is roughly equal to that of males.

dosage mapping A technique for mapping genes in which excess or deficient gene product is correlated with a chromosomal duplication or deletion.

double helix Describes the "twisted ladder" shape of the double-stranded DNA molecule.

duplication The presence of an extra copy of chromosome material. Compare with **deletion.**

dysmorphology The study of abnormal physical development.

dysplasia A defect in which cells are abnormally organized into tissue. Example: bone dysplasia.

electrophoresis A technique in which charged molecules are placed in a medium and exposed to an electrical field, causing them to migrate through the medium at different rates, according to charge, length, or other attributes.

electrophoresis, denaturing gradient gel (**DGGE**) A method of mutation detection in which DNA fragments are electrophoresed through a gel in which there is a changing denaturing factor, such as temperature.

empirical risk Risk estimate based upon direct observation of data.

endocytosis Process in which molecules are transported into the interior of cells.

enhancer Regulatory DNA sequence that interacts with promoters to increase the transcription of genes.

equational division The second major cycle of meiosis; also called meiosis II. Compare with **reduction division.**

equatorial plane The middle of the cell's spindle, along which homologous chromosomes are arranged during metaphase.

erythroblast A nucleated red blood cell; precursors of erythrocytes.

erythrocyte A red blood cell.

euchromatin Chromatin that is light-staining during interphase and tends to be transcriptionally active. Compare with **heterochromatin.**

eukaryotes Organisms whose cells have true nuclei.

euploid Cells whose chromosome number is a multiple of 23 (in humans).

exon Portions of genes that encode amino acids and are retained after the primary mRNA transcript is spliced. Compare with **intron.**

expanded repeat A type of mutation in which a tandem trinucleotide repeat increases in number. Example: Huntington disease.

false negative A test result in which an affected individual is incorrectly identified as being unaffected with the disease in question. Compare with **false positive.**

false positive A test result in which an unaffected individual is incorrectly identified as being affected with the disease in question. Compare with **false negative.**

fetoscopy A fetal visualization technique in which an endoscope is inserted through the abdominal wall. Sometimes used in prenatal diagnosis.

fibrillin Connective tissue component; mutations in the fibrillin gene can cause Marfan syndrome.

flow cytometry A technique in which chromosomes can be individually sorted.

fluorescence in situ hybridization (**FISH**) A molecular cytogenetic technique in which labelled probes are hybridized with chromosomes and then visualized under a fluorescence microscope.

frameshift mutation An alteration of DNA in which a duplication or deletion occurs that is not a multiple of three base pairs.

fusion gene A gene that results from a combination of two genes, or parts of two genes.

gamete The haploid germ cell (sperm and ova).

gametogenesis The process of gamete formation.

gene The fundamental unit of heredity.

gene-environment interaction A mutual phenotypic effect of a gene and an environmental factor that is greater than the single effect of either factor alone. Example: the effect of α_1-antitrypsin deficiency and cigarette smoking on pulmonary emphysema.

gene family A group of genes that are similar in DNA sequence and have evolved from a single common ancestral gene; may or may not be located in the same chromosome region.

gene flow The exchange of genes between different populations.

gene frequency In a population, the proportion of chromosomes that contain a specific gene.

gene therapy The insertion of normal genes into a cell to correct a disease.

gene therapy, germline Gene therapy that alters all cells of the body, including the germ line. Compare with **gene therapy, somatic cell.**

gene therapy, somatic cell Gene therapy that alters somatic cells but not cells of the germ line. Compare with **gene therapy, germline.**

genetic code The combinations of mRNA **codons** that specify individual amino acids.

genetic counseling The delivery of information about genetic diseases (risks, natural history, and management) to patients and their families.

genetic drift An evolutionary process in which gene frequencies change, as a result of random fluctuations in the transmission of genes from one generation to the next. Drift is greater in smaller populations.

genetic engineering The alteration of genes; typically involves **recombinant DNA** techniques.

genetic mapping The ordering of genes on chromosomes according to recombination frequency. Compare with **physical mapping.**

genetic screening The large-scale testing of defined populations for a genetic disease or disease-causing gene.

genome The totality of an organism's DNA.

genomic library A collection of DNA fragments from an organism's entire genome. Includes cDNA as well as noncoding DNA. Compare with **cDNA library.**

genotype An individual's allelic constitution at a locus.

genotype frequency The proportion of individuals in a population that carry a specific genotype.

germ line Cells responsible for the production of gametes.

Giemsa A type of staining that produces G-bands in chromosomes.

globin Major component of the hemoglobin molecule. Globin is also found in the vertebrate myoglobin molecule.

growth factor A substance capable of stimulating cell proliferation.

growth factor receptor Structures on cell surfaces to which growth factors can bind.

guanine One of the four DNA bases. (abbrev.: G).

guanosine diphosphate (GDP) Partially dephosphorylated form of **guanosine triphosphate.**

guanosine triphosphate (GTP) A molecule required for the synthesis of peptide bonds during translation.

haploid Cells having one copy of each chromosome, the typical state for gametes. In humans, the haploid number is 23.

haplotype The allelic constitution of multiple loci on a single chromosome. Derived from "haploid genotype".

Hardy-Weinberg principle Specifies an equilibrium relationship between gene frequencies and genotype frequencies in populations.

heavy chain A major structural component of an antibody molecule, having a higher molecular weight than the other major component, the light chain. There are five major types of heavy chains in the human, γ, μ, α, δ, and ϵ.

helper T lymphocyte A type of T lymphocyte whose receptors bind to a complex of MHC Class II molecule and foreign peptide on the surfaces of antigen presenting cells. Part of the cellular immune system.

heme Iron-containing component of the hemoglobin molecule; binds with oxygen.

hemizygous A gene present in only a single copy. Most commonly refers to genes on the single male X chromosome, but can refer to other genes in the haploid state, such as the genes homologous to a deleted region of a chromosome.

heritability The proportion of population **variance** in a trait that can be ascribed to genetic factors.

heterochromatin Dark-staining chromatin that is usually transcriptionally inactive and consists mostly of repetitive DNA. Compare with **euchromatin.**

heterochromatin, constitutive Heterochromatin that consists of **satellite DNA**; located near centromeres and on the short arms of acrocentric chromosomes.

heterodisomy The presence in a cell of two chromosomes derived from a single parent and none from the other parent (disomy). In *hetero*disomy, the two chromosomes are the nonidentical homologous chromosomes. Compare with **isodisomy.**

heterogeneity, allelic Describes conditions in which different alleles at a locus can produce varying expression of a disease. Depending on phenotype definition, allelic heterogeneity may cause two distinct diseases, as in Duchenne and Becker muscular dystrophy.

heterogeneity, locus Describes diseases in which mutations at distinct loci can produce the same disease phenotype. Example: osteogenesis imperfecta.

heteromorphism Variation in the microscopic appearance of a chromosome.

heteroplasmy The existence of differing DNA sequences at a locus within a single cell. Often seen in mitochondrial genes.

heterotetramer A molecule consisting of four (tetra) subunits, at least one of which differs from the others. Compare with **homotetramer.**

heterozygote An individual who has two different alleles at a locus. Compare with **homozygote.**

high-resolution banding Chromosome banding using prophase or prometaphase chromosomes, which are more extended than metaphase chromosomes and thus yield more bands and greater resolution.

histone The protein core around which DNA is wound in a chromosome.

holandric Y-linked inheritance; a transmission exclusively from father to son.

homologous 1. DNA or amino acid sequences that are highly similar to one another. 2. Describes chromosomes that pair during meiosis, one derived from the individual's father and the other derived from the mother.

homologs Chromosomes that are **homologous.**

homotetramer Molecule consisting of four (tetra) identical subunits. Compare with **heterotetramer.**

homozygote An individual in whom the two alleles at a locus are the same. Compare with **heterozygote.**

human leukocyte antigen (HLA) Older term for **major histocompatibility complex (MHC).**

humoral immune system The B-cell component of the adaptive immune system, termed humoral because antibodies are secreted into the circulation.

immunodeficiency disease A class of diseases characterized by insufficiencies in the immune response. Example: severe combined immune deficiency, SCID.

immunogenetics The study of the genetic basis of the immune system.

immunoglobulin Receptor found on the surfaces of B cells. When secreted into the circulation by B cells that have matured into plasma cells, immunoglobulins are known as **antibodies.**

imprinting Describes process in which genetic material is expressed differently when inherited from the mother than when inherited from the father.

in situ hybridization Molecular gene mapping technique in which labeled probes are hybridized to stained metaphase chromosomes and then exposed to X-ray film to reveal the position of the probe.

in vitro fertilization (IVF) diagnosis A form of genetic diagnosis in which DNA from a single blastomere cell, obtained by IVF, is amplified by PCR so that disease-causing mutations can be tested.

incest The mating of closely related individuals, usually describing the union of first-degree relatives.

independence A principle, often invoked in statistical analysis, indicating that the occurrence of one event has no effect on the probability of the occurrence of another. (adj.: independent)

independent assortment One of Mendel's fundamental principles; dictates that alleles at different loci are transmitted independently of one another.

index case See **proband.**

indirect diagnosis A form of genetic diagnosis in which the disease-causing mutation is not directly observed; usually refers to diagnosis using linked markers. Compare with **direct diagnosis.**

innate immune system Portion of the immune system that does not change its characteristics to respond to infections. Part of the initial immune response. Compare with **adaptive immune system.**

insert A DNA sequence that is placed into a vector, such as a plasmid or cosmid, using recombinant DNA techniques.

interphase Portion of the cell cycle that alternates with **meiosis** or **mitosis.** DNA is replicated and repaired during this phase.

intraclass correlation coefficient A statistical measure that varies between -1 and 1 and specifies the degree of similarity of two quantities in a sample or population.

intron DNA sequence found between two **exons.** Transcribed into primary mRNA but spliced out in the formation of the mature mRNA transcript.

inversion A structural rearrangement of a chromosome in which two breaks occur, followed by the reinsertion of the chromosome segment, but in reversed order. May be either paracentric or pericentric. See also **inversion, paracentric** and **inversion, pericentric.**

inversion, paracentric An inversion that does not include the centromere.

inversion, pericentric An inversion that includes the centromere.

isochromosome A structural chromosome rearrangement caused by the division of a chromosome along an axis perpendicular to the usual axis of division; results in chromosomes with either two short arms or two long arms.

isodisomy The presence in a cell of two identical chromosomes derived from one parent and none from the other parent. Compare with **heterodisomy.**

isotype Classes of immunoglobulin molecules, e.g., IgA, IgE and IgG, determined by the type of heavy chain present in the molecule.

joint probability The probability of two events *both* occurring.

karyotype A display of chromosomes, ordered according to length.

kilobase (kb) One thousand DNA base pairs.

light chain A major structural component of the antibody molecule, consisting of either a κ or a λ chain. The light chain has a lower molecular weight than the other major component, the heavy chain.

likelihood A statistic that measures the probability of an event or a series of events.

LINEs **(long interspersed elements)** A class of dispersed repetitive DNA in which each repeat is relatively long, up to 7 kb. Compare with **SINEs.**

linkage Describes two loci that are located close enough on the same chromosome that their **recombination frequency** is less than 50%.

linkage disequilibrium Nonrandom association of alleles at linked loci in populations. Compare with **linkage equilibrium.**

linkage equilibrium Lack of preferential association of alleles at linked loci. Compare with **linkage disequilibrium.**

linkage phase The arrangement of alleles of linked loci on chromosomes.

locus The chromosome location of a specific gene. (pl.: loci) *locus control region* DNA sequence in the 5' region of the globin gene clusters that is involved in transcription regulation.

LOD score Common logarithm of the ratio of the likelihood of linkage at a specific recombination fraction to the likelihood of no linkage.

loss of heterozygosity Describes a locus or loci at which a deletion or other process has converted the locus from heterozygosity to homozygosity or hemizygosity.

Lyon hypothesis A proposal (now verified) that one X chromosome is randomly inactivated in each somatic cell of the normal female embryo (Lyonization).

macrophage A type of **phagocyte** that ingests foreign microbes and displays them on its surface for recognition by T-cell receptors.

major gene A single locus responsible for a trait (sometimes contrasted with a polygenic component).

major histocompatibility complex (MHC), class I A membrane-spanning glycoprotein, found on the surfaces of nearly all cells, that presents antigen for recognition by cytotoxic T lymphocytes. Compare with **MHC class II.**

major histocompatibility complex (MHC), class II A membrane-spanning glycoprotein, found on the surfaces of **antigen-presenting cells,** that presents antigen for recognition by helper T cells.

malformation A primary morphologic defect resulting from an intrinsically abnormal developmental process. Example: polydactyly.

malignant Describes a tumor that is capable of invading surrounding tissue and metastasizing to other sites in the body. Compare with **benign.**

manifesting heterozygote An individual who is heterozygous for a recessive trait, but displays the trait. Most often used to describe females heterozygous for an X-linked trait who display the trait.

markers Polymorphisms, such as RFLPs, VNTRs, microsatellite repeats, and blood groups, that are linked to a disease locus.

maternal serum alpha-fetoprotein (MSAFP) Alpha-fetoprotein present in the serum of pregnant women; used in the prenatal screening of fetal disorders such as neural tube defects and Down syndrome.

mature transcript Describes mRNA after the introns have been spliced out. Prior to splicing, the mRNA is referred to as a primary transcript.

maximum likelihood estimate A statistical procedure in which the likelihoods of a variety of parameter values are estimated and then compared to determine which likelihood is the largest. Used, for example, in evaluating LOD scores to determine which recombination frequency is the most likely.

megabase (mb) One million base pairs.

meiosis Cell division process in which haploid gametes are formed from diploid germ cells.

meiotic failure Aberrant **meiosis** in which a diploid gamete is produced rather than the normal haploid gamete.

memory cells A class of high-affinity-binding B cells that remains in the body after an immune response has ended; provides a relatively rapid, high-affinity response should the same disease microbe be encountered a second time.

mendelian Referring to Gregor Mendel, describes a trait that is attributable to a single gene.

messenger RNA (**mRNA**) RNA molecule that is formed from the **transcription** of DNA. Prior to intron splicing, mRNA is termed a primary transcript; after splicing, the mature transcript (or mature mRNA) proceeds to the cytoplasm where it is translated into an amino acid sequence.

metacentric A chromosome in which the centromere is located approximately in the middle of the chromosome arm.

metaphase A stage of mitosis and meiosis in which homologous chromosomes are arranged along the equatorial plane, or metaphase plate, of the cell. This is the mitotic stage at which chromosomes are maximally condensed and most easily visualized.

metastasis The spread of malignant cells from one site in the body to another. (v.: metastasize)

methylation The attachment of methyl groups; in genetics, refers especially to the addition of methyl groups to cytosine bases, forming 5-methylcytosine. Methylation is correlated with reduced transcription of genes.

MHC restriction The limiting of immune response functions to MHC-mediated interactions; e.g., the binding of T-cell receptors is MHC-restricted, because it requires the presentation of antigen by MHC Class I or MHC Class II molecules.

microdeletion A chromosome deletion too small to be visible under a microscope. Examples: DiGeorge syndrome; Prader-Willi syndrome.

microsatellite A type of **satellite DNA** that consists of small repeat units, usually two, three or four bp, that occur in tandem.

microsatellite repeat polymorphism A type of genetic variation in populations consisting of differing numbers of microsatellite repeat units at a locus.

minisatellite A type of **satellite DNA** that consists of tandem repeat units that are each about 20-70 bp in length. Variation in the number of minisatellite repeats is the basis of VNTR polymorphisms.

mismatch The presence in one chain of double-stranded DNA of a base that is not complementary to the corresponding base in the other chain. Also known as mispairing.

missense A type of mutation that results in a single amino acid change in the translated gene product. Compare with **nonsense mutation.**

mitochondria Cytoplasmic organelles that are important in cellular respiration. The mitochondria have their own unique DNA.

mitosis Cell division process in which two identical progeny cells are produced from a single parent cell. Compare with **meiosis.**

mobile elements DNA sequences that are capable of inserting themselves into other locations in the genome.

modifier gene A gene that alters the expression of a gene at another locus.

molecular genetics Study of the structure and function of genes at the molecular level.

monoclonal A group of cells that consist of a single clone; i.e., all cells are derived from the same single ancestral cell.

monogenic Describing a single-gene, or mendelian, trait.

monosomy An aneuploid condition in which a specific chromosome is present in only single copy, giving the individual a total of 45 chromosomes.

monozygotic Describing a twin pair in which both members are derived from a single zygote. Synonymous with "identical" twin. Compare with **dizygotic.**

morphogenesis The process of development of a cell, organ, or organism.

mosaic The existence of two or more genetically different cell lines in an individual.

mosaic, germline A type of **mosaic** in which the germline of an individual contains an allele not present in the somatic cells.

multi-hit concept of carcinogenesis The principle that most tumors arise from a series of errors, or "hits," occurring in a cell.

multifactorial Describes traits or diseases that are the product of the interaction of multiple genetic and environmental factors. Example: neural tube defects.

multiplication rule A law of probability that states that the probability of occurrence of two or more independent events can be obtained by multiplying the individiual probabilities of each event.

multipoint mapping A type of genetic mapping in which the recombination frequencies among three or more loci are estimated simultaneously.

mutagen A substance that causes a **mutation.**

mutation An alteration in DNA sequence.

mutation, induced A mutation that is caused by an exogenous factor, such as radiation. Compare with **mutation, spontaneous.**

mutation, spontaneous A mutation that is not known to be the result of an exogenous factor. Compare with **mutation, induced.**

natural killer cells A type of lymphocyte that is involved in the early phase of defense against foreign microbes and tumors and is not MHC restricted.

natural selection An evolutionary process in which individuals with favorable genotypes produce relatively greater numbers of surviving offspring.

neoplasm or tumor A group of cells characterized by unregulated proliferation (may be **benign** or **malignant).**

neurofibromin The protein product of the neurofibromatosis type 1 gene.

new mutation An alteration in DNA sequence that appears for the first time in a family as the result of a mutation in one of the parents' germ cells.

nondirectiveness Describes genetic counseling approach in which information is provided to a family, while leaving decisions about reproduction to the family.

nondisjunction Failure of homologous chromosomes (in mitosis or meiosis I) or sister chromatids (in meiosis II) to separate properly into different progeny cells. Can produce aneuploidy.

nonsense mutation A type of mutation in which an mRNA stop codon is produced or removed, resulting respectively in premature termination of translation or an elongated protein product. Compare with **missense mutation.**

Northern blotting A gene expression assay in which mRNA on a blot is hybridized with a labeled probe.

nucleosome A structural unit of chromatin in which 140 to 150 bp of DNA are wrapped around a core unit of eight histone molecules.

nucleotide A basic unit of DNA or RNA, consisting of one deoxyribose (or ribose in the case of RNA), one phosphate group, and one nitrogenous base.

obligate carrier An individual who is known to possess a disease-causing gene, usually on the basis of pedigree examination, but may or may not be affected with the disease phenotype.

occurrence risk The probability that a couple will produce a child with a genetic disease. Refers to couples who have not yet produced a child with the disease in question. Compare with **recurrence risk.**

oligonucleotide DNA sequence consisting of a small number of nucleotide bases.

oncogene A gene that can transform cells into a highly proliferative state, causing cancer.

oogenesis The process in which ova are produced.

oogonium The diploid germline stem cell from which ova are ultimately derived.

palindrome A DNA sequence whose complementary sequence is the same if read backwards; e.g., 5' AATGCGCATT 3'.

panmixia Describes a population in which individuals mate at random with respect to a specific genotype.

partial trisomy Chromosome abnormality in which a portion of a chromosome is present in three copies; may be produced by reciprocal translocation or unequal crossover. See also **translocation, reciprocal** and **crossover, unequal.**

pedigree A diagram that describes family relationships, gender, disease status, and other attributes.

penetrance In a population, the proportion of individuals possessing a disease-causing genotype who express the disease phenotype. When this proportion is less than 100%, the disease genotype is said to have reduced or incomplete penetrance.

percutaneous umbilical blood sampling (PUBS) Prenatal diagnostic technique in which fetal blood is obtained by puncturing the umbilical cord. Also called cordocentesis.

phagocyte A cell that engulfs foreign particles.

phenotype The observed characteristics of an individual, produced by the interaction of genes and environment.

Philadelphia chromosome A reciprocal translocation between the long arms of chromosomes 9 and 22 in somatic cells; produces chronic myelogenous leukemia.

physical mapping The determination of physical distances between genes using cytogenetic and molecular techniques. Compare with **genetic mapping,** in which recombination frequencies are estimated.

plasma cell Mature B lymphocyte capable of secreting antibodies.

plasmid Circular double-stranded DNA molecule found in bacteria; capable of independent replication. Plasmids are often used as cloning vectors in recombinant DNA techniques.

pleiotropy Describes genes that have multiple phenotypic effects. Examples: Marfan syndrome, cystic fibrosis. (adj.: pleiotropic)

polar body Cell produced during oogenesis that has a nucleus but very little cytoplasm.

polar body diagnosis Prenatal diagnostic technique in which DNA from a polar body is subjected to PCR amplification and assayed using molecular methods.

poly-A tail The addition of several adenine nucleotides to the 3' end of a primary mRNA transcript.

polygenic Describes a trait caused by the combined additive effects of multiple genes.

polymerase chain reaction (**PCR**) A technique for amplifying a large number of copies of a specific DNA sequence flanked by two oligonucleotide primers. The DNA is alternately heated and cooled in the presence of DNA polymerase and free nucleotides so that the specified DNA segment is denatured, hybridized with primers, and extended by DNA polymerase.

polymorphism A locus in which two or more alleles have gene frequencies greater than 0.01 in a population. When this criterion is not fulfilled, the locus is monomorphic.

polypeptide A series of amino acids linked together by peptide bonds.

polyploidy Chromosome abnormality in which the number of chromosomes in a cell is a multiple of 23 but is greater than the diploid number [examples are **triploidy** (69 chromosomes in the human) and **tetraploidy** (92 chromosomes in the human)].

population genetics Branch of genetics dealing with genetic variation and genetic evolution of populations.

population screening The large-scale testing of populations for a disease.

positional cloning The isolation and cloning of a disease gene after determining its approximate physical location; the gene product is subsequently determined. Formerly termed "reverse genetics".

positive predictive value Among the individuals identified by a test as having a disease, the proportion that actually have the disease.

posterior probability In Bayesian analysis, the final probability of an event after taking into account prior, conditional, and joint probabilities.

posttranslational modification Various types of additions to and alterations of a polypeptide that take place after the mature mRNA transcript is translated into a polypeptide; e.g., hydroxylation, glycosylation, cleavage of portions of the polypeptide.

prenatal diagnosis The identification of a disease in a fetus or embryo.

presymptomatic diagnosis The identification of a disease before the phenotype is clinically observable.

primary oocyte The diploid product of an oogonium. All primary oocytes are produced in the female during prenatal development; they undergo meiosis I to produce secondary oocytes when ovulation begins.

primary spermatocyte The diploid progeny cell of a spermatogonium, which then undergoes meiosis I to produce secondary spermatocytes.

primary transcript The mRNA molecule directly after transcription from DNA. A mature mRNA transcript is formed from the primary transcript when the introns are spliced out.

primer An oligonucleotide sequence that flanks either side of the DNA to be amplified by **PCR.**

primer extension Part of the **PCR** process, in which DNA polymerase extends the DNA sequence beginning at an oligonucleotide primer.

prior probability In Bayesian analysis, the probability that an event will occur *before* any additional information, such as a biochemical carrier test, is incorporated.

probability The proportion of times that a specific event occurs in a series of trials.

proband The first person in a pedigree to be identified clinically as having the disease in question. Synonymous with **propositus** and **index case.**

probe In molecular genetics, a labelled substance, such as a DNA segment, that is used to identify a gene, mRNA transcript, or gene product, usually through hybridization of the probe with the target.

promoter A DNA sequence located 5' of a gene to which RNA polymerase binds in order to begin transcription of the DNA into mRNA.

proofreading The correction of errors that occur during replication, transcription, or translation.

prophase The first stage of mitosis and meiosis.

propositus See **proband.**

protein electrophoresis A technique in which amino acid variations are identified on the basis of charge differences that cause differential mobility of polypeptides through an electrically charged medium.

protein kinase An enzyme that phosphorylates serine, threonine, or tyrosine residues in proteins.

proto-oncogene A gene whose protein product is involved in the regulation of cell growth. When altered, a proto-oncogene can become a cancer-causing **oncogene.**

pseudoautosomal region The distal tip of the Y chromosome short arm, which undergoes crossover with the distal tip of the X chromosome short arm during meiosis in the male.

pseudogene A gene that is highly similar in sequence to another gene or genes but has been rendered transcriptionally or translationally inactive by mutations.

pseudomosaicism A false indication of fetal mosaicism, caused by an artifact of cell culture.

pulsed field gel electrophoresis A type of electrophoresis suitable for relatively large DNA fragments; the fragment is moved through a gel by alternating pulses of electricity across fields that are 90 degrees from one another in orientation.

Punnett square A table specifying the genotypes that can arise from the gametes contributed by a mating pair of individuals.

purine The two DNA (also RNA) bases, adenine and guanine, that consist of double carbon-nitrogen rings. Compare with **pyrimidine.**

pyrimidine The bases (cytosine and thymine in DNA, and cytosine and uracil in RNA) that consist of single carbon-nitrogen rings. Compare with **purine.**

quantitative trait Characteristics that can be measured on a continuous scale; e.g., height, weight.

quantitative trait locus method A method for finding genes underlying complex multifactorial traits; involves crosses in experimental animals, linkage analysis, and gene cloning.

quasidominant A pattern of inheritance that appears to be autosomal dominant but is actually autosomal recessive. Usually the result of a mating between an affected homozygote and a heterozygote.

Quinacrine banding **(Q-banding)** Chromosome staining technique in which a fluorochrome dye (quinacrine compound) is added to chromosomes, which are then viewed under a fluorescence microscope.

radiation, ionizing A type of energy emission that is capable of removing electrons from their orbits, thus causing ion formation. Example: X-rays.

radiation, non-ionizing A type of energy emission that does not remove electrons from atoms, but can change their orbits. Example: ultraviolet radiation.

random mating See **panmixia.**

receptor A cell-surface structure that binds to extracellular particles.

recessive An allele that is phenotypically expressed only in the homozygous or hemizygous state. The recessive allele is masked by a dominant allele when the two occur together in a heterozygote. Compare with **dominant.**

recognition site See **restriction site.**

recombinant DNA A DNA molecule that consists of components from more than one parent molecule; e.g., a human DNA insert placed in a plasmid vector.

recombinase An enzyme that helps to bring about somatic recombination in B and T lymphocytes.

recombination The occurrence among offspring of new combinations of alleles, resulting from crossovers that occur during parental meiosis.

recombination frequency The proportion of meioses in which recombinants between two loci are observed. Used to estimate genetic distances between loci. *See also* **centiMorgans.**

recombination hot spot A region of a chromosome in which the recombination frequency is elevated.

recurrence risk The probability that another affected offspring will be produced in families in which one or more affected offspring have already been produced. Compare with **occurence risk.**

reduction division The first stage of meiosis (meiosis I), in which the chromosome number is reduced from diploid to haploid.

repetitive DNA DNA sequences that are found in multiple copies in the genome. They may be dispersed or repeated in **tandem.**

replication The process in which the double-stranded DNA molecule is duplicated.

replication bubble Replication structures that occur in multiple locations on a chromosome, allowing replication to proceed more rapidly.

replication origin The point at which replication begins on a DNA strand; in eukaryotes, each chromosome has numerous replication origins.

replicative segregation Refers to changes in the proportions of mitochondrial DNA alleles as the mitochondria reproduce.

restriction digest Process in which DNA is exposed to a restriction enzyme, causing it to be cleaved into **restriction fragments.**

restriction endonuclease Bacterial enzyme that cleaves DNA at a specific DNA sequence (restriction site).

restriction fragment A piece of DNA that has been cleaved by a restriction endonuclease.

restriction fragment length polymorphism (RFLP) Variations in DNA sequence in populations, detected by digesting DNA with a restriction endonuclease, electrophoresing the resulting restriction fragments, transferring the fragments to a solid medium (blot), and hybridizing the DNA on the blot with a labelled probe.

restriction site A DNA sequence that is cleaved by a specific restriction endonuclease.

restriction site polymorphism A variation in DNA sequence that is due to the presence or absence of a restriction site. This type of polymorphism is the basis for most traditional RFLPs.

retrovirus A type of RNA virus that can reverse transcribe its RNA into DNA for insertion into the genome of a host cell; useful as a vector for gene therapy.

reverse banding (R-banding) A chromosome banding technique in which chromosomes are heated in a phosphate buffer; produces dark and light bands in patterns that are the reverse of those produced by G-banding.

reverse transcriptase An enzyme that transcribes RNA into DNA (hence "reverse").

ribonucleic acid (RNA) A single-stranded molecule that consists of a sugar (ribose), phosphate group, and a series of bases (adenine, cytosine, guanine, and uracil). There are three basic types of RNA: **messenger RNA, ribosomal RNA,** and **transfer RNA.**

ribosomal RNA (rRNA) In conjunction with protein molecules, composes the **ribosome.**

ribosome The site of translation of mature messenger RNA into amino acid sequences.

ring chromosome A structural chromosome abnormality formed when both ends of a chromosome are lost and the new ends fuse together.

RNA polymerase Enzyme that binds to a promoter site and synthesizes messenger RNA from a DNA template.

satellite DNA A portion of the DNA that differs enough in base composition so that it forms a distinct band on a cesium chloride gradient centrifugation; usually contains highly repetitive DNA sequences.

secondary oocyte A cell containing 23 double-stranded chromosomes, produced from a primary oocyte after meiosis I in the female.

secondary spermatocyte A cell containing 23 double-stranded chromosomes, produced from a primary spermatocyte after meiosis I in the male.

segregation The distribution of genes from homologous chromosomes to different gametes during meiosis.

sensitivity The proportion of affected individuals who are correctly identified by a test (true positives). Compare with **specificity.**

sequence (formerly "anomalad") A primary defect with secondary structural changes in development. Examples: oligohydramnios sequence, Pierre-Robin sequence.

sex chromatin See **Barr body.**

sex chromosomes The X and Y chromosomes in humans. Compare with **autosomes.**

sex-influenced A trait whose expression is modified by the gender of the individual possessing the trait.

sex-limited A trait that is expressed only in one sex or the other.

signal transduction Process in which biochemical messages are transmitted from the cell surface to the nucleus.

silent substitution DNA sequence change that does not alter the amino acid sequence because of the degeneracy of the genetic code.

SINEs (short interspersed elements) A class of dispersed repetitive DNA in which each repeat is relatively short. Compare with **LINEs.**

Single strand conformation polymorphism (SSCP) A technique for detecting variation in DNA sequence by running single-stranded DNA fragments through a nondenaturing gel. Fragments with differing secondary structure (conformation) caused by sequence variation will migrate at different rates.

single-copy DNA DNA sequences that occur only once in the genome. Compare with **repetitive DNA.**

single-gene disorder or trait A feature or disease that is caused by a single gene. Compare with **polygenic** and **multifactorial.**

sister chromatid exchange Crossover between **sister chromatids;** can occur either in the sister chromatids of a tetrad during meiosis or between sister chromatids of a duplicated somatic chromosome.

sister chromatids The two identical strands of a duplicated chromosome, joined by a single centromere.

solenoid A structure of coiled DNA, consisting of approximately six **nucleosomes.**

somatic cell Cells other than those of the gamete-forming germline. In humans, most somatic cells are diploid.

somatic cell hybridization A physical gene mapping technique in which somatic cells from two different species are fused and allowed to undergo cell division. Chromosomes from one species are selectively lost, resulting in clones with only one or a few chromosomes from one of the species.

somatic hypermutation An extreme increase in the mutation rate of somatic cells, observed in B lymphocytes as they achieve increased binding affinity for a foreign antigen.

somatic recombination The exchange of genetic material between homologous chromosomes during mitosis in somatic cells; much rarer than meiotic recombination.

Southern transfer (also, **Southern blot**) Laboratory procedure in which DNA fragments that have been electrophoresed through a gel are transferred to a solid membrane, such as nitrocellulose. The DNA can then be hybridized with a labeled probe and exposed to X-ray film. *See also* **autoradiogram.**

specificity The proportion of unaffected individuals who are correctly identified by a test (true negatives). Compare with **sensitivity.**

spermatid One of the four haploid cells formed from a primary spermatocyte during spermatogenesis. Spermatids mature into spermatozoa.

spermatogenesis The process of male gamete formation.

spermatogonia Diploid germline stem cells from which sperm cells (spermatozoa) are ultimately derived.

spindle fiber One of the microtubular threads that form the spindle in a cell.

splice site mutation DNA sequence alterations in **donor** or **acceptor sites** or in the consensus sites near them. Produces altered intron splicing, such that portions of exons are deleted or portions of introns are included in the mature mRNA transcript.

sporadic The occurrence of a disease in a family with no apparent genetic transmission pattern, often the result of a new mutation.

stop codon mRNA base triplets that specify the point at which translation of the mRNA ceases.

structural genes Genes that encode protein products.

submetacentric A chromosome in which the centromere is located closer to one end of the chromosome arm than the other. Compare with **metacentric** and **acrocentric.**

synapsis The pairing of homologous chromosomes during prophase I of meiosis.

syndrome A pattern of multiple primary malformations or defects all due to a single underlying cause. Examples: Down syndrome, Marfan syndrome.

syntenic Describes two loci located on the same chromosome; they may or may not be linked.

T lymphocyte or **T cell** A component of the adaptive immune system whose receptors bind to a complex of MHC molecule and foreign antigen (also known as B cell). There are two major classes of T lymphocytes, **helper T lymphocytes** and **cytotoxic T lymphocytes.**

tandem repeat DNA sequences that occur in multiple copies located directly next to one another. Compare with **dispersed repetitive DNA.**

telomere The tip of a chromosome.

telophase The final major stage of mitosis and meiosis, in which daughter chromosomes are located on opposite edges of the cell and new nuclear envelopes form.

template A strand of DNA that serves as the model for replication of a new strand. Also denotes the DNA strand from which mRNA is transcribed.

teratogen A substance in the environment that can cause a birth defect.

teratology The study of environmental factors that cause birth defects or congenital malformations.

termination sequence DNA sequence that signals the cessation of transcription.

tetrad The set of four homologous chromatids (two sister chromatids from each homologous chromosome) observed during meiotic prophase I and metaphase I. Synonymous with **bivalent.**

tetraploidy A polyploid condition in which the individual has four copies of each chromosome in each cell, for a total of 92.

thymine One of the four DNA bases, abbreviated T.

tissue-specific mosaic A **mosaic** in which the mosaicism is confined only to specific tissues of the body.

transcription The process in which an mRNA sequence is synthesized from a DNA template.

transcription factor Substance that binds to DNA to influence and regulate transcription.

transfection The transfer of a DNA sequence into a cell.

transfer RNA (**tRNA**) A class of RNA that helps to assemble a polypeptide chain during translation. The anticodon portion of the tRNA binds to a complementary mRNA codon, and the 3' end of the tRNA molecule attaches to a specific amino acid.

transformation The oncogenic conversion of a normal cell to a state of unregulated growth.

translation The process in which an amino acid sequence is assembled according to the pattern specified by the mature mRNA transcript.

translocation The exchange of genetic material between nonhomologous chromosomes.

translocation, reciprocal A translocation resulting from breaks on two different chromosomes and a subsequent exchange of material. Carriers of reciprocal translocations maintain the normal number of chromosomes and normal amount of chromosome material.

translocation, Robertsonian A translocation in which the long arms of two acrocentric chromosomes are fused at the centromere; the short arms of each chromosome are lost. The translocation carrier has 45 chromosomes instead of 46 but is phenotypically normal because the short arms contain no essential genetic material.

transposon See **mobile element.**

triploidy A polyploid condition in which the individual has three copies of each chromosome in each cell, for a total of 69.

trisomy An aneuploid condition in which the individual has an extra copy of one chromosome, for a total of 47 chromosomes in each cell.

true negative Individual who is correctly identified by a test as not having a disease. *See also* **specificity.**

true positive Individual who is correctly identified by a test as having a disease. *See also* **sensitivity.**

tumor See **neoplasm.**

tumor suppressor A gene whose product helps to control cell growth and proliferation; mutations in tumor suppressors can lead to cancer. Example: retinoblastoma gene, *RB.*

two-hit model A model of carcinogenesis in which both copies of a gene must be altered before a neoplasm can form.

ultrasonography A technique for fetal visualization in which sound waves are transmitted through the fetus and their reflection patterns displayed on a monitor.

unequal crossover Crossing over between improperly aligned DNA sequences; produces deletions or duplications of genetic material.

uninformative mating A mating in which **linkage phase** cannot be established.

uniparental disomy Condition in which two copies of one chromosome are derived from a single parent, and no copies are derived from the other parent. May be either **heterodisomy** or **isodisomy.**

variable expression A trait in which the same genotype may produce phenotypes of varying severity or expression. Example: neurofibromatosis type 1.

variable number of tandem repeats (VNTR) A type of polymorphism created by variations in the number of minisatellite repeats in a defined chromosome region.

variance Statistical measure of variation in a quantity: estimated as the sum of the squared differences from the average value.

vector The vehicle used to carry a DNA insert; e.g., phage, plasmid, cosmid, or YAC.

X inactivation Process in which genes from one X chromosome in each cell of the female embryo are rendered transcriptionally inactive.

X inactivation center The location on the X chromosome from which the X inactivation signal is transmitted. Includes the *XIST* gene.

X-linked Refers to genes that are located on the X chromosome.

yeast artificial chromosome (YAC) A synthesized yeast chromosome capable of carrying a large DNA insert (approximately 1,000 kb).

zygote The diploid fertilized ovum.

Appendix

■ SLICE OF LIFE BAR CODES

Apply a bar code reader to each bar code to retrieve
the Slice of Life (*SOL*) illustration. The first number
under each bar code is the *SOL* reference used in
the text. The second number under the bar code is
the *SOL* frame number for the illustration.

1
18255
type III OI: arm bowing

2
45500
type III OI: old fractures and bowing

3
45510
OI: radial fracture

4
49473
OI: blue sclerae

5
8449
sickle cell disease: infarcted spleen

270

6
45613
sickle cell disease: collapsed femoral head

7
45637
sickle cell disease: "hair on end" skull appearance

8
45693
sickle cell disease: sclerotic lesions of knee

9
13472
NF1: dermal neurofibroma and freckling

10
13474
NF1: axillary freckling

11
27883
NF1: plexiform neurofibroma on left eyelid

12
27892
NF1: Lisch nodules

13
37726
NF1: dermal neurofibromas

14
16396
NF2: vestibular schwannoma

15
9847
retinoblastoma: tumor mass

16
22140
retinoblastoma: tumor observable in retina

17
22149
untreated retinoblastoma

18
27773
untreated retinoblastoma

19
49611
retinoblastoma: tumor mass

20
31625
Huntington disease: brain atrophy

21
37335
normal caudate

22
37336
caudate atrophy in Huntington disease

23
37338
normal brain; atrophy in Huntington disease

24
25688
achondroplasia: proximal shortening of limbs

25
6809
Marfan syndrome: dilated and normal aortic roots

26
39124
Marfan syndrome: dolichostenomelia, pectus excavatum

27
14491
myotonic dystrophy: open mouth, expressionless face

28
53755
myotonic dystrophy: long, expressionless face

29
20078
cystic fibrosis: meconium ileus

30
29255
cystic fibrosis: lung pathology

31
42657
Tay-Sachs disease: cytoplasmic accumulations

32
45509
hemophilia A: secondary arthritis

33
45513
hemophilia A: joint lesions secondary to hemoarthrosis

34
14443
Duchenne muscular dystrophy: calf hypertrophy

35
14452
Duchenne muscular dystrophy: lordosis of spine

36
14470
Becker muscular dystrophy

37
13442
Down syndrome: Brushfield spots in iris

38
53767
Down syndrome: flat mid-facial region

39
13443
Down syndrome: simian crease

40
31575
Down syndrome: brain atrophy

41
15602
trisomy 18: prominent occiput; ear abnormality

42
15731
trisomy 18: overriding fingers, clenched hand

43
15732
trisomy 18: rocker-bottom feet

44
20103
trisomy 18: horseshoe kidney

45
11000
trisomy 13: bilateral cleft lip, camptodactyly

46
16617
trisomy 13: postaxial polydactyly

47
20099
trisomy 13: ventricular septal defect

48
20105
Turner syndrome: gonadal dysgenesis

49
16982
adult polycystic kidney disease: cysts

50
16983
adult polycystic kidney disease; kidney section

51
39166
Ellis van Creveld syndrome: postaxial polydactyly

52
49415
hydrops fetalis

53
17660
ataxia telangiectasia: cerebellar atrophy

54
26762
Alzheimer disease: neurofibrillary tangle

55
37296
Alzheimer disease: amyloid plaque

56
49619
Alzheimer disease: gyrate atrophy

57
18241
galactosemia: cataract

58
18
Wilson disease: liver cirrhosis

59
21992
Wilson disease: Kayser-Fleischer ring

60
41145
Leber hereditary optic neuropathy

61
22074
retinitis pigmentosa: pigmentation deposits

62

24587

Wilms tumor and normal kidney

63

12219

xanthoma on Achilles tendon

64

9741

eyelid xanthoma

65

40232

bilateral cleft lip

66

40233

bilateral cleft lip

67

12143

epidermolysis bullosa: skin blisters

68

10091

Potter sequence: large ears, depressed nasal tip

69

39148

Potter sequence: depressed nasal tip, small jaw

70
16518
chronic myelogenous leukemia

71
49198
Hirschsprung disease: megacolon

72
11985
systemic lupus erythematosus: discoid lesions

73
25645
systemic lupus erythematosus: skin lesions

74
3278
ventricular septal defect

75
37552
anencephaly

76
37554
anencephaly

77
39172
anencephaly

78
39175
anencephaly

79
12424
lumbar meningomyelocele

80
13398
lumbar meningomyelocele

81
24834
large parietal-occipital encephalocele

82
49634
frontal encephalocele

83
22038
diabetes mellitus: retinopathy

84
48075
diabetes mellitus: gangrenous lesions

85
8597
atrioventricular canal

86
11533
atrioventricular canal

87
8495
atrial septal defect

88
8507
atrial septal defect

89
37657
massive untreated obstructive hydrocephalus

Index

NOTES

NOTES

NOTES

NOTES

NOTES

NOTES

NOTES

NOTES

NOTES

NOTES

NOTES

NOTES

NOTES

NOTES

NOTES

NOTES

NOTES

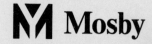 **Mosby**

Dedicated to Publishing Excellence

WE WANT TO HEAR FROM YOU!

To help us publish the most useful materials for students, we would appreciate your comments on this book. Please take a few moments to complete the form below, and then tear it out and mail to us. Thank you for your input.

Jorde: *MEDICAL GENETICS*

1. What courses are you using this book for?

___medical school   ___1st year
___osteopathic school   ___2nd year
___dental school   ___3rd year
___pharmacy school   ___4th year
___physician assistant program   ___other _____
___nursing school
___undergrad
___other _____

2. Was this book useful for your course? Why or why not?

____ yes ____ no _____
_____
_____

3. What features of textbooks are important to you? (*check all that apply*)

___color figures   ___text summaries
___summary tables and boxes   ___self-assessment questions
___price
___other _____
_____

4. What influenced your decision to buy this text? (*check all that apply*)

___required/recommended by instructor   ___bookstore display
___recommended by student   ___journal advertisement

___other _____

5. What other instructional materials did/would you find useful in this course?

___computer-assisted instruction   ___slides
___case studies book

___other _____

Are you interested in doing in-depth reviews of our basic science textbooks?   ____yes ____no

NAME:_____

ADDRESS:_____

_____

TELEPHONE:_____

THANK YOU!

A Times Mirror Company

NO POSTAGE
NECESSARY
IF MAILED
IN THE
UNITED STATES

BUSINESS REPLY MAIL

FIRST CLASS MAIL   PERMIT No. 135   St. Louis, MO.

POSTAGE WILL BE PAID BY ADDRESSEE

CHRIS REID
MEDICAL EDITORIAL
MOSBY–YEAR BOOK, INC.
11830 WESTLINE INDUSTRIAL DRIVE
ST.LOUIS, MO 63146-9987

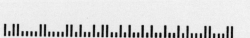